Prostate Biopsy Interpretation:
An Illustrated Guide

Rajal B. Shah • Ming Zhou
Authors

Prostate Biopsy Interpretation: An Illustrated Guide

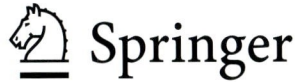

Authors

Rajal B. Shah, M.D.
Director, Urologic Pathology
Caris Life Sciences
6655 North MacArthur Boulevard
Irving, Texas 75039
USA
rshah@carisls.com

Ming Zhou, M.D., Ph.D.
Associate Professor
Director of Surgical Pathology, Tisch Hospital
Director of Genitourinary Pathology, Tisch Hospital
New York University
550 First Avenue
New York, NY 10016
USA
Ming.zhou@nyumc.org

ISBN 978-3-642-21368-7   e-ISBN 978-3-642-21369-4
DOI 10.1007/978-3-642-21369-4
Springer Heidelberg Dordrecht London New York

Library of Congress Control Number: 2011937719

© Springer-Verlag Berlin Heidelberg 2012

This work is subject to copyright. All rights are reserved, whether the whole or part of the material is concerned, specifically the rights of translation, reprinting, reuse of illustrations, recitation, broadcasting, reproduction on microfilm or in any other way, and storage in data banks. Duplication of this publication or parts thereof is permitted only under the provisions of the German Copyright Law of September 9, 1965, in its current version, and permission for use must always be obtained from Springer. Violations are liable to prosecution under the German Copyright Law.

The use of general descriptive names, registered names, trademarks, etc. in this publication does not imply, even in the absence of a specific statement, that such names are exempt from the relevant protective laws and regulations and therefore free for general use.

Product liability: The publishers cannot guarantee the accuracy of any information about dosage and application contained in this book. In every individual case the user must check such information by consulting the relevant literature.

Cover design: eStudioCalamar, Figueres/Berlin

Printed on acid-free paper

Springer is part of Springer Science+Business Media (www.springer.com)

To my wife, Ami Shah, and sons Ansh and Alay, for their unconditional love, support, and constantly reminding me that there is life beyond work.
To my parents, Bipin Shah and Sharmishtha Shah, for their genes, sacrifice, and motivation.

Rajal B. Shah, M.D.

To my wife, Lan Zhou, and daughters Grace and Rebecca, for their unwavering support.

Ming Zhou, M.D., Ph.D.

Preface

This book is the product of a prostate biopsy course that we taught at several national pathology meetings over a period of 5 years. After the lectures, attendees of different levels – residents, fellows, pathologists in private practice and academia – came to us to compliment the practicality and timeliness of our course and encouraged us to turn it into a handy reference book. When Melissa Ramondetta, Executive Editor at Springer, approached us for writing a book on prostate biopsy, we enthusiastically agreed to her proposal.

Prostate needle biopsy specimens constitute a significant portion of a surgical pathologist's daily work. However, prostate biopsy specimens are not every pathologist's darling. There is a significant error rate on diagnosing prostate cancer in needle biopsy, slow adoption of the modified Gleason grading system, and considerable variation in reporting. This book aims to cover all the practical issues related to interpretation of prostate biopsies in day-to-day practice, including diagnosis of limited cancer and its distinction from common benign mimickers; diagnosis and the clinical significance of "atypical glands suspicious for cancer" and high-grade prostatic intraepithelial neoplasia; prostate cancers mimicking benign lesions and other variant histologies of prostate cancer; recently described new entities; contemporary approaches to Gleason grading; application of immunohistochemical and emerging molecular markers in diagnosis and differential diagnosis of prostate cancer; and reporting of prostate biopsy. In addition, we discuss several other timely topics and issues, including prostate biopsy sampling techniques and its impact on pathologic diagnosis; molecular biology of prostate cancer; and specimen handling, processing, and quality assurance measures.

This book is structured in a way that engages its readers. Chapters are comprehensive yet concise, with numerous illustrations of real cases. Many algorithms, flow charts, and tables are used to illustrate the thought and decision-making process during sign-out of prostate biopsies. Dr. Levin, one of our reviewers, agrees: "I feel like I am on my microscope and signing out those difficult prostate biopsies when I am reading this book."

It is our hope that readers will not only use this book to look up a specific prostate lesion but also to learn the most effective way to evaluate a prostate biopsy and formulate a diagnostic approach upon encountering a specific clinical and pathological problem.

Irving, Texas, USA   Rajal B. Shah, M.D.
New York City, New York, USA   Ming Zhou, M.D., Ph.D.

Acknowledgments

The authors wish to express their profound appreciation to Dr. Howard Levin, Cleveland, Ohio, and Dr. Kirk Wojno, Royal Oak, Michigan, for their critical reading, and to many of their colleagues who have generously provided material presented in this book. Dr. Huiying He, Beijing, China, photographed many images used in this book. The secretarial support of Ms. Margaret LaPlaca and Ms. Georgene Hockey shall also be gratefully acknowledged.

Our thanks are also extended to Lee Klein for his stellar administrative assistance, and to Melissa Ramondetta, who saw the value of putting a practical prostate biopsy atlas on busy practicing pathologists' desks and initiated this project.

About the Authors

Rajal B. Shah is Director of Urologic Pathology at Caris Life Sciences in Dallas, Texas. Previously, he served as Clinical Associate Professor of Pathology and Urology, Director of the Urologic Pathology Division and Director of Urologic Pathology Fellowship program at the University of Michigan in Ann Arbor, MI. Dr. Shah's clinical expertise and research focus include prostate, bladder, kidney, testis, and penile neoplasms. He has been active in translational research and frequently presents at national and international meetings on urologic pathology. He has authored more than 100 peer-reviewed journal publications and book chapters and was among a group of scientists awarded the inaugural "Team Science Award" from the American Association of Cancer Research for the discovery of recurrent gene fusions in prostate cancer.

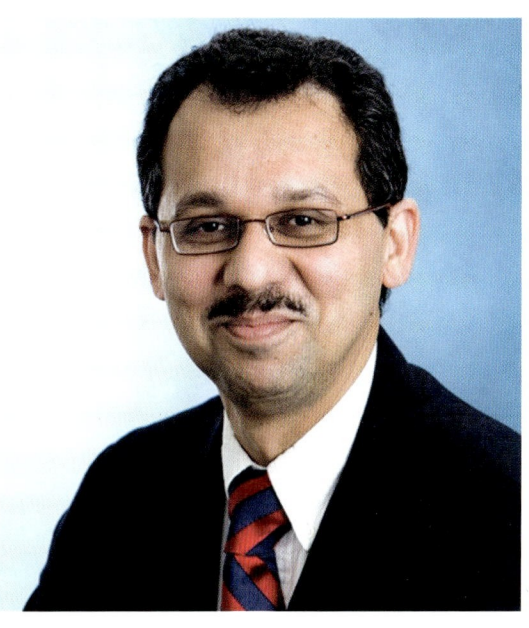

Ming Zhou is an Associate Professor and Director of Surgical Pathology and Genitourinary Pathology, Tisch Hospital, New York University, New York, USA. He was previously at the Pathology and Laboratory Medicine Institute, Cleveland Clinic, Ohio. As an expert in genitourinary pathology, Dr. Zhou has authored more than 100 research articles and 12 book chapters, and he also co-edits a textbook, *Genitourinary Pathology*. He frequently lectures at national and international meetings on urological pathology, and currently serves on several editorial boards, including those for *Modern Pathology* and *Advances in Anatomic Pathology*.

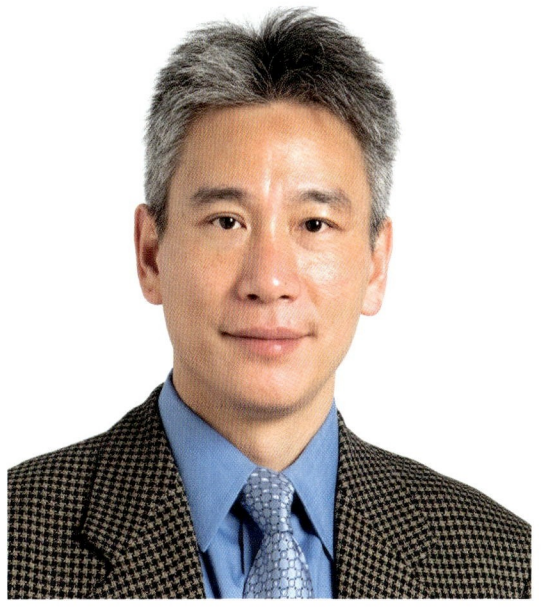

Contents

1 Anatomy and Normal Histology of the Prostate Pertinent to Biopsy Practice 1
  1.1 Anatomy of Normal Prostate 1
  1.2 Anatomy and Disease Preference of Three Zones of the Prostate 1
  1.3 Histology of Normal Prostate 2
  1.4 Immunophenotype of Prostate Glandular Cells 5
  1.5 Histology of Three Zones of Normal Prostate Glands, Other Intraprostatic Structures, and Their Mimics 6
  1.6 Histologic Variations of Normal Prostate Tissue 8
  References 9

2 Prostate Needle Biopsy Sampling Techniques: Impact on Pathological Diagnosis 11
  2.1 Biopsy Techniques for Prostate Cancer Detection and Its Impact on Pathological Diagnosis 11
  2.2 Transrectal and Transperineal Biopsy Approaches for Prostate Cancer Detection 12
  2.3 Biopsy Parameters That Impact Prostate Cancer Detection Rate in Prostate Needle Biopsy 13
  2.4 Future Trends in Prostate Biopsy Sampling and Its Clinical Applications 13
  References 13

3 Diagnosis of Limited Cancer in Prostate Biopsy 15
  3.1 General Approach to Prostate Needle Biopsy Evaluation 15
  3.2 Histological Features Considered Specific for and Diagnostic of Cancer 15
  3.3 Major and Minor Histological Features of Prostate Cancer in Biopsy 17
  3.4 Benign Conditions That Cause Architectural and Cytological Atypia 23
  3.5 Quantitative Threshold for Diagnosing Limited Cancer in Biopsy 24
  3.6 Histological Features For and Against Cancer Diagnosis in Biopsy 26
  3.7 A Practical Approach to Diagnosis of Limited Cancer in Needle Biopsy 26
  References 27

4 Immunohistochemistry in Prostate Biopsy Evaluation 29
  4.1 Commonly Used Immunohistochemical Markers for Diagnosis of Prostate Cancer in Biopsy 29
  4.2 Basal Cell Markers 30
  4.3 α-Methyacyl-coA-Racemase (AMACR, P504S) 34
  4.4 ERG Protein 37
  4.5 Antibody Cocktails 38
  4.6 Differential Diagnosis of Prostate Cancer by Immunohistochemistry 38

4.7	Practical Guideline for Using Immunohistochemistry in Workup of Prostate Biopsies	39
References		39

5 Contemporary Approach to Gleason Grading of Prostate Cancer ... 41
5.1	Significance of Gleason Grading in Prostate Cancer Management	42
5.2	Prostate Cancer Nomograms Recurrence Categories and Prediction Models	42
5.3	Current Concepts of Gleason Grading	44
5.4	Contemporary Gleason Pattern 1	44
5.5	Contemporary Gleason Pattern 2	44
5.6	Contemporary Gleason Pattern 3	45
5.7	Contemporary Gleason Pattern 4	46
5.8	Gleason Grading of Cribriform Carcinomas	48
5.9	Contemporary Gleason Pattern 5	48
5.10	Gleason Grading of Unusual "Variant" Histology Types and Patterns	49
5.11	Gleason Grading in the Setting of Multiple Cores with Prostate Cancer of Different Gleason Patterns	52
5.12	Tertiary Pattern 5 in Prostate Biopsy	52
5.13	Recommendations for Gleason Grading in the Post-therapy Setting	52
5.14	Impact of ISUP-modified Gleason Grading System	52
5.15	Problem Areas in Gleason Grading and Future Trends	54
References		54

6 Histologic Variants of Prostate Carcinoma ... 57
6.1	Histological Variants of Prostate Carcinoma	57
6.2	Histologic Variants of Prostate Carcinoma Mimicking Benign Lesions	57
6.3	Foamy Gland Carcinoma	57
6.4	Pseudohyperplastic Carcinoma	59
6.5	Prostate Adenocarcinoma with Atrophic Features	61
6.6	Prostate Adenocarcinoma with Glomeruloid Features	63
6.7	Ductal Adenocarcinoma	64
6.8	Mucinous (Colloid) Carcinoma	66
6.9	Small Cell Neuroendocrine Carcinoma	68
6.10	Approach to Neuroendocrine Differentiation in Prostate Cancer	70
6.11	Sarcomatoid Carcinoma (Carcinosarcoma)	71
6.12	Urothelial Carcinoma	72
6.13	Squamous and Adenosquamous Cell Carcinoma	73
6.14	Signet Ring Cell Carcinoma	75
6.15	Adenoid Cystic Basal Cell Carcinoma	76
References		77

7 Benign Mimics of Prostate Carcinoma ... 79
7.1	Classification of Benign Mimics of Prostate Carcinoma using Architectural Pattern-Based Approach	80
7.2	Histological Features Commonly Associated with Benign Mimics	81
7.3	Atypical Morphological Features Commonly Encountered in Various Benign Mimics of Prostate Cancer	82
7.4	Seminal Vesicle/Ejaculatory Duct Epithelium	82
7.5	Verumontanum Mucosal Gland Hyperplasia	83
7.6	Cowper's Glands	84
7.7	Mesonephric Remnant Hyperplasia	85

7.8	Mucinous Metaplasia	86
7.9	Morphologic Classification of Focal Atrophy Lesions	86
7.10	Partial Atrophy	88
7.11	Postatrophic Hyperplasia	90
7.12	Adenosis (Atypical Adenomatous Hyperplasia)	92
7.13	Basal Cell Hyperplasia	94
7.14	Diagnostic Approach to Prostate Basal Cell Lesions	97
7.15	Postradiation Atypia in Benign Prostate Glands	98
7.16	Nephrogenic Adenoma	100
7.17	Cribriform Proliferations in the Prostate Gland	102
7.18	Central Zone Glands	102
7.19	Clear Cell Cribriform Hyperplasia	103
7.20	Differential Diagnosis of Prostate Cribriform Lesions	104
7.21	Nonspecific Granulomatous Prostatitis	105
7.22	Malakoplakia	107
7.23	Sclerosing Adenosis	108
7.24	Paraganglia	109
7.25	Xanthomatous Infiltrate	110
7.26	Benign Mimics of Prostate Cancer: Take-Home Messages	111
	References	111

8 Atypical Cribriform Lesions of the Prostate Gland: Emerging Concepts of Intraductal Carcinoma of the Prostate (IDC-P) ... 115

8.1	Intraductal Carcinoma of the Prostate	116
8.2	General Approach to the Workup of Atypical Cribriform Lesions in Prostate Needle Biopsy	119
8.3	Comparisons of Clinical, Morphological and Molecular characteristics between cribriform High Grade PIN and IDC-P	119
8.4	Pathologic features of IDC-P	120
8.5	Reporting Recommendations for IDC-P	120
	References	120

9 High-Grade Prostatic Intraepithelial Neoplasia (HGPIN) ... 121

9.1	Histological Features of Prostatic Intraepithelial Neoplasia (PIN)	121
9.2	Diagnostic Criteria for HGPIN	122
9.3	Clinical Significance of HGPIN	127
9.4	Differential Diagnosis of HGPIN	127
9.5	Reporting of PIN	130
	References	130

10 Atypical Glands Suspicious for Cancer (ATYP) ... 131

10.1	Histological Features Resulting in ATYP	131
10.2	Working up Cases with Atypical Diagnosis	137
10.3	Clinical Significance of ATYP	137
	References	138

11 Spindle Cell Lesions of the Prostate Gland ... 139

11.1	Classification of Spindle Cell Lesions of the Prostate	139
11.2	Specialized Stromal Tumors of the Prostate Gland	140
11.3	Clinical, Morphologic, and Immunohistochemical Features Suggestive of Prostate Origin of the Spindle Cell Lesions	141
11.4	Diagnostic Approach to Spindle Cell Lesions of the Prostate	144

11.5	Immunohistochemical Characteristics of Select Spindle Cell Lesions of the Prostate.	145
References		145

12 Treatment Effect in Benign and Malignant Prostate Tissue ... 147
12.1	Treatment Modalities for Prostate Lesions.	147
12.2	Androgen Pathway and Anti-androgen Therapy for Prostate Lesions	148
12.3	Histologic Changes Following Androgen-deprivation Therapy in Benign and Malignant Prostate Tissue	149
12.4	Histological Changes Associated with Radiation Therapy	151
	12.4.1 Histological Changes Following Radiation Therapy in Benign and Malignant Prostate Tissue	151
	12.4.2 Significance of Postradiotherapy Prostate Biopsy	151
12.5	Histological Changes Associated with Cryotherapy	154
12.6	Histological Changes Associated with Hyperthermia	155
References		155

13 Molecular Biology of Prostate Cancer and Emerging Diagnostic and Prognostic Biomarkers ... 157
13.1	Types of Prostate-Specific Antigen (PSA) Measurements in Clinical Practice	158
13.2	Multistep Model of Prostate Cancer Progression	158
13.3	Emerging Biomarkers for the Diagnosis and Prognosis of Prostate Cancer	159
13.4	Genes Involved in the Chromosomal Translocations in Prostate Cancer	171
13.5	A Model of Molecular Basis of Prostate Cancer Progression Demonstrating Potential Role of *ETS* Gene Fusions	165
References		166

14 Biopsy Specimen Handling, Processing, Quality Assurance Program ... 169
14.1	Best Practices for Submission, Handling, and Processing of Prostate Biopsies	170
14.2	Recommendations for tissue submission of transurethral resection specimens	172
14.3	Quality assurance measures known to improve prostate biopsy practice	172
References		172

15 Reporting of Prostate Biopsy ... 173
15.1	Benign Diagnosis	173
15.2	High-grade Prostatic Intraepithelial Neoplasia and Atypical Glands Suspicious for Cancer	173
15.3	Adenocarcinoma of the Prostate	174
References		180

Index ... 181

Anatomy and Normal Histology of the Prostate Pertinent to Biopsy Practice

In an adult man without significant prostatic hyperplasia, the prostate gland is shaped like an inverted cone and weighs 30–40 g. It is located within the pelvis, with its base proximally at the bladder neck and its apex distally at the urogenital diaphragm. It lies anterior to the rectum, with the urethra running through its center and serving as an important reference landmark. Therefore, the prostate is amenable to transrectal needle biopsy and transurethral resection. Anatomically, it comprises three zones with different volume, histology, and disease preference [1].

1.1 Anatomy of Normal Prostate

Table 1.1 Anatomy of the prostate gland

Average weight 30–40 g
Inverted cone-shaped, with the base at the bladder neck and apex at the urogenital diaphragm (*see* Fig. 1.1)
Prostatic urethra runs though the center of the gland with a 35° anterior bend at the verumontanum
Divided into three zones: peripheral zone, central zone, and transition zone (*see* Fig. 1.1 and 1.2)
Anterior fibromuscular stroma covers anteromedial surface
Peripheral and central zones collectively referred to as *outer prostate*; transition zone and anterior fibromuscular layer termed *inner prostate* [2]

1.2 Anatomy and Disease Preference of Three Zones of the Prostate

Table 1.2 Anatomy and disease preference of three zones of the prostate

	Peripheral zone	Central zone	Transition zone
Anatomic landmarks			
Intraprostatic location	Horseshoe-shaped region extending posterolaterally around central zone proximally and distal prostatic urethra distally	Inverted cone-shaped area surrounding ejaculatory ducts. Its base at the bladder neck and apex at verumontanum	Anterolateral to proximal prostatic urethra
Disease preference			
Atrophy	Frequent	Infrequent	Variable
Benign prostatic hyperplasia	Infrequent	Rare	Frequent
Inflammation	Frequent	Infrequent	Variable
Carcinoma (% of total cancer)	70%	10%	20%
Tissue-sampling techniques			
Transrectal needle biopsy	Good	Good	Poor
Transurethral resection	Poor	Poor	Good

Fig. 1.1 Anatomy of the prostate. Using the prostatic urethra and ejaculatory ducts as reference landmarks, the prostate comprises three principal zones and an anterior fibromuscular layer. The central zone, about 25% of the prostate volume, is an inverted cone surrounding ejaculatory ducts and forms part of the prostate base. The transition zone lies anterolateral to the proximal prostatic urethra. The peripheral zone, about 70% of the prostate volume, extends posterolaterally around the central zone and distal prostatic urethra. Peripheral and central zones are collectively referred to as *outer prostate*, whereas the transition zone and anterior fibromuscular layer are termed *inner prostate*

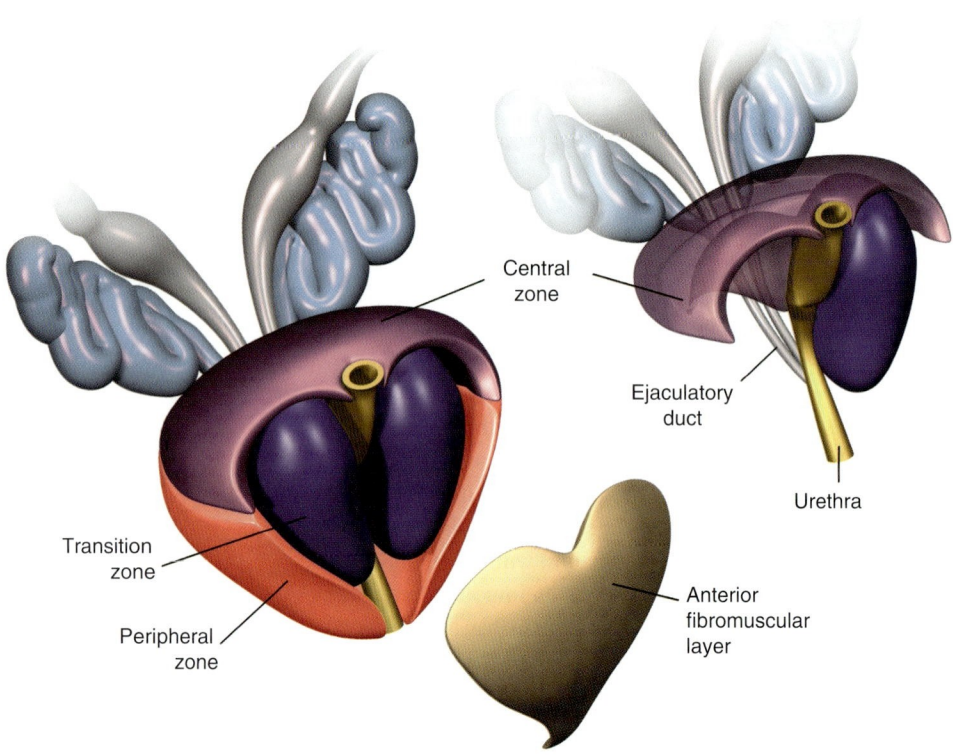

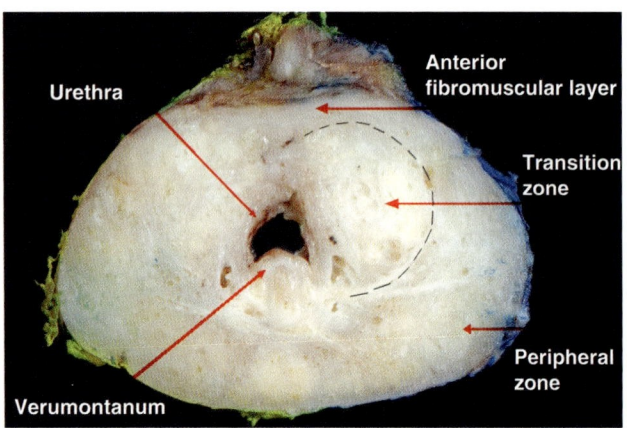

Fig. 1.2 Coronal section of the prostate showing the location of the peripheral zone and transition zone in relation to the proximal urethral and verumontanum

1.3 Histology of Normal Prostate

Table 1.3 Histology of the normal prostate gland

Prostate glands medium to large in size and forming lobulated architecture with intervening fibromuscular stroma (*see* Fig. 1.3)
Irregular contour with luminal undulation and papillary infoldings (*see* Fig. 1.4)
Glands lined mainly with two major types of cells: secretory cells and basal cells, and several cell types intermediate between basal and secretory cells
Prostate epithelial cells represent a continuum of differentiation from stem cells (basal cells) to fully mature luminal cells (secretory cells)
Secretory cells with clear to pale cytoplasm and reddish granular chromatin (*see* Fig. 1.5)
Basal cells situated at the periphery with blue-grayish, smooth nuclei (*see* Fig. 1.5)
Intermediate cells represent intermediate steps in basal to secretory cell differentiation with distinct immunophenotype (*see* Table 1.4)
Epithelial cells with neuroendocrine differentiation rarely seen (*see* Fig. 1.6)
Corpora amylacea within the glandular lumens (*see* Fig. 1.7)
Lipofuscin pigment may be seen in secretory cells (*see* Fig. 1.8)
Small nodules may be seen in stroma (*see* Fig. 1.9)
Prostate glands of central zone morphologically distinct from peripheral and transition zones glands (*see* Fig. 1.10)

1.3 Histology of Normal Prostate

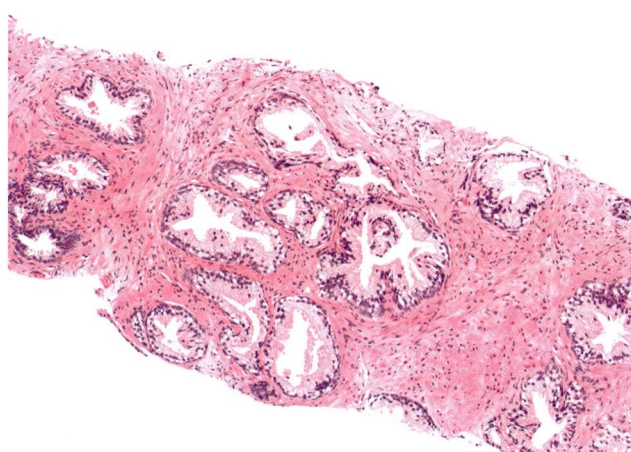

Fig. 1.3 Benign prostatic tissue. At scanning power, prostate glands are medium to large in size and form lobulated architecture with intervening fibromuscular stroma

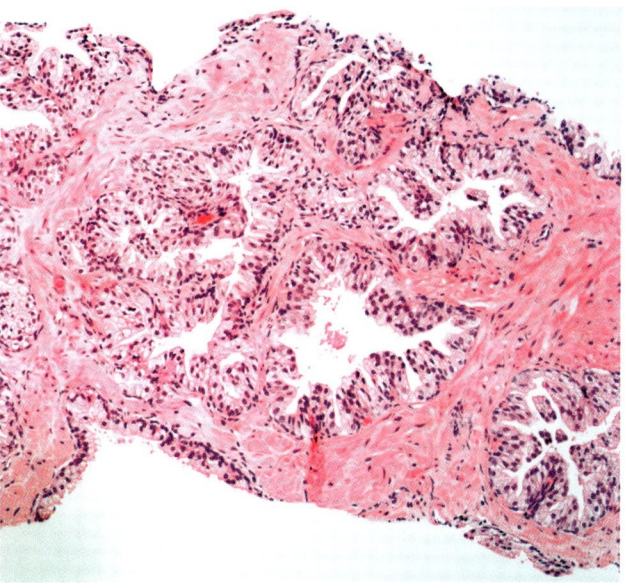

Fig. 1.4 Normal prostate glands have irregular contour with luminal undulation and papillary infoldings

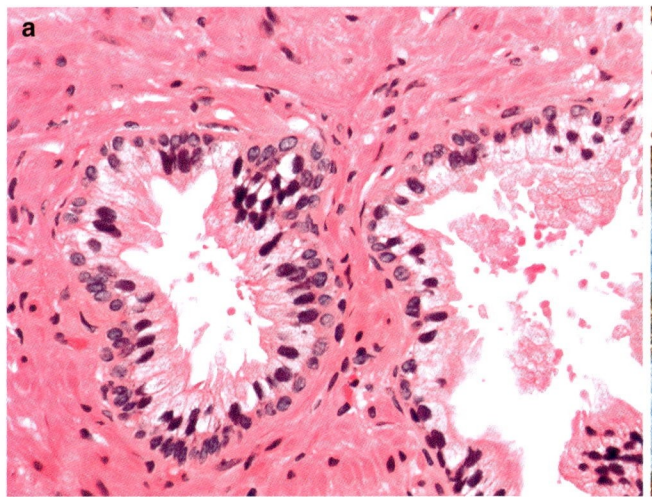

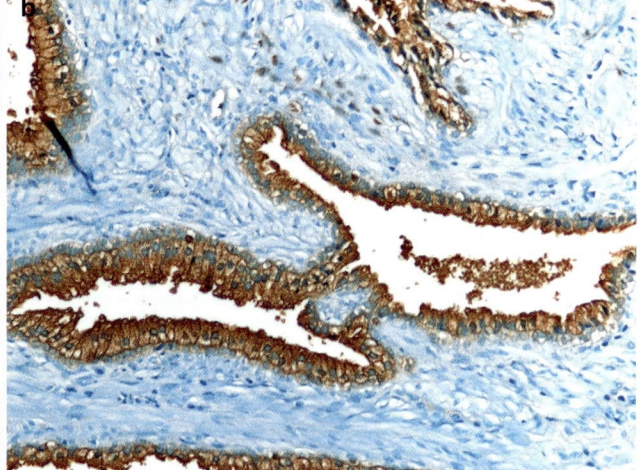

Fig. 1.5 Normal prostate glands comprise two main types of cells: secretory cells and basal cells. Secretory cells are cuboidal or columnar-shaped with clear to pale cytoplasm and pseudostratified nuclei. Basal cells are situated at the periphery of the gland beneath the secretory cells. They are spindle-shaped and parallel to the basement membrane. Basal cells may be difficult to distinguish from secretory cells or stromal fibroblasts on routine hematoxylin–eosin stain slide. However, secretory and basal cell nuclei exhibit some tinctorial difference on a well-stained slide: Secretory cells have reddish granular chromatin, while basal cells have blue-grayish, semi-transparent chromatin (**a**). Secretory cells are considered to be terminally differentiated and are positive for prostate-lineage specific markers such as prostate-specific antigen (PSA) (**b**), prostate-specific acid phosphatase (PAP) (**c**), prostate-specific membrane antigen (PSMA) (**d**) [3], and Nkx-3.1 (**e**) [4]. Basal cells are prostate stem cells and less differentiated [5]. They are negative for prostate-specific markers but positive for high molecular weight cytokeratin (34βE12 or cytokeratin 5/6) (**f**) and p63 (**g**) [6, 7]

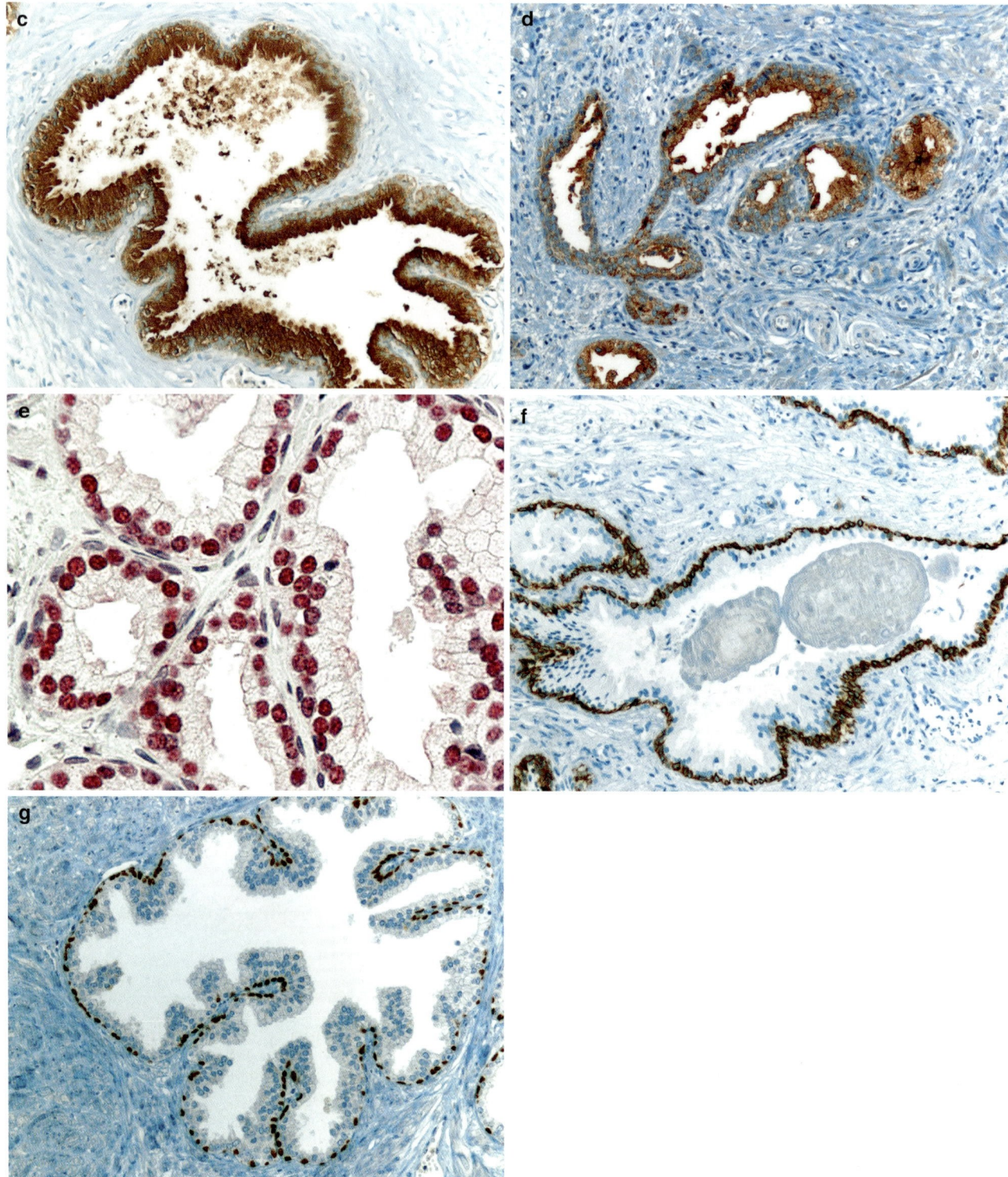

Fig. 1.5 (continued)

1.4 Immunophenotype of Prostate Glandular Cells

Table 1.4 Immunophenotype of prostate epithelial cell types (Modified from van Leenders et al. [8])

Markers	Prostate glandular cell			
	Basal	Basal intermediate	Secretory intermediate	Secretory
p63	++	++	–	–
Cytokeratin 14	++	–	–	–
Cytokeratin 5	++	++	++	–
C-Met	+/–	+/–	+/–	–
Cytokeratin 8	+	+	+	++
Cytokeratin 18	+	+	+	++
Androgen receptor	–/+	–/+	+/–	++

+: weak nearly homogeneous staining; ++: strong nearly homogeneous staining; +/–: weak to strong heterogeneous staining; –/+: weak heterogeneous staining; –: no staining

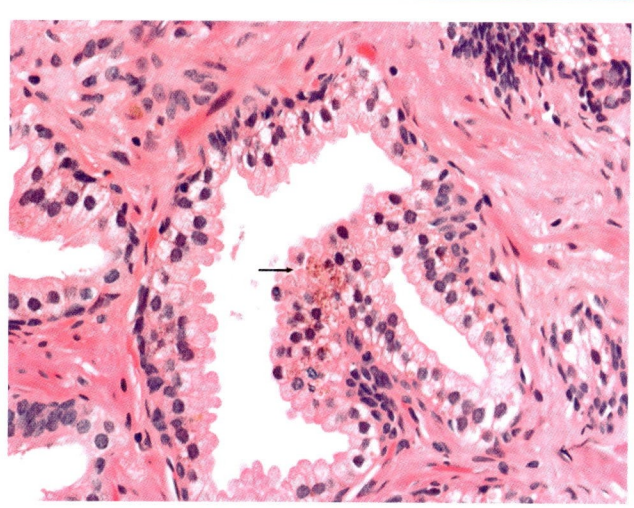

Fig. 1.8 Lipofuscin pigment in benign prostate glands. It is considered "wear and tear" products in aging cells. Rarely seen in prostate cancer, its presence usually mitigates against a cancer diagnosis [10]

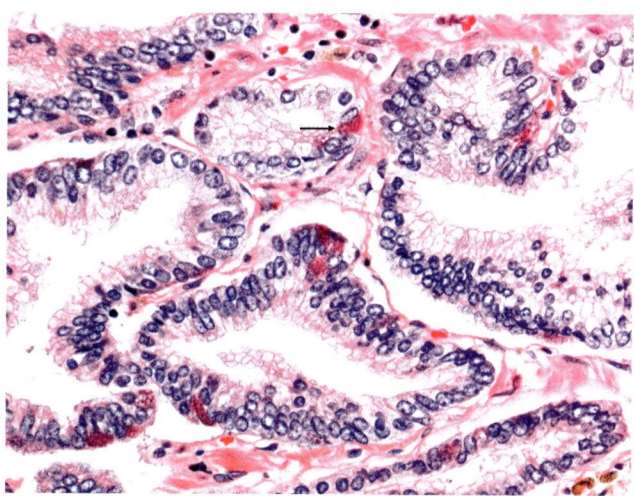

Fig. 1.6 Prostate glands with neuroendocrine cells and red cytoplasmic granules (*arrow*). Although rare, the neuroendocrine cells have the largest number in the prostate gland among genitourinary organs

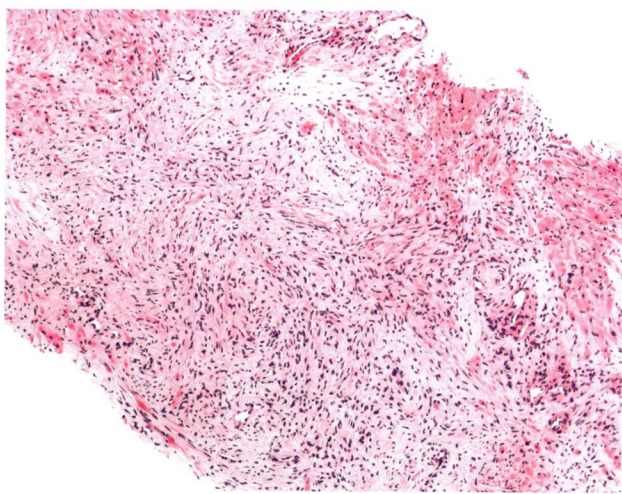

Fig. 1.9 Hyperplastic stromal nodule. Prostate stroma comprises skeletal and smooth muscle fibers, fibroblasts, nerves, and vessels. Stromal nodules can be seen in biopsies taken from all three zones and do not correlate with clinical symptomatology of benign prostatic hyperplasia [11]

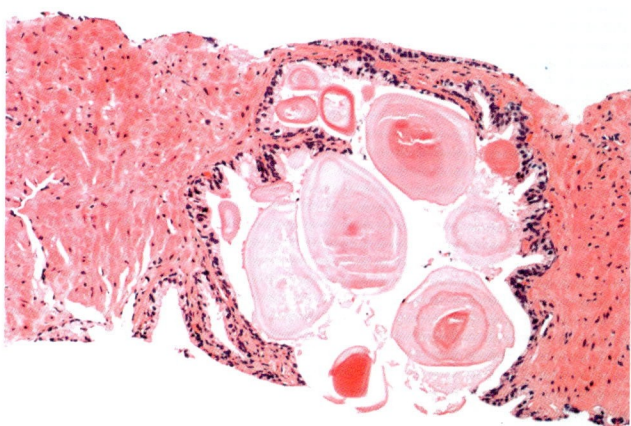

Fig. 1.7 Benign prostate glands with corpora amylacea, which are round, concentrically laminated structures within lumens. Rarely seen in prostate cancer, their presence usually mitigates against a cancer diagnosis [9]

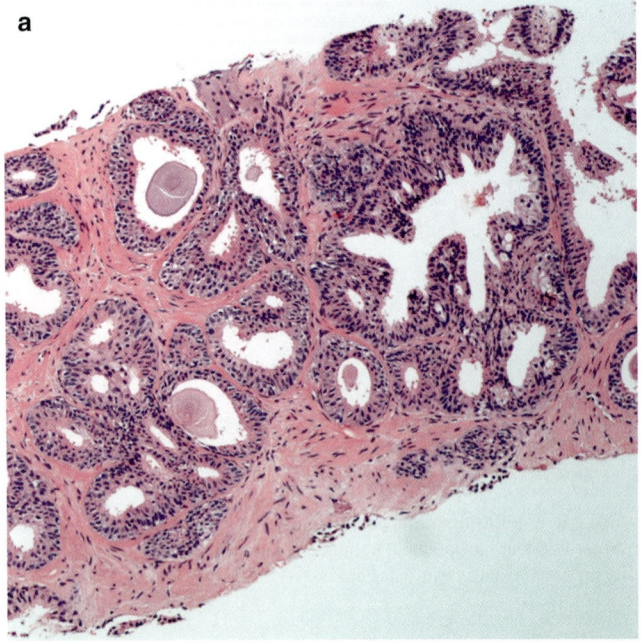 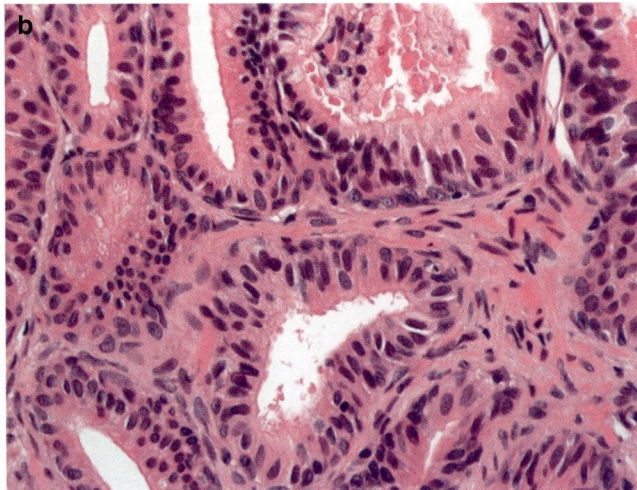

Fig. 1.10 Central zone prostate glands are large complex acini with cribriform and intraluminal ridges with dense stroma (**a**). The secretory cells have eosinophilic cytoplasm, stratified nuclei, and prominent basal cell layer (**b**). Central zone glands may be mistaken for HGPIN [13]. Unlike HGPIN, central zone glands lack significant nuclear atypia, including nuclear enlargement and prominent nucleoli

1.5 Histology of Three Zones of Normal Prostate Glands, Other Intraprostatic Structures, and Their Mimics

Table 1.5 Histology of three zones of normal prostate glands, other intraprostatic structures, and their mimickers (*see* Chap. 7)

	Architectural features	Cytological features	Mimics
Peripheral zone	Small simple acini Lobular configuration Loose stroma	Clear cytoplasm	–
Central zone [12] (*see* Fig. 1.10)	Large complex acini with cribriform and intraluminal ridges Dense stroma	Eosinophilic cytoplasm Stratified nuclei Prominent basal cell layer	High-grade prostatic intraepithelial neoplasia (HGPIN)
Transition zone [13]	Small simple acini Conspicuous nodular configuration Dense stroma	Clear cytoplasm	Adenosis
Seminal vesicle/ejaculatory ducts (*see* Fig. 1.11)	Central irregular lumen with surrounding clusters of smaller glands	Scattered cells showing prominent degenerative nuclear atypia Golden brown lipofuscin pigment	HGPIN Prostate carcinoma
Verumontanum mucosal gland hyperplasia (*see* Fig. 1.12)	Closely packed small acini beneath urethral mucosa Orange-brown dense luminal secretion	Lipofuscin pigment Basal cells	Prostate carcinoma
Cowper's glands (*see* Fig. 1.13)	Noninfiltrative, lobular pattern Dimorphic population of ducts and mucinous acini Intermixed with skeletal muscle fibers	Acini with voluminous, pale cytoplasm	Foamy gland carcinoma Prostate glands with mucinous metaplasia
Paraganglia (*see* Fig. 1.14)	Small clusters or nests of clear cells with prominent vascular pattern Intimately associated with nerve Most common in periprostatic soft tissue	Clear or amphophilic, granular cytoplasm Inconspicuous nucleoli	High-grade prostate carcinoma

1.5 Histology of Three Zones of Normal Prostate Glands, Other Intraprostatic Structures, and Their Mimics

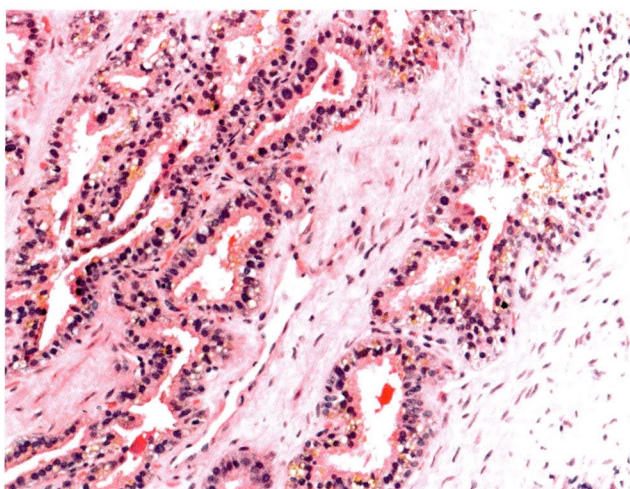

Fig. 1.11 Seminal vesicle/ejaculatory ducts. On prostate biopsies, the two structures cannot be distinguished reliably as they have similar morphology. They have a central irregular lumen with surrounding clusters of smaller glands whose cells display scattered but prominent degenerative nuclear atypia and golden brown pigment in cytoplasm and prostate carcinoma. They may be mistaken for HGPIN, radiation-induced changes [14]

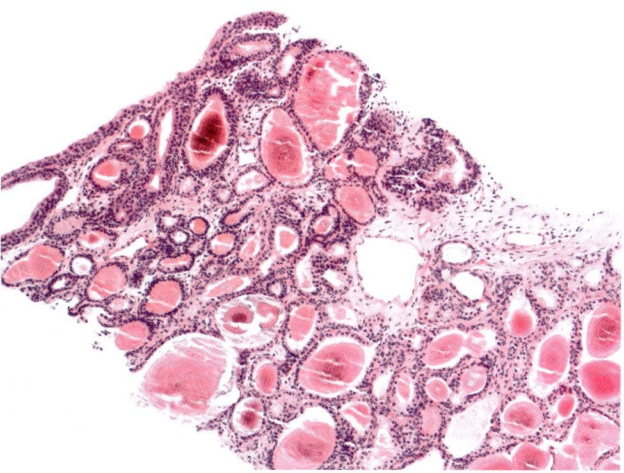

Fig. 1.12 Verumontanum mucosal gland hyperplasia. Rarely sampled in needle biopsy, it comprises closely packed small acini beneath the urethral mucosa. Orange-brown dense secretion is found in glandular lumens [15]

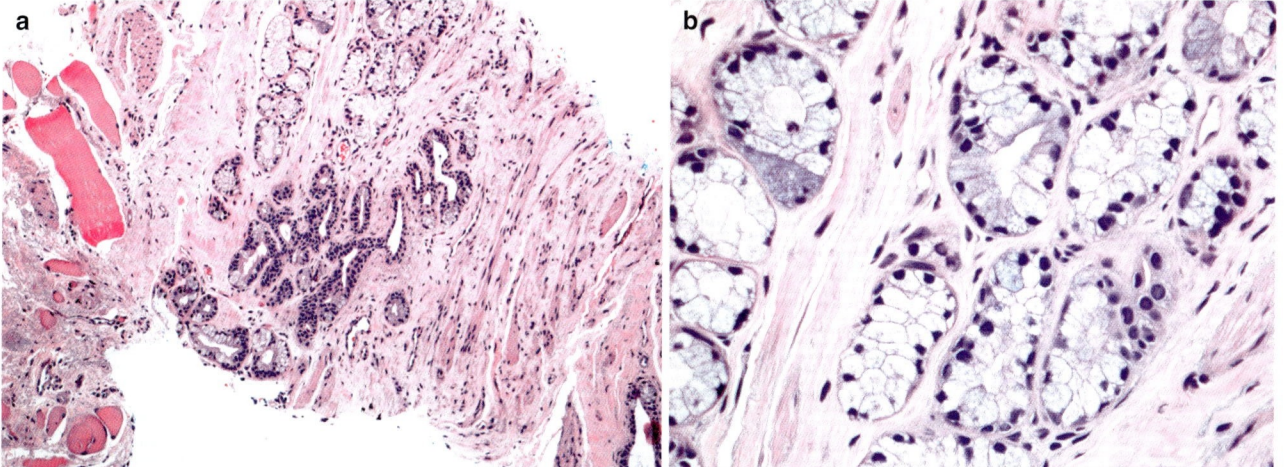

Fig. 1.13 Cowper's glands. They are extraprostatic structures found within the urogenital diaphragm, and therefore are rarely sampled in the biopsy from the apex. They are composed of a dimorphic population of ducts and mucinous acini intermixed with skeletal muscle fibers (**a** and **b**) [16]

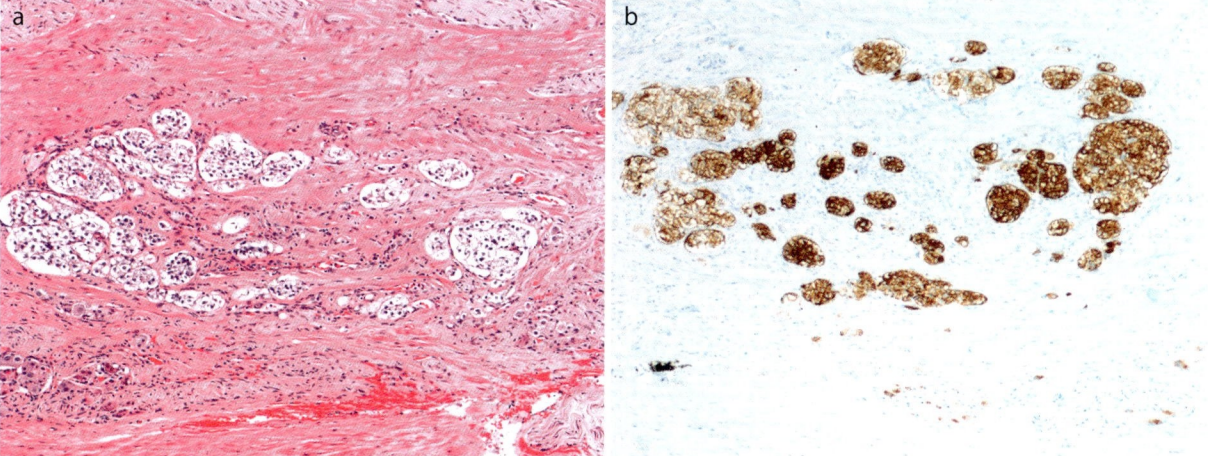

Fig. 1.14 Paraganglia are found most commonly in periprostatic soft tissue. They are composed of small clusters or nests of clear cells with a prominent vascular pattern and are intimately associated with nerves (**a**). Cells are positive for neuroendocrine markers such as synaptophysin (**b**) [17]

1.6 Histologic Variations of Normal Prostate Tissue

Table 1.6 Histologic variations of normal prostate tissue

Atrophy (see Fig. 1.15)
Basal cell hyperplasia (see Fig. 1.16)
Urothelial metaplasia (see Fig. 1.17)
Perineural abutment (see Fig. 1.18)
Glands within skeletal muscle fibers (see Fig. 1.19)
Irregular prostate–periprostatic interface (see Fig. 1.20)

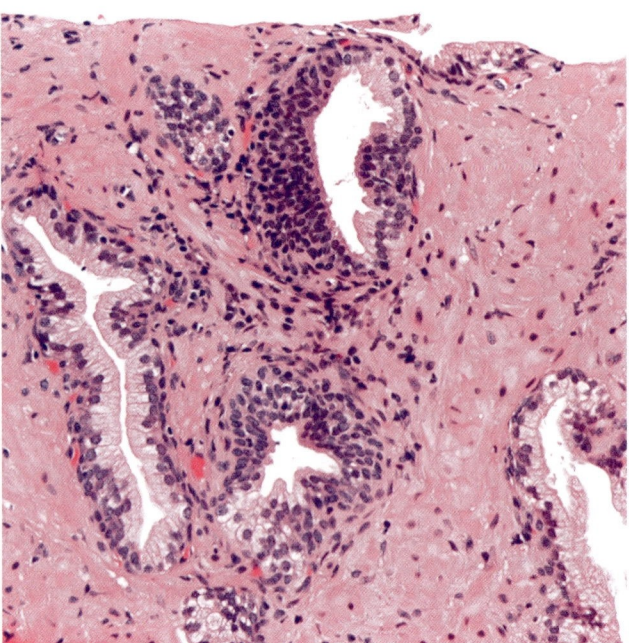

Fig. 1.17 Urothelial metaplasia. A form of basal cell hyperplasia, urothelial metaplasia consists of stratified basal cells with longitudinal nuclear grooves arranged perpendicular to the basement membrane

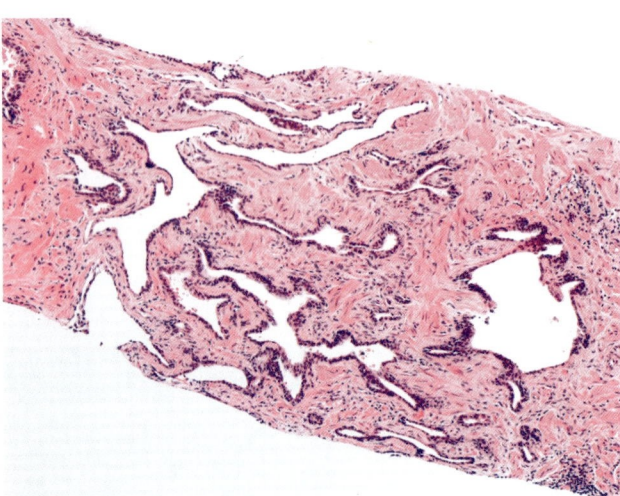

Fig. 1.15 Atrophic prostate glands retain lobulated architecture. Cystic dilatation is common. Glands appear dark due to reduced cytoplasm. There are several distinct histologic variants of atrophy. It is very common and affects patients of a wide age range, including men in their early twenties [18, 19]

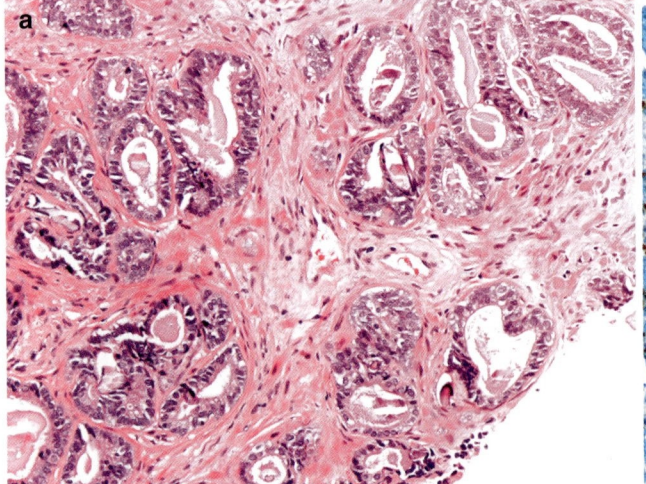 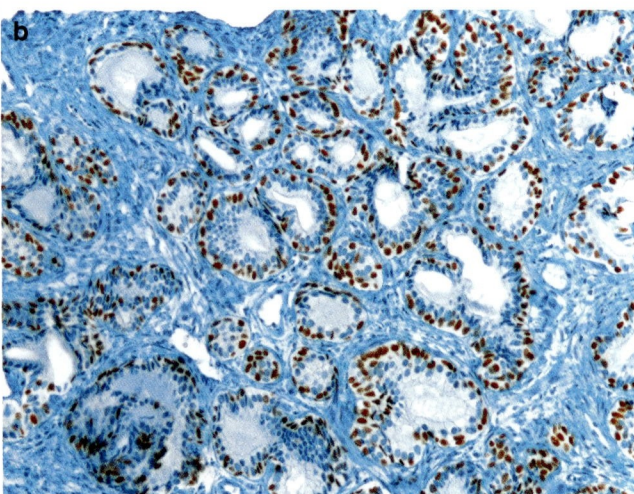

Fig. 1.16 Basal cell hyperplasia. Prostate glands are rimmed with one or several layers of basal cells (**a**). Basal cells have scant cytoplasm and round-to-oval hyperchromatic nuclei. They are positive for basal cell markers such as p63 (**b**). Some basal cells are stratified and have prominent nucleoli and may be mistaken for HGPIN. Calcification can also be seen [20]

References

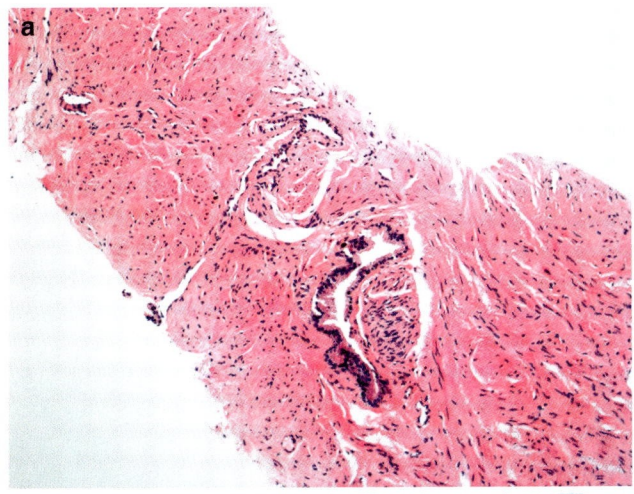

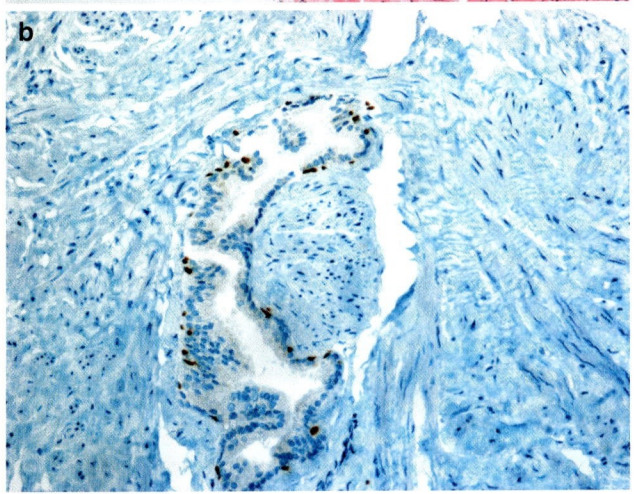

Fig. 1.18 Perineural abutment. A benign prostate gland abuts and loosely encircles a nerve fiber (**a**). It is critical to distinguish it from perineural invasion by prostate cancer. In difficult cases, immunostains for basal cells, such as p63, can be used to confirm the benign nature of the glands (**b**) [21]

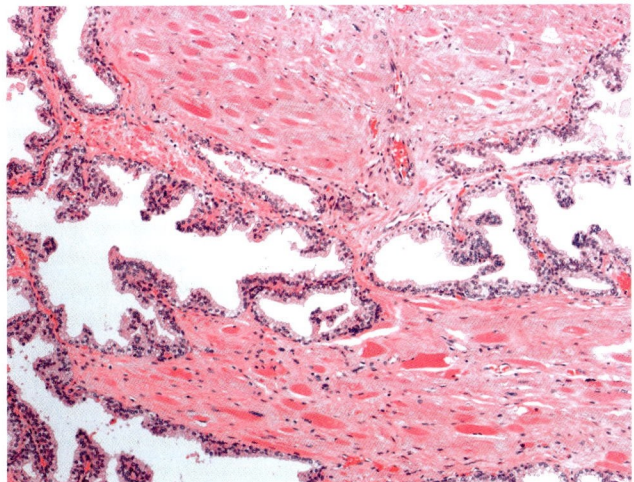

Fig. 1.19 Prostate glands within skeletal muscle fibers. Skeletal muscle can be found intraprostatically, usually in the apex and anterior fibromuscular layer. Prostate glands can be found within the skeletal muscle fibers [22]; therefore, finding cancer glands within the skeletal muscle fibers should not be interpreted as extraprostatic extension

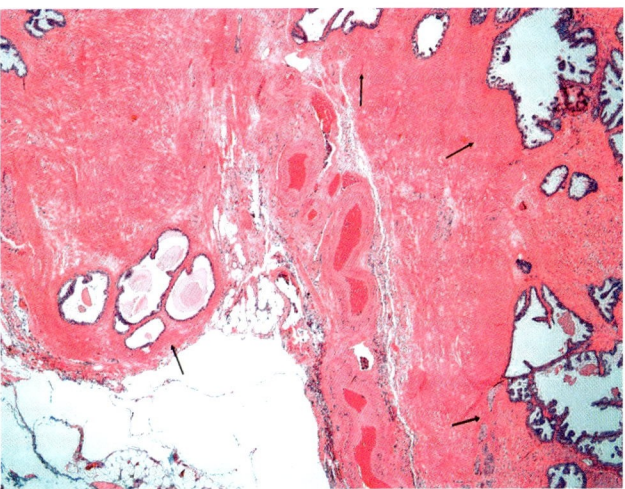

Fig. 1.20 Irregular prostate–periprostatic interface. The prostate does not have a true capsule. To determine if cancer glands have extended outside the prostate gland, one could draw an imaginary prostate–periprostatic interface that forms a smooth contour and encompasses all the prostate glands. However, the prostate–periprostatic interface is often irregular and jagged at the anterior aspect and the base of the gland (*arrows*). The determination of extraprostatic extension at these sites is difficult and requires finding cancer glands within fat, as it is exceedingly rare to find fat within the prostate gland; therefore, cancer glands intermixed with fat in needle biopsy can be safely interpreted as extraprostatic extension by cancer

References

1. McNeal J (2006) In: Mills S (ed) Prostate, 3rd edn. Lippincott Williams & Wilkins, Philadelphia, pp 997–1097
2. Bostwick D (1997) Normal anatomy and histology. In: Bostwick D, Dundore P (eds) Biopsy pathology of the prostate. Chapman & Hall, London, pp 1–26
3. Marker PC, Donjacour AA, Dahiya R, Cunha GR (2003) Hormonal, cellular, and molecular control of prostatic development. Dev Biol 253:165–174
4. Bieberich CJ, Fujita K, He WW, Jay G (1996) Prostate-specific and androgen-dependent expression of a novel homeobox gene. J Biol Chem 271:31779–31782
5. Signoretti S, Loda M (2006) Defining cell lineages in the prostate epithelium. Cell Cycle 5:138–141
6. Signoretti S, Waltregny D, Dilks J et al (2000) p63 is a prostate basal cell marker and is required for prostate development. Am J Pathol 157:1769–1775
7. Zhou M, Shah R, Shen R, Rubin MA (2003) Basal cell cocktail (34betaE12 + p63) improves the detection of prostate basal cells. Am J Surg Pathol 27:365–371
8. van Leenders GJ, Gage WR, Hicks JL et al (2003) Intermediate cells in human prostate epithelium are enriched in proliferative inflammatory atrophy. Am J Pathol 162:1529–1537
9. Christian JD, Lamm TC, Morrow JF, Bostwick DG (2005) Corpora amylacea in adenocarcinoma of the prostate: incidence and histology within needle core biopsies. Mod Pathol 18:36–39
10. Brennick JB, O'Connell JX, Dickersin GR et al (1994) Lipofuscin pigmentation (so-called "melanosis") of the prostate. Am J Surg Pathol 18:446–454
11. Viglione MP, Potter S, Partin AW et al (2002) Should the diagnosis of benign prostatic hyperplasia be made on prostate needle biopsy? Hum Pathol 33:796–800

12. Srodon M, Epstein JI (2002) Central zone histology of the prostate: a mimicker of high-grade prostatic intraepithelial neoplasia. Hum Pathol 33:518–523
13. Babinski MA, Chagas MA, Costa WS, Sampaio FJ (2003) Prostatic epithelial and luminal area in the transition zone acini: morphometric analysis in normal and hyperplastic human prostate. BJU Int 92:592–596
14. Amin MB, Bostwick DG (1996) Pigment in prostatic epithelium and adenocarcinoma: a potential source of diagnostic confusion with seminal vesicular epithelium. Mod Pathol 9:791–795
15. Gagucas RJ, Brown RW, Wheeler TM (1995) Verumontanum mucosal gland hyperplasia. Am J Surg Pathol 19:30–36
16. Cina SJ, Silberman MA, Kahane H, Epstein JI (1997) Diagnosis of Cowper's glands on prostate needle biopsy. Am J Surg Pathol 21:550–555
17. Kawabata K (1997) Paraganglion of the prostate in a needle biopsy: a potential diagnostic pitfall. Arch Pathol Lab Med 121:515–516
18. Gardner WA Jr, Culberson DE (1987) Atrophy and proliferation in the young adult prostate. J Urol 137:53–56
19. Postma R, Schroder FH, van der Kwast TH (2005) Atrophy in prostate needle biopsy cores and its relationship to prostate cancer incidence in screened men. Urology 65:745–749
20. Cleary KR, Choi HY, Ayala AG (1983) Basal cell hyperplasia of the prostate. Am J Clin Pathol 80:850–854
21. Ali TZ, Epstein JI (2005) Perineural involvement by benign prostatic glands on needle biopsy. Am J Surg Pathol 29:1159–1163
22. Kost LV, Evans GW (1964) Occurrence and significance of striated muscle within the prostate. J Urol 92:703–704

Prostate Needle Biopsy Sampling Techniques: Impact on Pathological Diagnosis

The clinicopathological characteristics of newly diagnosed prostate cancer have significantly changed due to widespread prostate-specific antigen (PSA) screening after its introduction in the late 1980s. The most remarkable change has been "stage migration" toward smaller volume disease at younger age. The diagnosis of prostate cancer now is mostly triggered by an elevated or rising PSA rather than an abnormal digital rectal examination, resulting in a significant increase in the percentage of nonpalpable cancers (stage T1c) between 1988 and 1996 from 10% to 73% [1]. With this trend, the prostate biopsy application and sampling techniques have also rapidly evolved. In 1989, the sextant prostate biopsy was introduced and rapidly became the standard over directed biopsies of hypoechoic lesions and palpable nodules [2]. In recent years, it has become increasingly evident that sextant biopsies could miss a significant number (up to 30%) of cancers because only a small percentage of prostates has a tumor distribution detectable with the paramedian template utilized by the sextant approach [3, 4]. Furthermore, sextant protocol tends to undersample certain areas of the prostate, such as "anterior horns" and the lateral aspects of the peripheral zone, where the majority of prostate cancer arises [5–7].

Recent studies suggested moving the biopsies more laterally to better sample the lateral aspects and anterior horns of the peripheral zones [8]. This recommendation was supported by the zonal anatomy of the prostate as well as the origin of the tumor [9]. Because approximately 70–80% of prostate cancers originate in the peripheral zone, alternative systemic biopsy techniques that more extensively sample this region could improve the cancer detection rate. In addition to improved cancer detection, these extended biopsy techniques have also impacted day-to-day pathologic diagnoses, most notably in the reduction of the predictive value for cancer of focal high-grade prostatic intraepithelial neoplasia (HGPIN) diagnosed in needle biopsies (< 2 cores) and improving biopsy and radical prostatectomy Gleason grade correlation [10–18]. This chapter discusses the application of various biopsy sampling methods and their impact on day-to-day practice.

2.1 Biopsy Techniques for Prostate Cancer Detection and Its Impact on Pathological Diagnosis (Fig. 2.1)

Table 2.1 Comparisons of three biopsy techniques utilized for prostate cancer detection

Technique	Sextant biopsy	Extended biopsy	Saturation biopsy
Definition	Six cores from paramedian base, mid, apex of the prostate	Six cores from the sextant sites with additional ≥4 cores from the lateral aspect and anterior horns of prostate	≥14 cores (median, 24) targeted from lateral to median aspect of prostate
Approach	Paramedian, typically via transrectal route	Paramedian and lateral, usually via transrectal route	Lateral and paramedian, via transrectal or transperineal route
Indications	Traditionally first-time biopsy approach	Contemporary approach as first-time biopsy and repeat biopsy for both diagnosis and staging of minute focus of Gleason score 6 cancer (currently recommended by NCCN)	Primarily for staging minute focus of Gleason score 6 prostate cancer
Impact on pathologic diagnosis	Poor biopsy/prostatectomy Gleason score correlation (40–50% exact correlation)	Improves biopsy/prostatectomy Gleason score correlation Significantly improves prostate cancer detection Cancer risk of focal HGPIN (< 2 cores) significantly reduced (~20%)	Improves biopsy/prostatectomy Gleason score correlation Able to detect multifocal cancer with foci of high-grade component Improves prostate cancer detection
Disadvantages	High false-negative rate (30–70%)	None specifically	Requires general anesthesia

NCCN National Comprehensive Cancer Network

2.2 Transrectal and Transperineal Biopsy Approaches for Prostate Cancer Detection

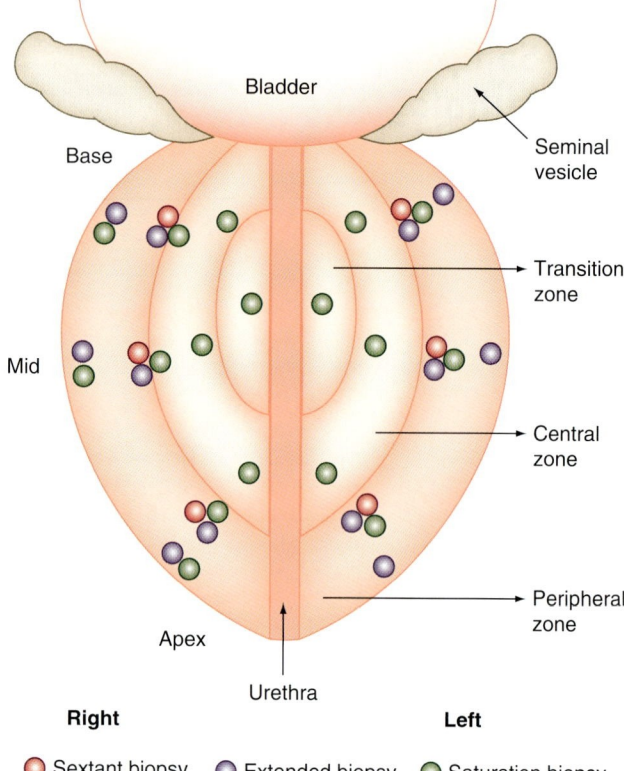

Fig. 2.1 Diagrammatic representation of sextant, extended, and saturation biopsy techniques in prostate cancer detection. Sextant biopsy protocol utilizes paramedian (parasagittal) plane sampling approach directed toward the base, mid, and apex of the prostate bilaterally. In comparison, contemporary extended biopsy approach utilizes various laterally directed biopsies in addition to the standard sextant biopsies to improve the detection of peripherally located prostate cancer. This approach is supported by the zonal anatomy of the prostate and the origin of the tumor. As shown in this diagram, the NCCN recommends an extended 12-core biopsy that includes a standard sextant sampling of the apex, midgland, and base of both the right and left sides of the prostate, as well as six additional cores from the lateral peripheral zone on each side. This technique has been validated in a study of more than 2,000 patients, with a cancer detection rate of 44% compared with approximately 20% with a standard sextant biopsies [19]. Saturation biopsy is an extensive sampling approach and is primarily utilized for staging minute focus of Gleason score 6 prostate cancer. Using an inward radial step approach, prostates are biopsied starting at the far lateral peripheral zone (anterior horn) and continuing until the midgland is reached. The process is repeated on the contralateral side. Transition zone of the prostate is also regularly sampled. On average, 23 (range, 14–45) biopsy cores are taken

Table 2.2 Comparisons of transrectal and transperineal biopsy approaches [20, 21]

Technique	Transrectal	Transperineal
Approach	Biopsies taken through transrectal approach	Biopsies taken through transperineum (anterior approach)
	Biopsy needle guided by transrectal ultrasound	Biopsy needle maintained exactly parallel to transrectal probe (parallel to rectum)
	Biopsies taken primarily from posterolateral area	Biopsies taken from the anterior to the distal part of the prostate
Indications	Most common biopsy approach	Commonly used in saturation biopsy protocol
Advantages	Ease of procedure	Every part of the prostate can be easily reached providing an effective technique for prostate cancer detection
	Widely accepted by urologists	
	Local anesthesia may not be required	Improves detection of anteriorly located (transverse zone) prostate cancer
		No passage through rectum; better approach for patients with proctitis
		Low incidence of infectious complications; does not require antibiotics use
		Low complication rates
Disadvantages	Traverses through rectum with higher rate of infectious complications; requires regular antibiotic use	Technically demanding; requires learning curve
	Higher chance of missing anteriorly located (transverse zone) tumors	Requires local anesthesia

2.3 Biopsy Parameters That Impact Prostate Cancer Detection Rate in Prostate Needle Biopsy

Table 2.3 Biopsy parameters that impact prostate cancer detection rate in prostate needle biopsy

Factors related to biopsy procedure and operator
Number of cores obtained
Laterality of the biopsy procedure (paramedian versus laterally directed biopsy approach)
Transrectal versus transperineal (anterior-based) approach
Operator experience and skill

Factors related to pathology laboratory practice
Number of needle cores embedded in cassette (ideal 1–2 core/cassette)
Tissue-sectioning protocol and number of levels examined
Histotechnologist's skill
Pathologist's skill and experience

2.4 Future Trends in Prostate Biopsy Sampling and Its Clinical Applications

Table 2.4 Future trends in prostate biopsy sampling and its clinical applications [22–28]

Future trends	Potential applications
Site-specific labeling with functional imaging technology and three-dimensional mapping of prostate biopsies	Aim to precisely detect prostate cancer location(s) and functional characteristics for potential focal therapy of prostate cancer (e.g., ablative therapy and cryotherapy)
Application of emerging molecular markers in needle biopsies (e.g., determination of status of *TMPRSS2:ERG* fusions and *PTEN* deletion)	To supplement Gleason grade for more precise personalized outcome predictions and improve the understanding of "clinically insignificant" prostate cancer
Application of advanced methods of database analysis; neural networks	Personalized outcome predictions

References

1. Catalona WJ, Richie JP, Ahmann FR et al (1994) Comparison of digital rectal examination and serum prostate specific antigen in the early detection of prostate cancer: results of a multicenter clinical trial of 6,630 men. J Urol 151:1283–1290
2. Hodge KK, McNeal JE, Terris MK, Stamey TA (1989) Random systematic versus directed ultrasound guided transrectal core biopsies of the prostate. J Urol 142:71–74; discussion 74–75
3. Norberg M, Egevad L, Holmberg L et al (1997) The sextant protocol for ultrasound-guided core biopsies of the prostate underestimates the presence of cancer. Urology 50:562–566
4. Norberg M, Egevad L, Holmberg L et al (1998) Incidence and clinical significance of false-negative sextant prostate biopsies. J Urol 159:1247–1250
5. Chen ME, Troncoso P, Tang K et al (1999) Comparison of prostate biopsy schemes by computer simulation. Urology 53:951–960
6. Egevad L, Frimmel H, Norberg M et al (1999) Three-dimensional computer reconstruction of prostate cancer from radical prostatectomy specimens: evaluation of the model by core biopsy simulation. Urology 53:192–198
7. Frimmel H, Egevad L, Bengtsson E, Busch C (1999) Modeling prostate cancer distributions. Urology 54:1028–1034
8. Stamey TA (1995) Making the most out of six systematic sextant biopsies. Urology 45:2–12
9. McNeal JE, Redwine EA, Freiha FS, Stamey TA (1988) Zonal distribution of prostatic adenocarcinoma. Correlation with histologic pattern and direction of spread. Am J Surg Pathol 12:897–906
10. Emiliozzi P, Maymone S, Paterno A et al (2004) Increased accuracy of biopsy Gleason score obtained by extended needle biopsy. J Urol 172:2224–2226
11. Epstein JI, Herawi M (2006) Prostate needle biopsies containing prostatic intraepithelial neoplasia or atypical foci suspicious for carcinoma: implications for patient care. J Urol 175:820–834
12. King CR, McNeal JE, Gill H, Presti JC Jr (2004) Extended prostate biopsy scheme improves reliability of Gleason grading: implications for radiotherapy patients. Int J Radiat Oncol Biol Phys 59:386–391
13. Presti JC Jr, O'Dowd GJ, Miller MC et al (2003) Extended peripheral zone biopsy schemes increase cancer detection rates and minimize variance in prostate specific antigen and age related cancer rates: results of a community multi-practice study. J Urol 169:125–129
14. San Francisco IF, DeWolf WC, Rosen S et al (2003) Extended prostate needle biopsy improves concordance of Gleason grading between prostate needle biopsy and radical prostatectomy. J Urol 169:136–140
15. Schlesinger C, Bostwick DG, Iczkowski KA (2005) High-grade prostatic intraepithelial neoplasia and atypical small acinar proliferation: predictive value for cancer in current practice. Am J Surg Pathol 29:1201–1207
16. Singh H, Canto EI, Shariat SF et al (2004) Improved detection of clinically significant, curable prostate cancer with systematic 12-core biopsy. J Urol 171:1089–1092
17. Siu W, Dunn RL, Shah RB, Wei JT (2005) Use of extended pattern technique for initial prostate biopsy. J Urol 174:505–509
18. Herawi M, Kahane H, Cavallo C, Epstein JI (2006) Risk of prostate cancer on first re-biopsy within 1 year following a diagnosis of high grade prostatic intraepithelial neoplasia is related to the number of cores sampled. J Urol 175:121–124
19. National Comphrehensive Cancer Network: NCCN prostate cancer early detection – 2010 practice guidelines in oncology. Available at http://www.nccn.org/professionals/physician_gls/f_guidelines.asp. Accessed 21 Jan 2010
20. Emiliozzi P, Corsetti A, Tassi B et al (2003) Best approach for prostate cancer detection: a prospective study on transperineal versus transrectal six-core prostate biopsy. Urology 61:961–966
21. Watanabe M, Hayashi T, Tsushima T et al (2005) Extensive biopsy using a combined transperineal and transrectal approach to improve prostate cancer detection. Int J Urol 12:959–963
22. Bahn DK, Lee F, Badalament R et al (2002) Targeted cryoablation of the prostate: 7-year outcomes in the primary treatment of prostate cancer. Urology 60:3–11
23. Bahn DK, Silverman P, Lee F Sr et al (2006) Focal prostate cryoablation: initial results show cancer control and potency preservation. J Endourol 20:688–692

24. Burke HB, Goodman PH, Rosen DB et al (1997) Artificial neural networks improve the accuracy of cancer survival prediction. Cancer 79:857–862
25. Onik G (2004) The male lumpectomy: rationale for a cancer targeted approach for prostate cryoablation. A review. Technol Cancer Res Treat 3:365–370
26. Schulte RT, Wood DP, Daignault S et al (2008) Utility of extended pattern prostate biopsies for tumor localization: pathologic correlations after radical prostatectomy. Cancer 113:1559–1565
27. Shah RB, Chinnaiyan AM (2009) The discovery of common recurrent transmembrane protease serine 2 (TMPRSS2)-erythroblastosis virus E26 transforming sequence (ETS) gene fusions in prostate cancer: significance and clinical implications. Adv Anat Pathol 16:145–153
28. Piert M, Park H, Khan A et al (2009) Detection of aggressive primary prostate cancer with 11C-choline PET/CT using multimodality fusion techniques. J Nucl Med 50:1585–1593

Diagnosis of Limited Cancer in Prostate Biopsy

With widespread prostate-specific antigen (PSA) screening, an increasing number of patients are diagnosed with limited, or small focus of, prostate carcinoma on prostate biopsies. Many of these patients were found to have clinically insignificant disease on radical prostatectomy. Pathologists, nevertheless, still need to evaluate prostate biopsies with due diligence and diagnose cancer that meet the accepted diagnostic criteria for several reasons. First, many patients have clinically significant disease even after a biopsy diagnosis of limited cancer and currently, there is no reliable way to predict which patient may have clinically significant disease. Second, the current medico-legal environment demands that pathologists render accurate diagnoses on prostate biopsies according to the standard of care.

Diagnosis of cancer in prostate biopsy is often challenging, especially when the cancer focus is minute. There are two main issues: (1) recognition of limited cancer to avoid underdiagnosis (false-negative), and (2) recognition of benign mimics of prostate cancer to avoid overdiagnosis (false-positive). Diagnosis of cancer in prostate needle biopsy requires a methodical approach using a constellation of architectural and cytological features of cancer glands and sometimes also requires ancillary immunohistochemistry [1, 2]. However, no two pathologists have the same threshold for diagnosing limited cancer in biopsy, and even one's own threshold changes with time and experience. It is therefore expected that pathologists may not always agree upon a diagnosis in some borderline cases. It is critical, however, to recognize these cases as being atypical and suspicious for cancer so that further workup will ensue. In this sense, the most critical issue in prostate biopsy interpretation is to identify prostate glands that are morphologically atypical and suspicious for cancer.

3.1 General Approach to Prostate Needle Biopsy Evaluation

Table 3.1 General approach to prostate needle biopsy evaluation

Use benign glands as reference and study their low-power architectural features and high-power cytological features (cytoplasmic characteristics, nuclear size and morphology, and nucleolar prominence in secretory and basal cells)

Scan biopsy cores to look for glands that appear different from and do not fit in with benign glands

Evaluate the architectural features at low power and cytological features at high power of atypical glands

Cancer diagnosis is made based on hematoxylin–eosin stain (H&E) examination; use ancillary immunohistochemistry prudently to support H&E impression

3.2 Histological Features Considered Specific for and Diagnostic of Cancer

Table 3.2 Histological features considered specific for and diagnostic of cancer

Three features have not, to date, been reported in benign glands and are considered specific for prostate cancer [3]:
  Mucinous fibroplasia (collagenous micronodules)
  Glomerulation
  Perineural invasion

Cancer diagnosis can be rendered when one of the three features is present in biopsy

Prudent to confirm the cancer diagnosis with basal cell marker immunostains when the focus is small and without other cancer-associated features

Table 3.3 Histological features specific for prostate cancer

Features	Histology	Gleason grade	Incidence in biopsy
Mucinous fibroplasia (collagenous micronodules) (*see* Fig. 3.1)	Acellular or hypocellular hyalinized stroma within or outside cancer glands	Based on the architecture of the glandular component, pattern 3 or 4	1–2% [4]
Glomeration (*see* Fig. 3.2)	Balls or tufts of cancer cells within glands, superficially resembling renal glomeruli	Small with rounded contour: pattern 3. Large: pattern 4	3–15% [5]
Perineural invasion (*see* Fig. 3.3)	Tight circumferential or near circumferential encircling of a nerve fiber by cancer glands	Based on the glandular component, pattern 3 or 4	22% [6]

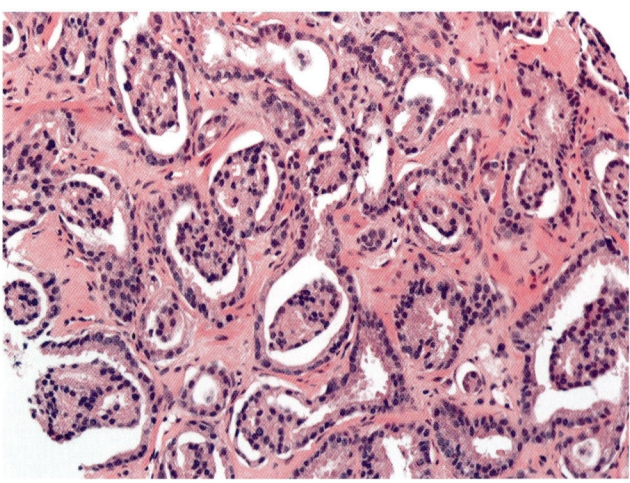

Fig. 3.2 Glomerulation: histological feature specific for prostate cancer. It results from the intraluminal proliferation of cancer cells that forms balls or tufts within cancer glands, superficially resembling renal glomeruli

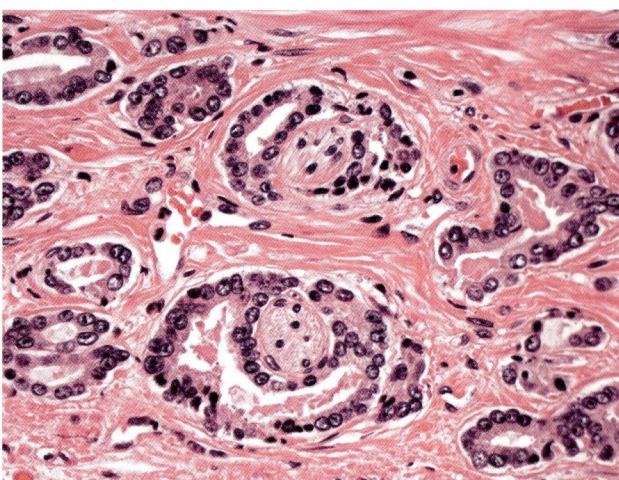

Fig. 3.3 Perineural invasion: histological feature specific for prostate cancer. It is defined as tight circumferential or near circumferential encircling of a nerve fiber by cancer glands. It should be distinguished from perineural abutment by benign glands (*see* Fig. 1.18)

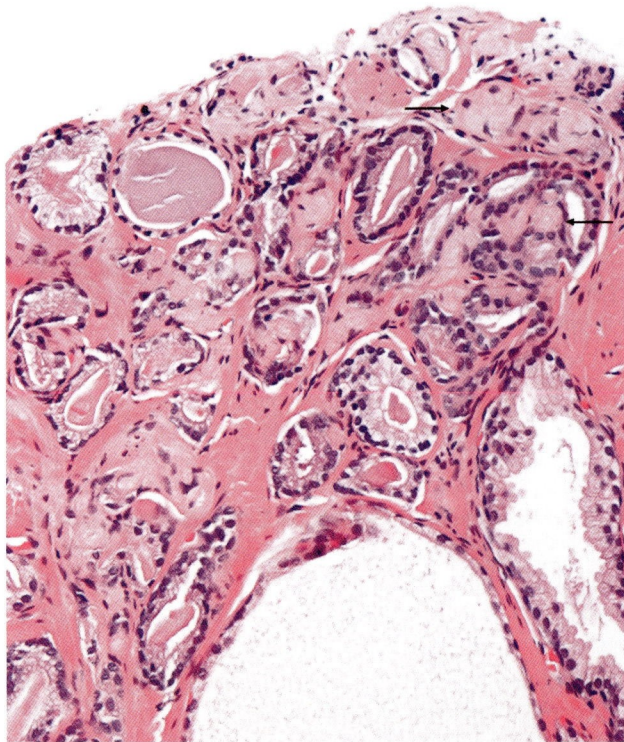

Fig. 3.1 Mucinous fibroplasia: histological feature specific for prostate cancer. It is acellular or hypocellular hyalinized stroma within or outside cancer glands (*arrows*), and results from hyalinization of extravasated mucin

3.3 Major and Minor Histological Features of Prostate Cancer in Biopsy

Table 3.4 Major and minor histological features of prostate cancer in biopsy. In the majority of prostate biopsies, the diagnosis of cancer relies on histological features other than mucinous fibroplasia, glomerulation, and perineural invasion. These features are categorized as major and minor features according to how strongly they are associated with cancer [7, 8]

Major features (strongly associated with cancer and rarely seen in noncancer lesions)

Abnormal architectural pattern [7, 8]	Infiltrative growth pattern (*see* Fig. 3.4)
	Large cribriform glands with irregular contour (*see* Fig. 3.7)
	Single or cords of atypical cells (*see* Fig. 3.8)
	Solid nests with or without comedo necrosis (*see* Fig. 3.9)
Absence of basal cells [7, 8]	Can be confirmed by basal cell marker immunohistochemistry (*see* Fig. 3.10–3.12)
Nuclear atypia [9–11]	Nuclear enlargement (*see* Fig. 3.13)
	Prominent nucleoli (*see* Fig. 3.14)
	Hyperchromasia (*see* Fig. 3.15)

Minor features (less strongly associated with cancer, may also be seen in noncancer lesions)

Cytoplasm	Cytoplasmic amphophilia (dark cytoplasm) (*see* Fig. 3.16) [12]
Intraluminal contents	Amorphous secretion (*see* Fig. 3.17) [12]
	Blue mucin (*see* Fig. 3.18) [13]
	Crystalloids (*see* Fig. 3.19) [14, 15]
Mitosis and apoptosis	More common in prostate cancer (*see* Fig. 3.20) [9, 16]
Adjacent high-grade prostatic intraepithelial neoplasia (HGPIN)	Cancer often associated with HGPIN (*see* Fig. 3.21)

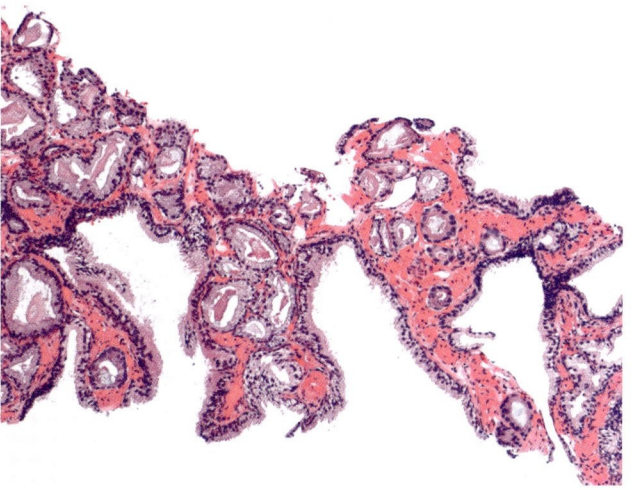

Fig. 3.4 Major histological feature 1: abnormal architectural pattern – infiltrative growth. This is the most characteristic growth pattern for prostate cancer, with cancer glands situated between and on both sides of the larger and paler benign glands. This growth pattern is indicative of invasion. The cancer glands are typically small with rigid round lumens as opposed to large benign glands with undulating luminal borders. Prostate cancer invariably exhibits some form of abnormal architectural features when compared to the adjacent benign glands (*see* Table 3.4). Some of the architectural features, such as infiltrative growth, large cribriform glands with infiltrative border and solid nests, are almost specific for cancer, whereas other features, such as crowded growth, are less strongly associated with cancer and may also be found in noncancer lesions

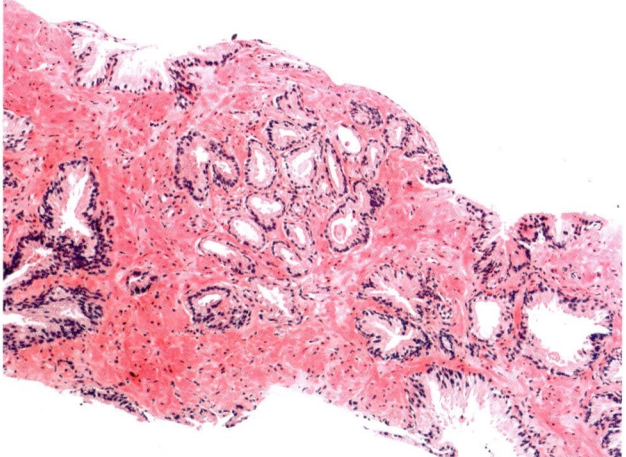

Fig. 3.5 Abnormal architectural pattern – crowded glands. Cancer glands are closely packed and more crowded than the adjacent benign glands, and are often circumscribed without infiltrative pattern. The presence of a focus of crowded glands should raise a suspicion for cancer. However, such growth pattern may also be seen in adenosis (atypical adenomatous hyperplasia), which should always be considered and ruled out before a cancer diagnosis is rendered

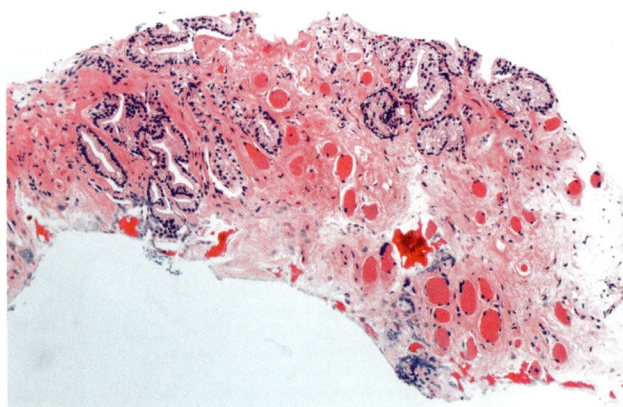

Fig. 3.6 Abnormal architectural pattern – haphazardly arranged glands without accompanying benign glands. The cancer glands grow in a haphazard fashion and dissect stroma and muscle bundles without accompanying benign glands

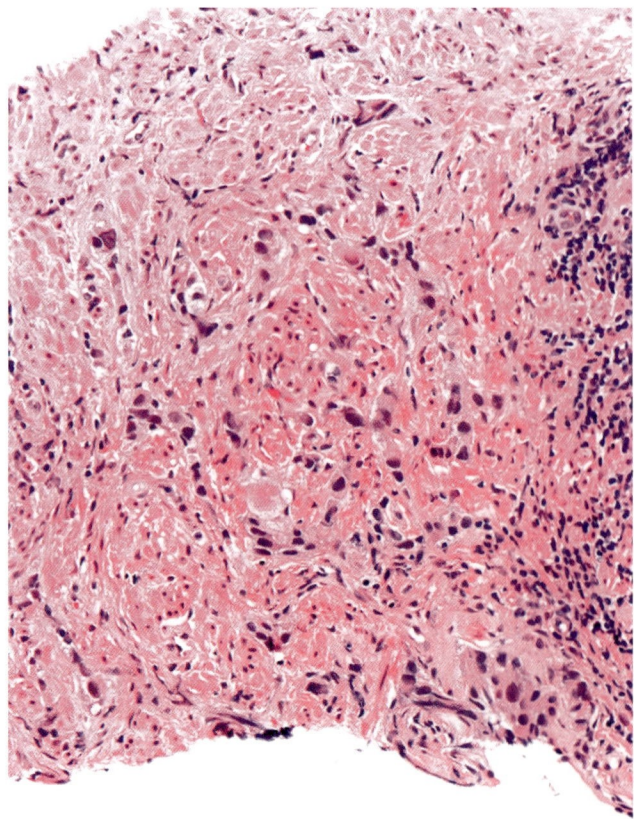

Fig. 3.8 Major histological feature 1: abnormal architectural pattern – single or cords of atypical cells. Single cancer cells infiltrate in the stroma. They also form short cords

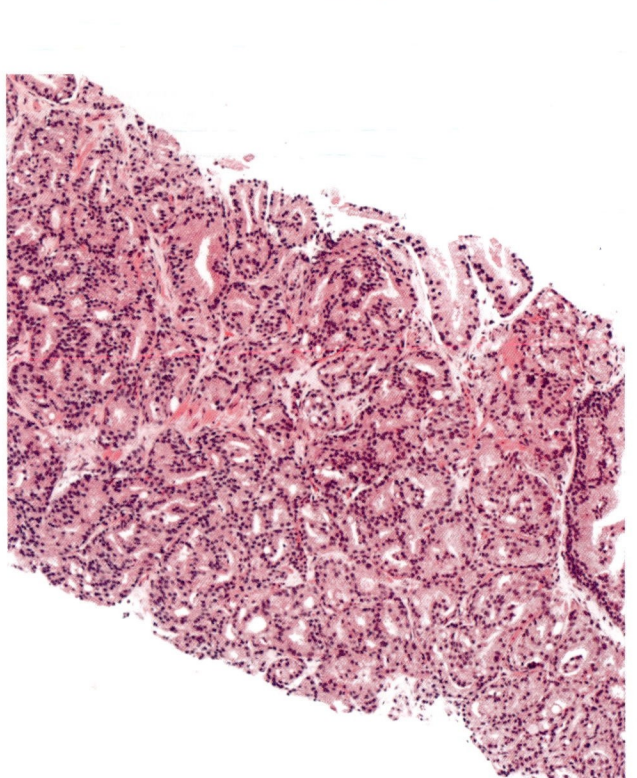

Fig. 3.7 Major histological feature 1: abnormal architectural pattern – irregular cribriform structure. Cancer glands demonstrate large cribriform architecture with irregular and infiltrative borders

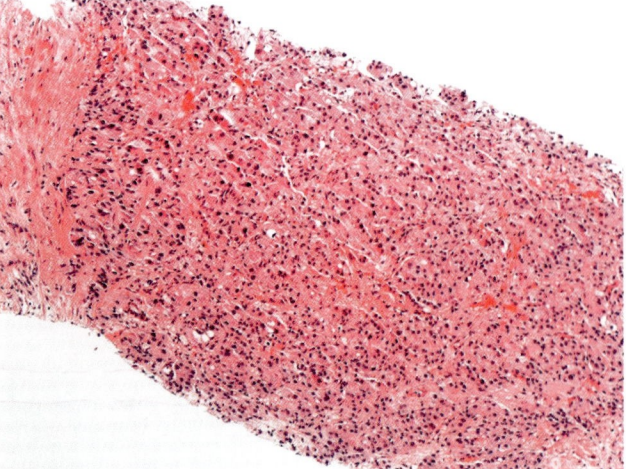

Fig. 3.9 Major histological feature 1: abnormal architectural pattern – solid nests. Cancer cells form solid nests without discernible lumens

3.3 Major and Minor Histological Features of Prostate Cancer in Biopsy

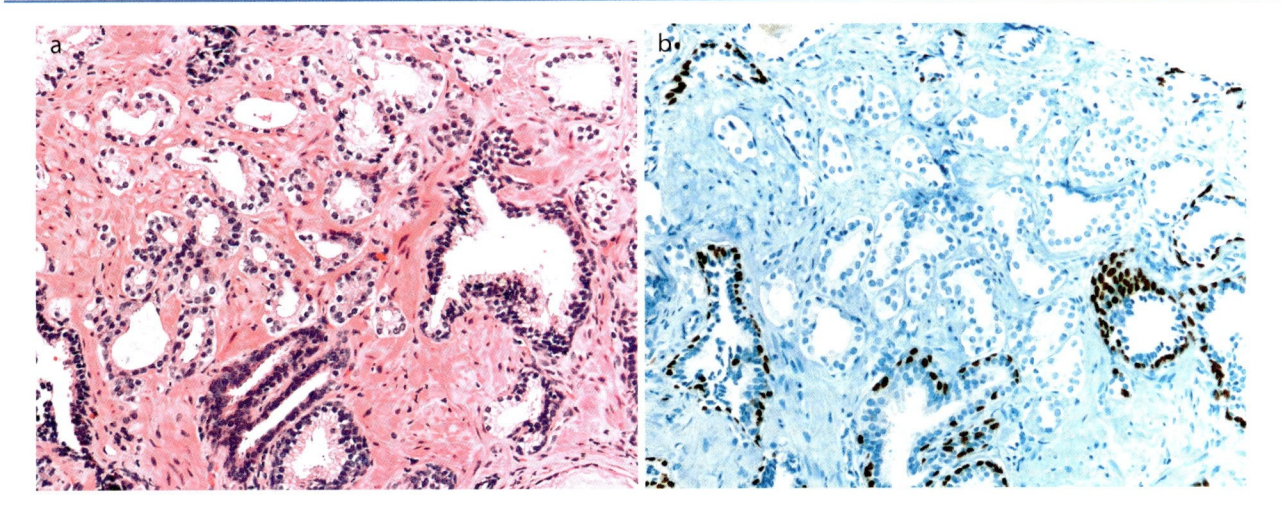

Fig. 3.10 Major histological feature 2: absence of basal cells. Cancer glands are devoid of basal cells on H&E examination (**a**), which is confirmed by immunostain for basal cell marker p63 (**b**)

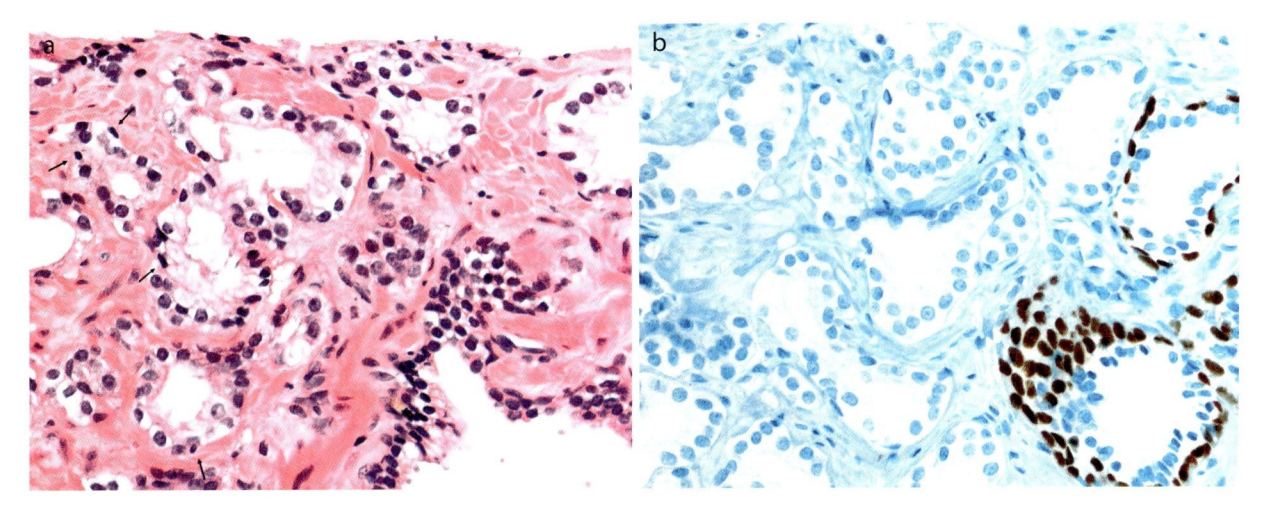

Fig. 3.11 Crushed cancer cells mimicking basal cells. Crushed cancer cells appear hyperchromatic (*arrows*) and different from other cancer cells and therefore may be mistaken for basal cells (**a**). Basal cells can assume a range of appearances and may be difficult to distinguish from stromal fibroblasts or crushed cancer cells on H&E examination [17, 18]. It is prudent to perform basal cell immunostains, p63 in this case, to confirm the absence of basal cells (**b**)

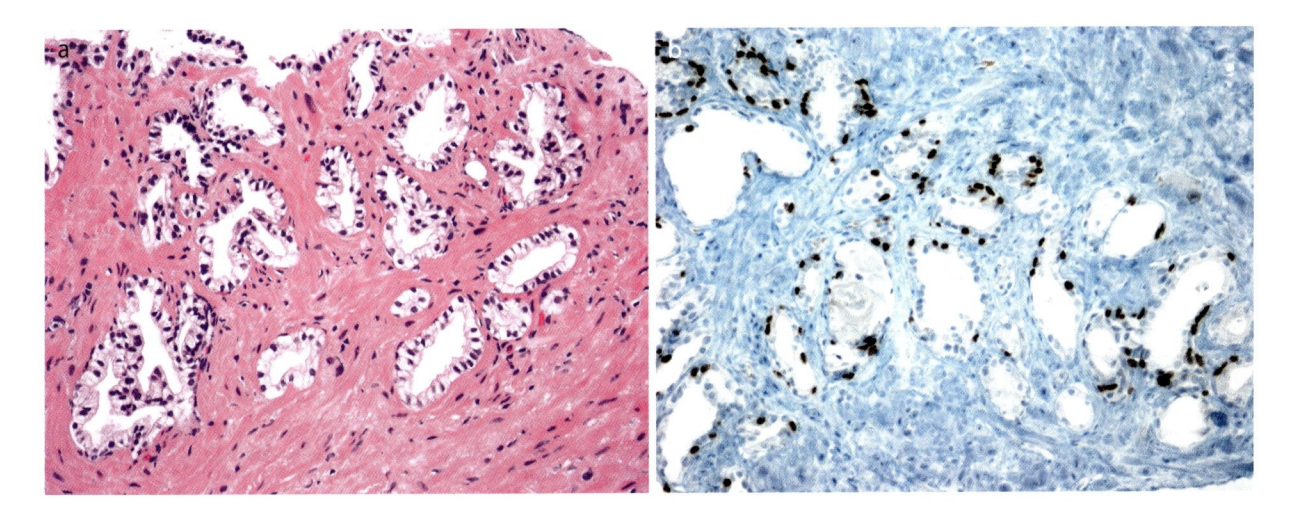

Fig. 3.12 Partial atrophy with patchy basal cells. Basal cells are not always present in all benign glands, such as partial atrophy (**a**). Basal cell immunostain for p63 demonstrates focal staining in some glands and complete absence of staining in other glands (**b**). However, glands with and without basal cell lining have identical cytological features. Other noncancerous lesions that often demonstrate patchy or absent basal cells include adenosis and HGPIN

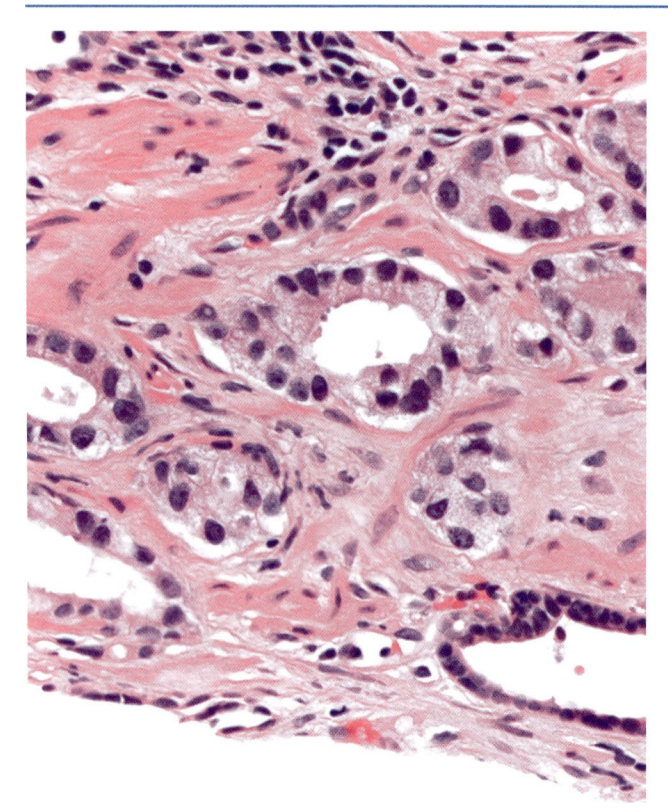

Fig. 3.13 Major histological feature 3: nuclear atypia – nuclear enlargement. Using the adjacent benign glands (right lower of the image) as reference, the cancer cells have significantly enlarged nuclei

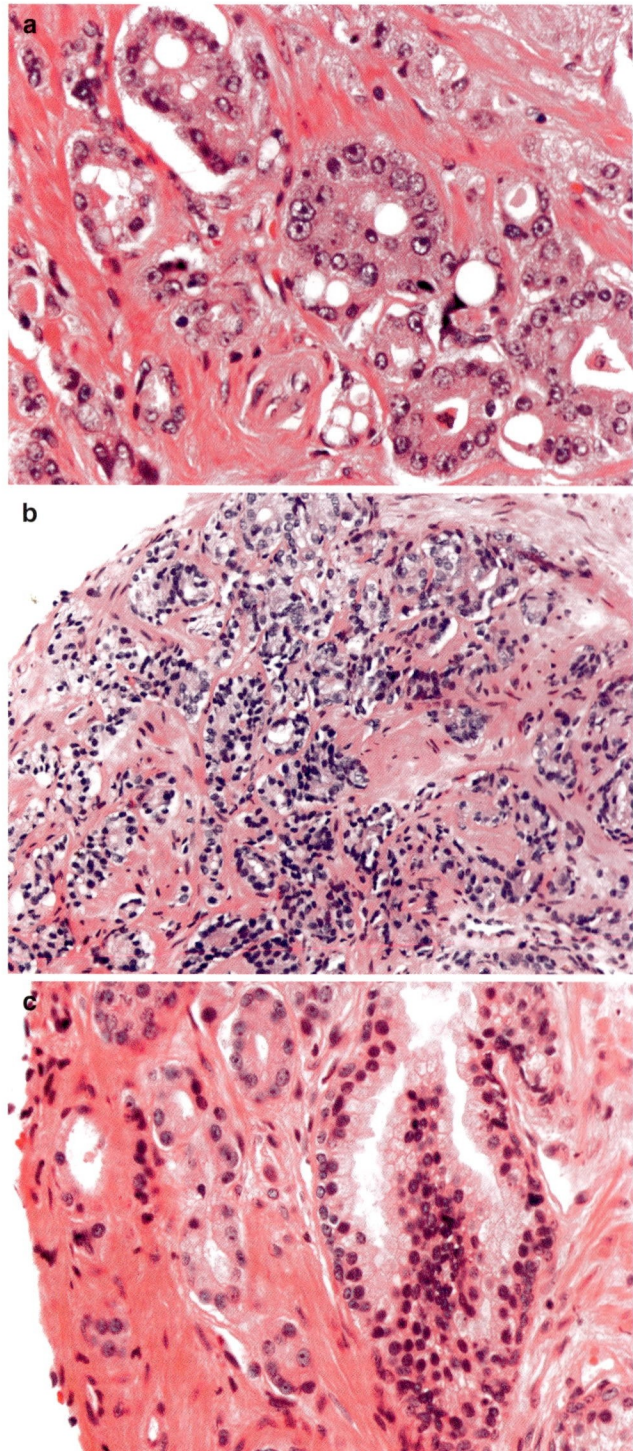

Fig. 3.14 Major histological feature 3: nuclear atypia – prominent nucleoli. Compared to the adjacent benign glands, the cancer cells have prominent nucleoli (**a**). However, nucleolar prominence depends on the several tissue processing factors, including fixation, tissue section thickness, and staining protocols. Alcohol-based fixatives often obscure the nuclear detail with blurred chromatin and inconspicuous nucleoli (**b**) whereas Hollandes fixative enhances nucleoli with visible nucleoli even in basal cells of benign glands (**c**)

3.3 Major and Minor Histological Features of Prostate Cancer in Biopsy

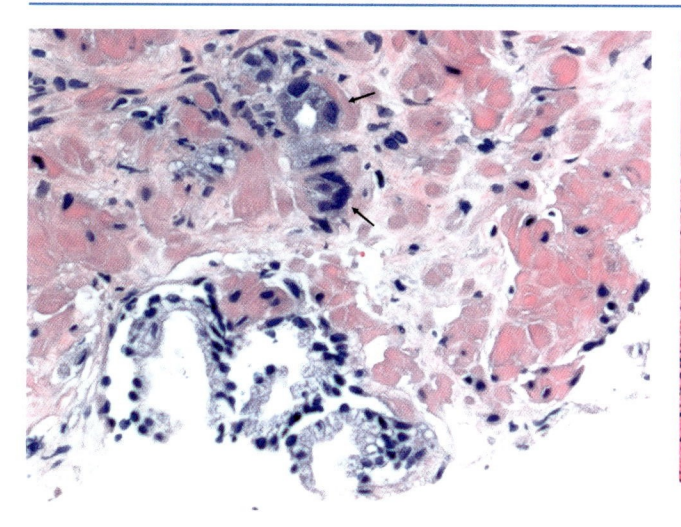

Fig. 3.15 Major histological feature 3: nuclear atypia – hyperchromasia. Compared to the adjacent benign glands, cancer cells can have larger hyperchromatic and pleomorphic nuclei (*arrows*)

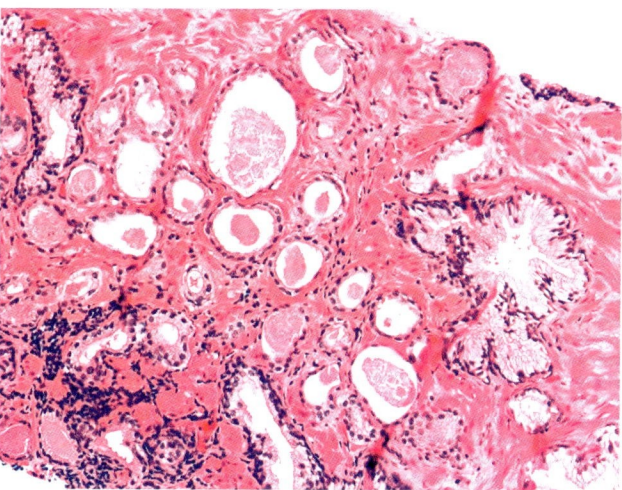

Fig. 3.17 Minor histological feature 2: amorphous intraluminal secretion. Cancer glands have eosinophilic amorphous material within their lumens. They are more common in cancer, but can also be found in some benign lesions

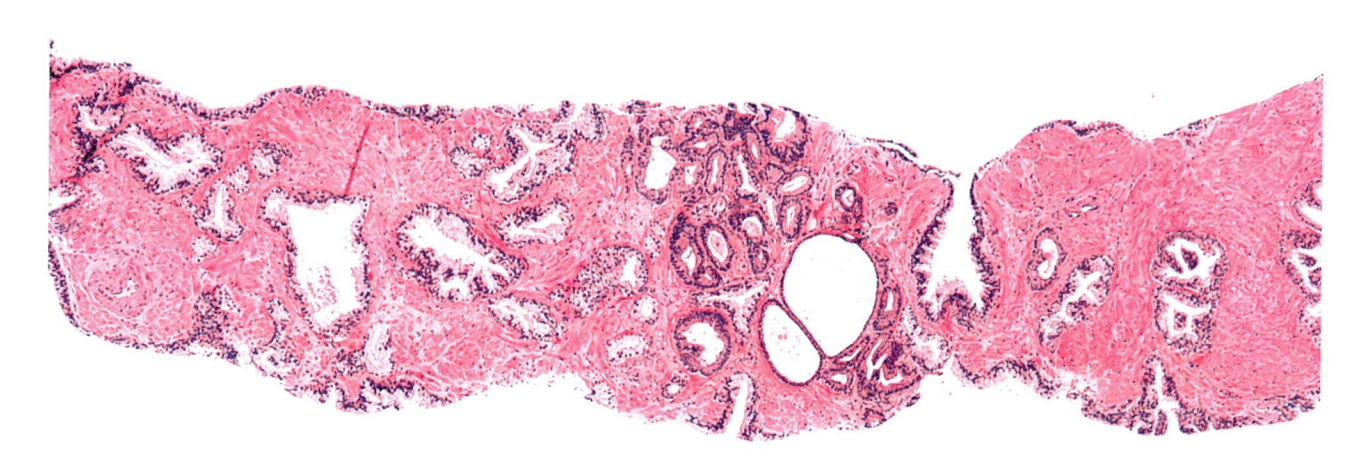

Fig. 3.16 Minor histological feature 1: amphophilic cytoplasm. Compared with benign glands with clear cytoplasm, cancer glands often have amphophilic, or dark, cytoplasm. This feature can be appreciated at low scanning power and, together with the infiltrative growth pattern, often provides the first clue to the presence of cancer in the biopsy. Although less strongly associated with cancer and may be seen in noncancer lesions, minor histological features associated with cancer are diagnostically very helpful as the atypical glands with these minor features usually appear significantly different and therefore stand out from the benign glands

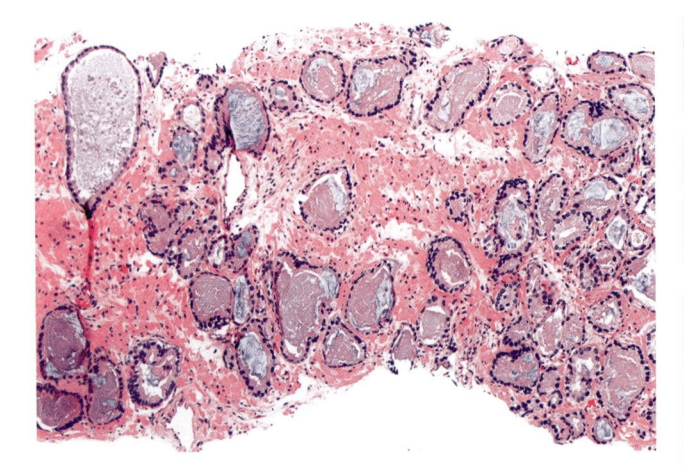

Fig. 3.18 Minor histological feature 3: blue mucin. Cancer glands have blue-tinged wisps of mucin, often together with dense pink secretion, within their lumens. They are more common in cancer, but can also be found in some benign lesions. Blue mucin depends on the H&E staining of the tissue section. If the tissue section is overstained, with rectal mucosa that is often present in prostate biopsies stained intensely blue, one should be cautious about the diagnostic utility of blue mucin

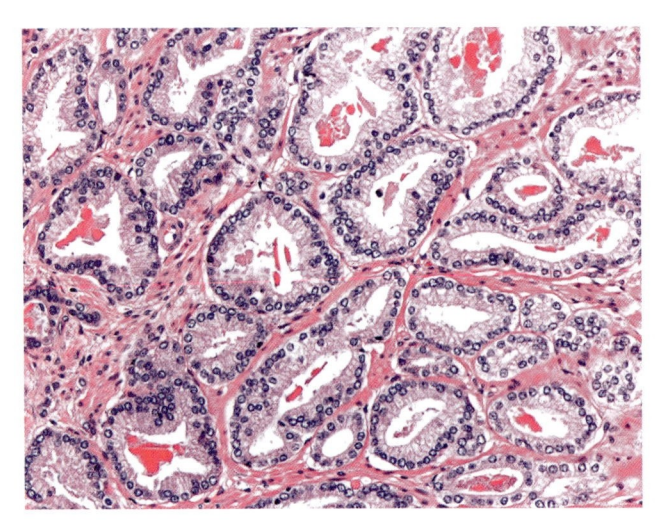

Fig. 3.19 Minor histological feature 4: crystalloids. Dense eosinophilic crystalloid structures that assume various shapes such as rhomboid and needle are in the lumens of the cancer glands. They are more common in cancer, but can also be found in some benign lesions

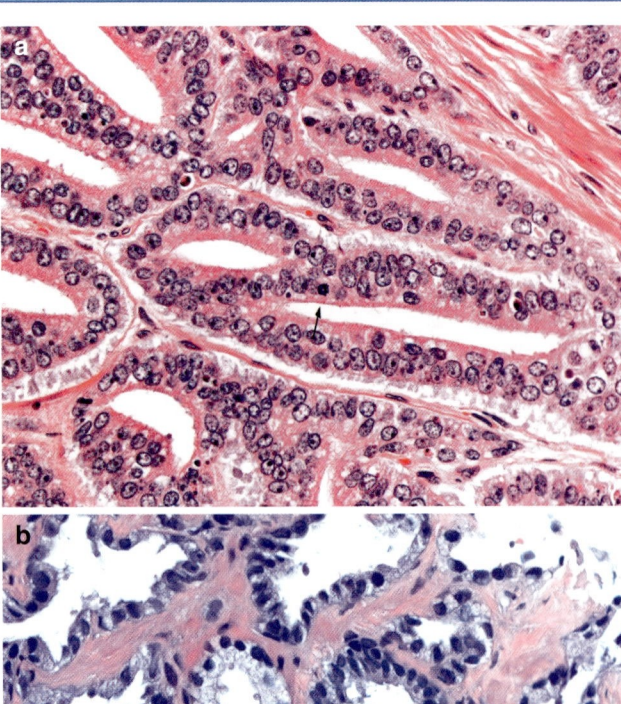

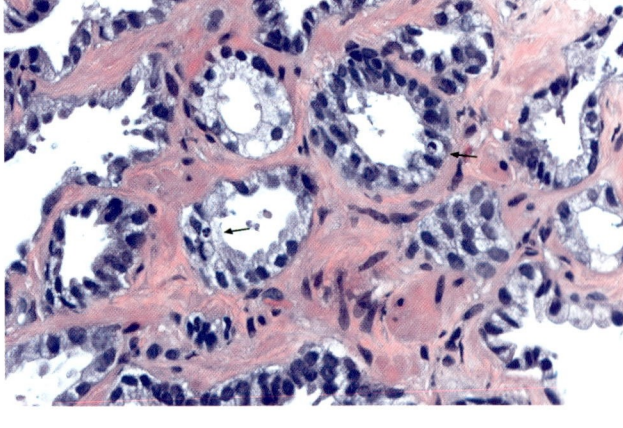

Fig. 3.20 Minor histological feature 5: mitosis and apoptosis. A mitotic figure (*arrow*, **a**) and apoptotic bodies (*arrows*, **b**) are found in cancer glands. Mitosis and apoptosis are more common in cancer cells

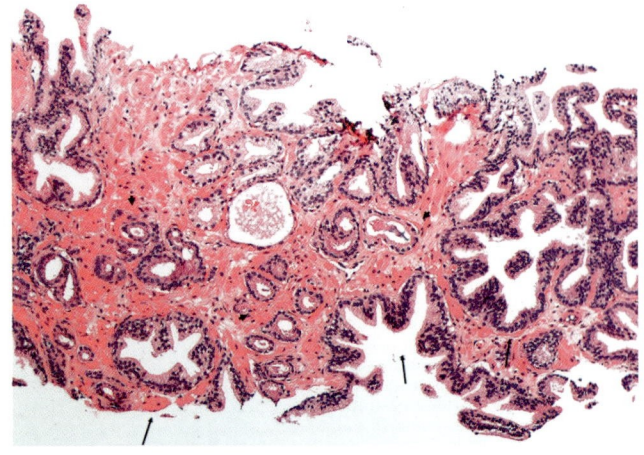

Fig. 3.21 Minor histological feature 6: cancer associated with HGPIN. Cancer glands (*arrowheads*) often intermingle with HGPIN glands (*arrows*). The presence of HGPIN should alert pathologists to look for cancer in the biopsy

3.4 Benign Conditions That Cause Architectural and Cytological Atypia

Table 3.5 Benign conditions that cause architectural and cytological atypia. Some benign processes may cause architectural and cytological atypia that is commonly associated with cancer. Each of these benign processes should be considered and ruled out before a cancer diagnosis is rendered (Also see Chapter 7)

Benign process	Atypical histological features
Inflammation (see Fig. 3.22)	Small, crowded or cribriform glands
	Significant nucleoli
Atrophy (see Fig. 3.23)	Haphazard and disorganized pattern, poorly formed glands, mild nuclear enlargement, and small nucleoli [19]
Adenosis (atypical adenomatous hyperplasia) (see Fig. 3.24)	Crowded glands [20, 21]
HGPIN with adjacent small focus of atypical glands (see Fig. 3.25)	A few atypical glands immediately adjacent to larger HGPIN glands (uncertain whether atypical glands represent micro invasive cancer or tangential sectioning and/or outpouching of HGPIN glands) [22]

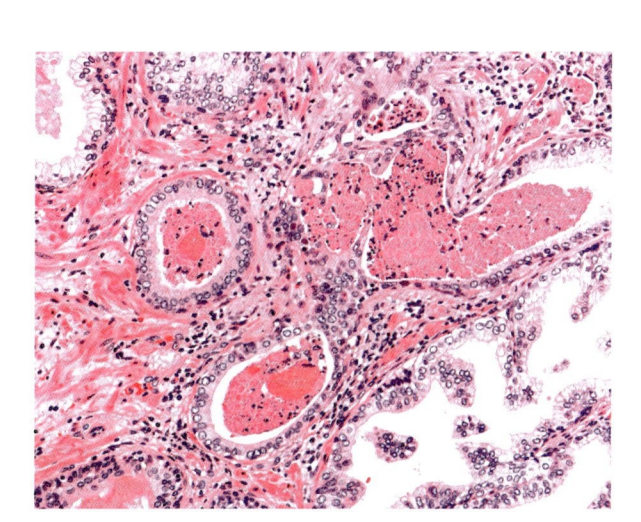

Fig. 3.22 Benign prostate glands with exuberant inflammation. The epithelial cells exhibit significant cytological atypia, including nuclear enlargement and small nucleoli. Cancer glands, however, can also be associated with inflammation

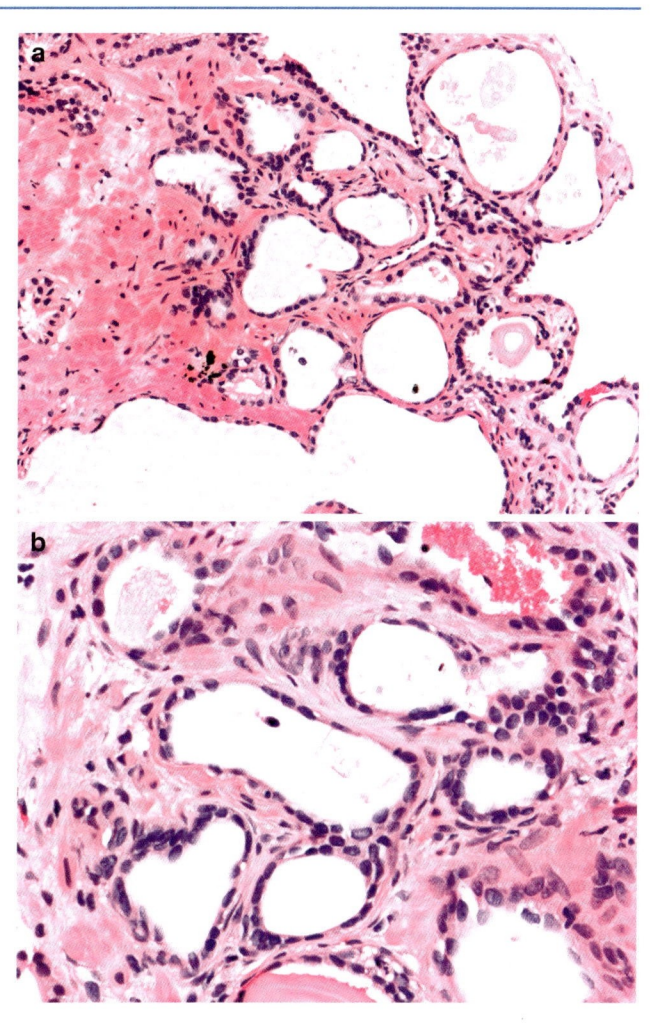

Fig. 3.23 Simple atrophy. Glands have lobulated architecture (**a**) and nuclei are slightly enlarged with small or inconspicuous nucleoli (**b**)

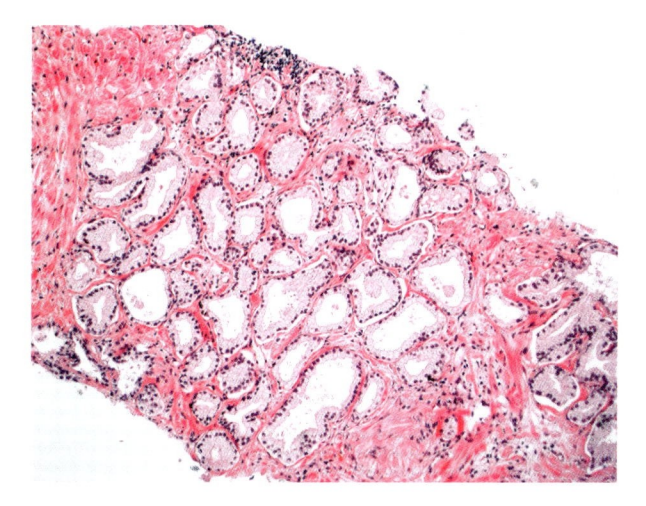

Fig. 3.24 Adenosis. Circumscribed, lobular collection of glands with variable sizes. Some glands are clearly benign with large irregular contour and undulating luminal borders. Smaller glands with rigid lumens are identical to larger benign glands cytologically

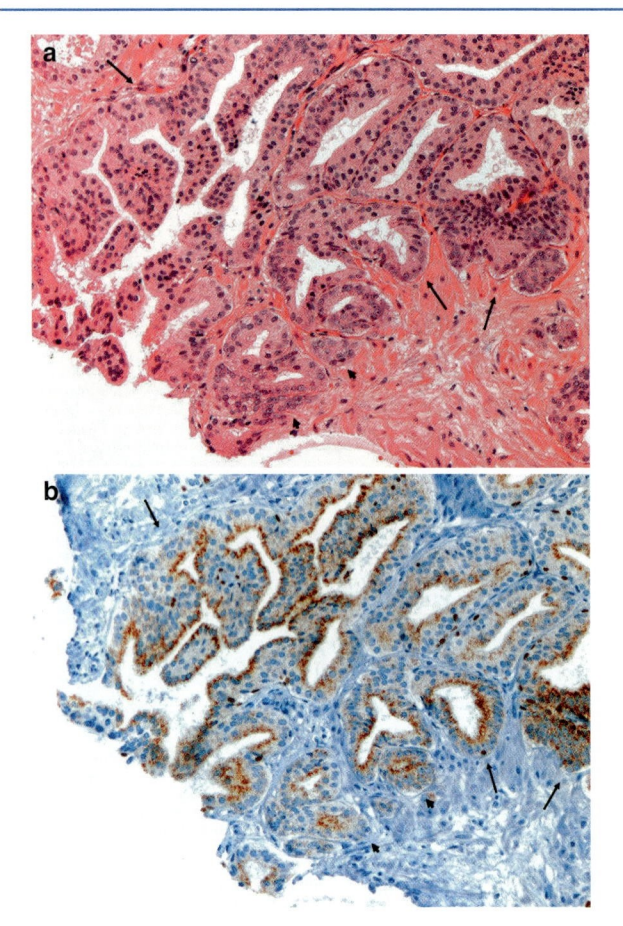

Fig. 3.25 HGPIN with adjacent small focus of atypical glands (PINATYP). A few atypical glands (*arrowhead*) lie immediately adjacent to larger HGPIN glands (*arrows*) (**a**) and are negative for basal cell marker p63 and positive for α-methylacyl-CoA racemase (AMACR) (**b**). Note the HGPIN glands are also positive for AMACR and are scarcely positive for p63. It is uncertain whether these atypical glands represent a microfocus of invasive cancer or tangential sectioning and/or outpouching of HGPIN glands. Such distinction may be made based on the number of the atypical glands and their distance to the adjacent HGPIN glands. If the atypical glands are more than a few and not immediately adjacent to the HGPIN glands, they are unlikely the result of tangential sectioning and/or outpouching of HGPIN glands

3.5 Quantitative Threshold for Diagnosing Limited Cancer in Biopsy

Table 3.6 Quantitative threshold for diagnosing limited cancer in biopsy

Depending on the architectural and cytological atypia: more atypia, fewer glands are required to make a cancer diagnosis (*see* Fig. 3.26) [4, 12, 23]
Most expert urological pathologists require at least three glands to make a cancer diagnosis, or more if there is no full-blown cancer-associated architectural and cytological features (*see* Fig. 3.26) [7]

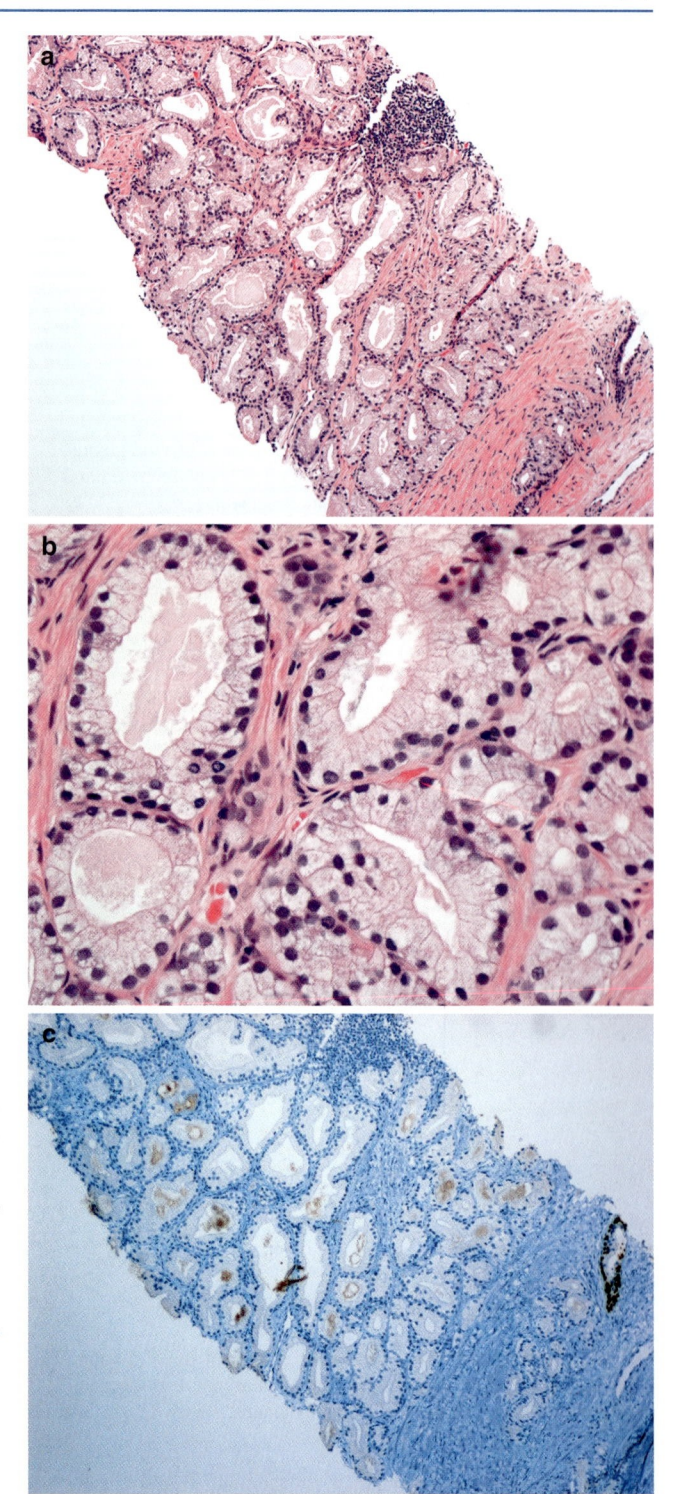

Fig. 3.26 Prostate cancer with subtle architectural and cytological atypia. In this case, the cancer glands display crowded growth pattern (**a**). The cancer cells have minimum nuclear enlargement and inconspicuous nucleoli (**b**). This focus is negative for basal cell marker p63 (**c**). The cancer diagnosis in such cases requires a substantial number of cancer glands and ancillary immunohistochemistry

Fig. 3.27 Limited prostate cancer. There are only five cancer glands present in one needle core. However, they display infiltrative growth pattern (**a**) and significant nuclear enlargement and hyperchromasia (**b**). These atypical glands are not inflamed or atrophic. These glands are negative for p63 (**c**). Ancillary immunostains are required to support a cancer diagnosis in such cases

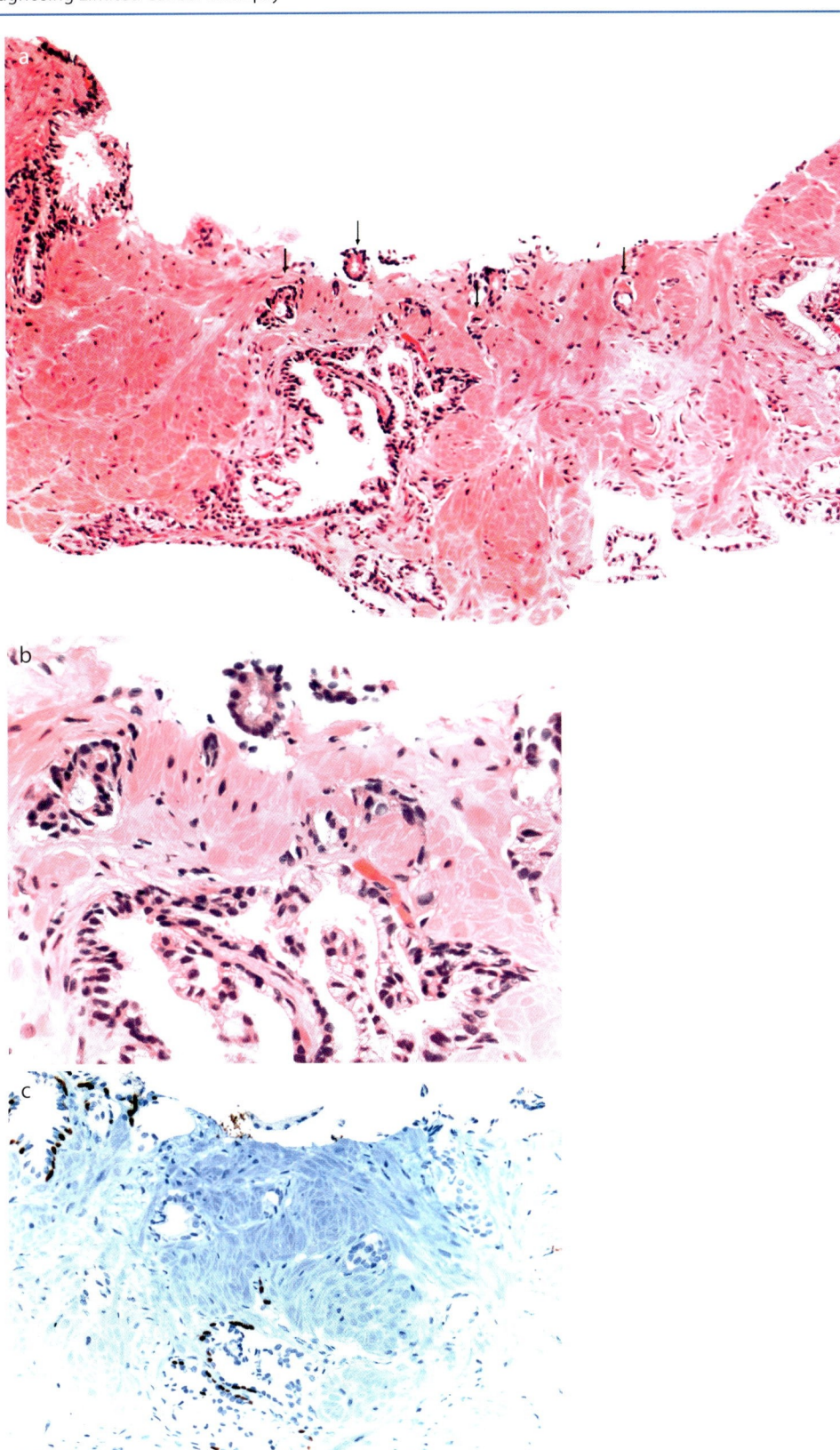

3.6 Histological Features For and Against Cancer Diagnosis in Biopsy

Table 3.7 Histological features favoring and against cancer diagnosis in biopsy

Favoring cancer	Against cancer
Architectural pattern	
Infiltrative growth pattern	Lobulated pattern
Glands with relatively uniform appearance	Small and large glands intermingle without cytological difference
Small glands with rigid luminal borders	Large glands with branching and papillary infolding
Nuclear features	
Enlargement	Nuclear atypia in the background of inflammation
Prominent nucleoli	Random nuclear atypia
Hyperchromasia	
Mitosis and apoptosis	
Cytoplasmic features	
Amphophilic (dark) cytoplasm	Pale-clear cytoplasm
	Atrophy
	Lipofuscin pigment
Intraluminal contents	
Blue mucin	Corpora amylacea
Amorphous secretion	Calcification
Crystalloids	
Stroma	
Desmoplasia and hemorrhage	Hyalinized stroma
Unaltered stroma	Cellular spindle cell stroma
Adjacent HGPIN	
Atypical glands are more than just a few in number or distant from HGPIN glands	A few atypical glands in close proximity to large HGPIN glands

Modified from Epstein and Netto [24]

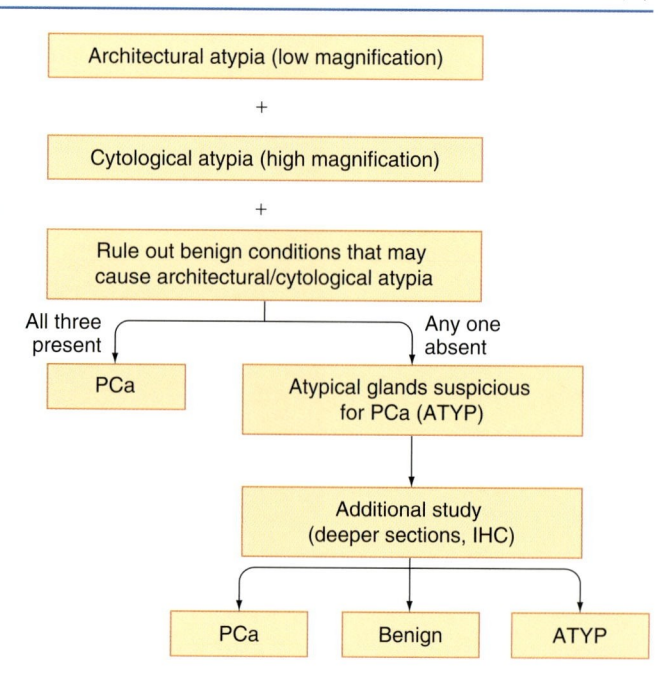

Fig. 3.28 A practical approach to the diagnosis of limited cancer in prostate biopsy. When evaluating atypical prostate glands, one should look for glands with atypical architectural and cytological features and consider and rule out all benign conditions that may cause such architectural and cytological atypia. A cancer diagnosis can be rendered only if all three criteria are satisfied. If any of these three criteria is missing, one should be very cautious about making a cancer diagnosis. Additional studies should be performed to clarify the diagnosis. *ATYP* atypical glands suspicious for cancer, *IHC* immunohistochemistry, *PCa* prostate cancer

3.7 A Practical Approach to Diagnosis of Limited Cancer in Needle Biopsy

Table 3.8 A practical approach to diagnosis of limited cancer in needle biopsy

Use benign glands as reference and evaluate the architectural and cytological features of atypical glands (*see* Table 3.4)

A definitive cancer diagnosis can be established only when all three criteria are met:

1. Atypical glands exhibiting major and/or minor architectural atypia
2. Atypical glands exhibiting cytological atypia
3. Benign processes that may cause architectural and cytological atypia are carefully considered and ruled out (*see* Fig. 3.28)

References

1. Epstein JI (2004) Diagnosis and reporting of limited adenocarcinoma of the prostate on needle biopsy. Mod Pathol 17:307–315
2. Humphrey PA (2007) Diagnosis of adenocarcinoma in prostate needle biopsy tissue. J Clin Pathol 60:35–42
3. Baisden BL, Kahane H, Epstein JI (1999) Perineural invasion, mucinous fibroplasia, and glomerulations: diagnostic features of limited cancer on prostate needle biopsy. Am J Surg Pathol 23:918–924
4. Thorson P, Vollmer RT, Arcangeli C et al (1998) Minimal carcinoma in prostate needle biopsy specimens: diagnostic features and radical prostatectomy follow-up. Mod Pathol 11:543–551
5. Pacelli A, Lopez-Beltran A, Egan AJM et al (1998) Prostate adenocarcinoma with glomeruloid features. Hum Pathol 29:543–546
6. Humphrey PA (2003) Prostate pathology. American Journal of Clinical Pathology Press, Chicago
7. Algaba F, Epstein JI, Aldape HC et al (1996) Assessment of prostate carcinoma in core needle biopsy – definition of minimal criteria for the diagnosis of cancer in biopsy material. Cancer 78:376–381
8. Totten RS, Heinemann MW, Hudson PB et al (1953) Microscopic differential diagnosis of latent carcinoma of prostate. AMA Arch Pathol 55:131–141
9. Aydin H, Zhou M, Herawi M, Epstein JI (2005) Number and location of nucleoli and presence of apoptotic bodies in diagnostically challenging cases of prostate adenocarcinoma on needle biopsy. Hum Pathol 36:1172–1177
10. Helpap B (1988) Observations on the number, size and localization of nucleoli in hyperplastic and neoplastic prostatic disease. Histopathology 13:203–211
11. Varma M, Lee MW, Tamboli P et al (2002) Morphologic criteria for the diagnosis of prostatic adenocarcinoma in needle biopsy specimens. A study of 250 consecutive cases in a routine surgical pathology practice. Arch Pathol Lab Med 126:554–561
12. Epstein JI (1995) Diagnostic criteria of limited adenocarcinoma of the prostate on needle biopsy. Hum Pathol 26:223–229
13. Epstein JI, Fynheer J (1992) Acidic mucin in the prostate: can it differentiate adenosis from adenocarcinoma? Hum Pathol 23:1321–1325
14. Henneberry JM, Kahane H, Humphrey PA et al (1997) The significance of intraluminal crystalloids in benign prostatic glands on needle biopsy. Am J Surg Pathol 21:725–728
15. Ro JY, Ayala AG, Ordonez NG et al (1986) Intraluminal crystalloids in prostatic adenocarcinoma. Immunohistochemical, electron microscopic, and x-ray microanalytic studies. Cancer 57:2397–2407
16. Vesalainen S, Lipponen P, Talja M, Syrjanen K (1995) Mitotic activity and prognosis in prostatic adenocarcinoma. Prostate 26:80–86
17. Cleary KR, Choi HY, Ayala AG (1983) Basal cell hyperplasia of the prostate. Am J Clin Pathol 80:850–854
18. Devaraj LT, Bostwick DG (1993) Atypical basal cell hyperplasia of the prostate. Immunophenotypic profile and proposed classification of basal cell proliferations. Am J Surg Pathol 17:645–659
19. Amin MB, Tamboli P, Varma M, Srigley JR (1999) Postatrophic hyperplasia of the prostate gland: a detailed analysis of its morphology in needle biopsy specimens. Am J Surg Pathol 23:925–931
20. Bostwick DG, Srigley J, Grignon D et al (1993) Atypical adenomatous hyperplasia of the prostate: morphologic criteria for its distinction from well-differentiated carcinoma. Hum Pathol 24:819–832
21. Gaudin PB, Epstein JI (1995) Adenosis of the prostate. Histologic features in needle biopsy specimens. Am J Surg Pathol 19:737–747
22. Kronz JD, Shaikh AA, Epstein JI (2001) High-grade prostatic intraepithelial neoplasia with adjacent small atypical glands on prostate biopsy. Hum Pathol 32:389–395
23. Iczkowski KA, Bostwick DG (2000) Criteria for biopsy diagnosis of minimal volume prostatic adenocarcinoma: analytic comparison with nondiagnostic but suspicious atypical small acinar proliferation. Arch Pathol Lab Med 124:98–107
24. Epstein JI, Netto GJ (2008) Diagnosis of limited adenocarcinoma of the prostate. In: Biopsy Interpretation of the prostate. Lippincott Williams and Wilkins, Philadelphia

Immunohistochemistry in Prostate Biopsy Evaluation

4

Immunohistochemistry has been widely used in the workup of difficult prostate biopsies [1, 2]. It is used in two clinical settings: to distinguish prostate cancer from benign lesions that mimic cancer and to distinguish poorly differentiated prostate cancer from other malignant tumors that can occasionally involve the prostate, including urothelial carcinoma and colonic adenocarcinoma (*see* Table 4.1). Immunohistochemistry, as an adjunct to histological examination, has had significant impact on the prostate biopsy evaluation. In the case of limited cancer or histological variants with deceptively bland morphology, immunohistochemistry is an indispensible part of the workup [2]. Use of immunohistochemistry has also significantly reduced the incidence of prostate biopsies with atypical diagnosis to establish a definitive diagnosis [3–5].

4.1 Commonly Used Immunohistochemical Markers for Diagnosis of Prostate Cancer in Biopsy

Table 4.1 Commonly used immunohistochemical markers for diagnosis of prostate cancer in biopsy

Markers to distinguish prostate carcinoma from its benign mimics
Basal cell markers
   High-molecular-weight cytokeratin (HMWCK)
   p63
Prostate cancer markers
   α-Methyl-CoA-racemase (AMACR, P504S)
   ERG

Markers to distinguish prostate carcinoma from nonprostatic malignancy secondarily involving prostate [6]
Cytokeratins
   Cytokeratin 7
   Cytokeratin 20
Prostate basal cell markers
   HMWCK
   p63
Prostate-specific markers
   Prostate-specific antigen (PSA)
   Prostate-specific acid phosphatase (PSAP)
   Prostate-specific membrane antigen (PSMA)
   Prostein (P501S)
Other Tissue lineage-specific lineage markers
   TTF-1
   CDX-2

4.2 Basal Cell Markers

Table 4.2 Basal cell markers commonly used in prostate biopsy workup

Basal cell markers in prostate biopsy work-up
Types of basal cell markers
HMWCK: cytoplasmic intermediate filaments detected by several antibody preparations (34βE12, CK5/6, CK14) (*see* Fig. 4.1)
p63: nuclear antigen (*see* Fig. 4.1)
Basal cell cocktail (34βE12+ p63) (*see* Fig. 4.1)
Staining pattern in prostate cancer
Prostate carcinoma lacks staining for basal cell markers (*see* Fig. 4.2)
HMWCK may rarely be positive in cancer cells, but not in basal cell distribution, due to excessive antigen retrieval and staining (*see* Fig. 4.4)
p63 can rarely be found in cancer cells with uniform and non-basal cell distribution (*see* Fig. 4.5)
Diagnostic utility
A negative basal cell marker staining in atypical glands morphologically suspicious for cancer supports a cancer diagnosis (*see* Fig. 4.3)
Pitfalls
Adenosis, partial atrophy, high-grade prostatic intraepithelial neoplasia (HGPIN) may have discontinuous or even absent basal cell lining (*see* Fig. 4.11)

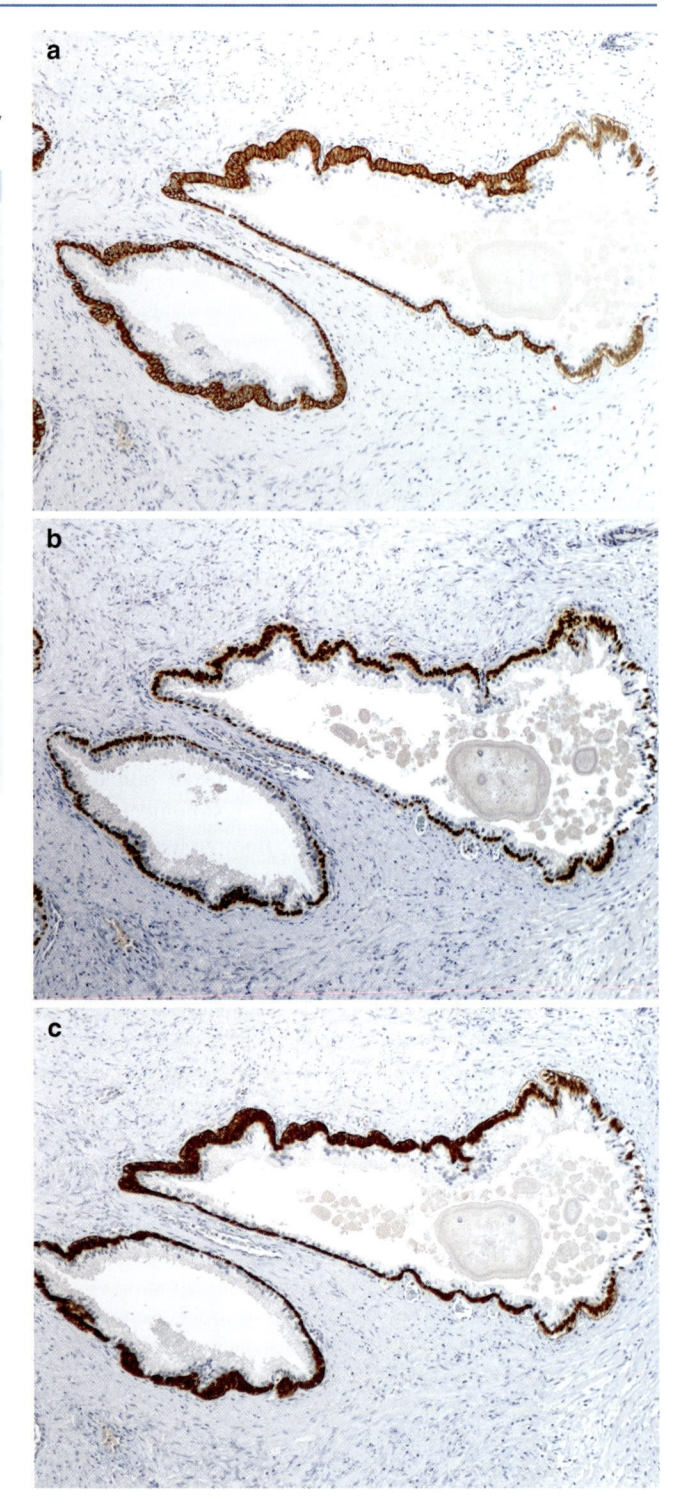

Fig. 4.1 Immunostains for basal cell markers in benign prostate glands, including HMWCK/34βE12 (**a**), p63 (**b**), and basal cell cocktail (34βE12 and p63) (**c**). The specificity of these basal cell markers is similar. However, the sensitivity for detecting basal cells varies, highest with basal cell cocktail and less with p63 and 34βE12, especially in transurethral resection specimens with significant cautery artifact [7–9]

4.2 Basal Cell Markers

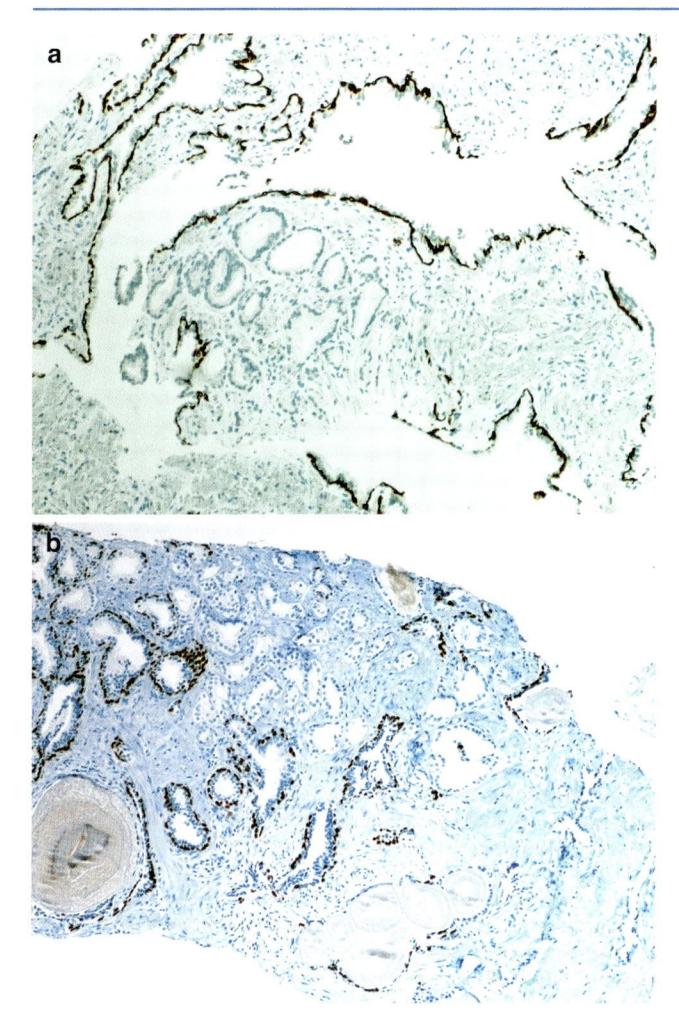

Fig. 4.2 Prostate cancer lacks basal cell marker HMWCK (**a**) and p63 (**b**). The basal cell marker immunoreactivity is affected by tissue fixation and staining protocols. For example, HMWCK antigenicity is affected by the duration of formalin fixation with progressive loss of immunoreactivity with increased fixation time [10]. It is therefore important to use the benign glands that are adjacent to cancer glands as the internal positive control

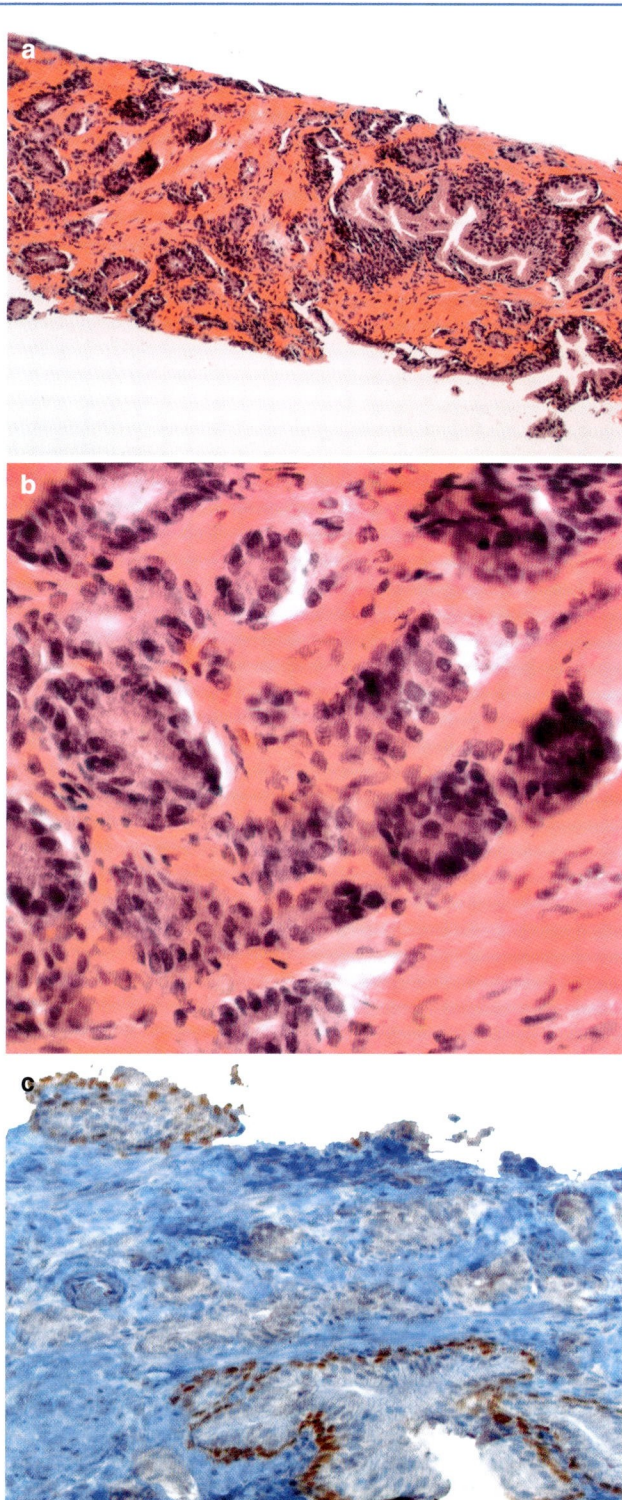

Fig. 4.3 Negative basal cell marker staining supports a cancer diagnosis. This biopsy contains many small crowded glands that exhibit infiltrative growth (**a**). Evaluation of the cytological features of these glands is hampered by the thick tissue sections (**b**). Without further workup, the diagnosis would be atypical glands suspicious for cancer. By immunohistochemistry, the atypical glands are negative for basal cell marker p63 (**c**). The final diagnosis is cancer

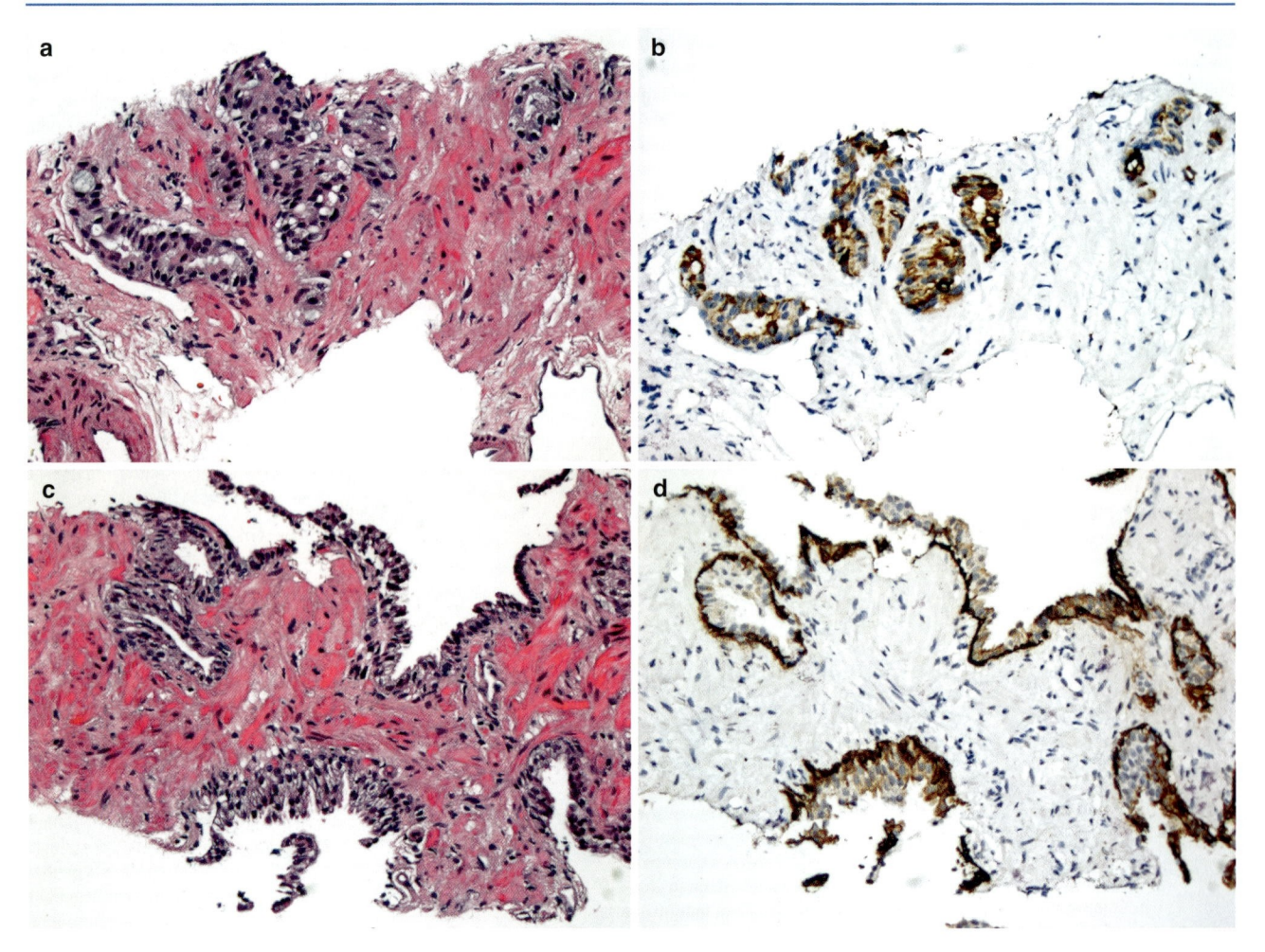

Fig. 4.4 Aberrant HMWCK staining in cancer glands. Cancer glands (**a**) have weak cytoplasmic staining (**b**) but not in a basal cell distribution. Benign glands in the same biopsy core (**c**) also have weak cytoplasmic staining in the secretory cells in addition to strong staining in basal cells (**d**). Such aberrant staining is due to excessive antigen retrieval and staining

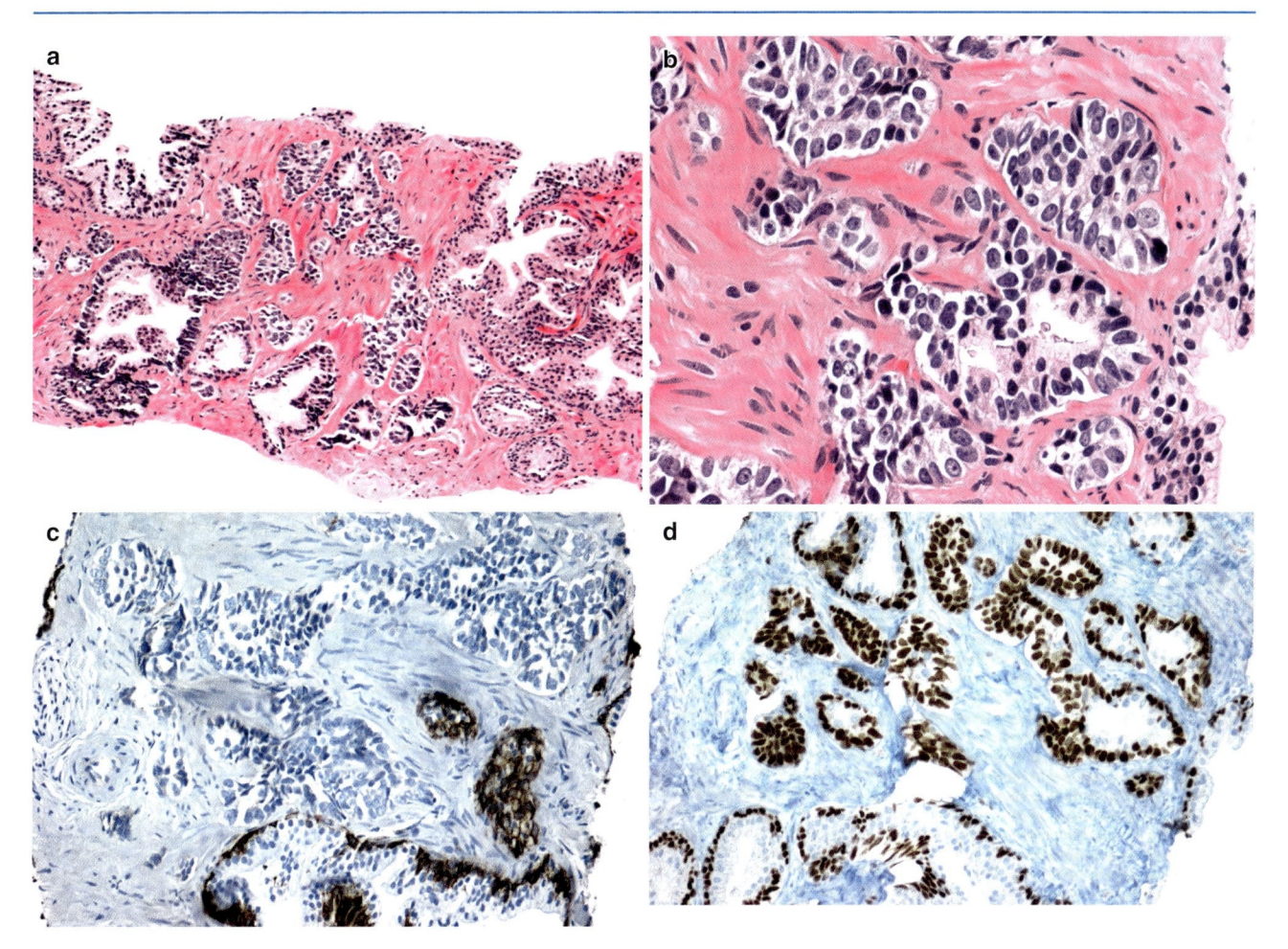

Fig. 4.5 Prostate cancer positive for p63. The cancer glands infiltrate between benign prostate glands (**a**). They are lined with several layers of cancer cells and some have poorly formed lumens. The nucleoli are prominent (**b**). All the cancer glands are negative for HMWCK (34βE12, **c**), but uniformly positive for p63 (**d**). Rather than being in basal cell distribution, the staining is found in all the cancer cells. Prostate cancer positive for p63 is exceedingly rare [11] and probably represents a form of prostate cancer with basal cell differentiation

4.3 α-Methylacyl-CoA-Racemase

Table 4.3 α-Methylacyl-CoA-Racemase (AMACR, P504S)

α-Methylacyl CoA Racemase (AMACR, P504S)
Types of antibodies
Monoclonal (P504S) and polyclonal, both with comparable sensitivity and specificity [12, 13]
Staining pattern in prostate cancer
Apical cytoplasmic granular staining (see Fig. 4.6)
Diagnostic utility
1. Positive AMACR staining in atypical glands morphologically suspicious for cancer supports a cancer diagnosis
2. Positive AMACR may convert an ATYP to cancer diagnosis where morphology is suspicious for but not diagnostic of cancer and basal cell markers are negative (see Fig. 4.8) [5, 12]
Pitfalls
Staining intensity often heterogeneous in cancer glands (see Fig. 4.7) [5]
Positive in 80% of prostate carcinomas diagnosed on needle biopsy [14–16]
Lower positive rate in several prostate carcinoma histologic variants (foamy gland, atrophic and pseudohyperplastic) (see Fig. 4.9) [13]
Positive in 91% of irradiated prostate carcinomas [17]; expression reduced in hormone-deprived cancer (see Fig. 4.10) [18]
Also positive in >90% HGPIN, 20% adenosis, some partial atrophy, occasional morphologically benign glands
Also expressed in nonprostatic tumors (urothelial carcinoma, colon cancer, renal cell carcinoma) [19], nephrogenic adenoma (see Fig. 4.11) [20–23]

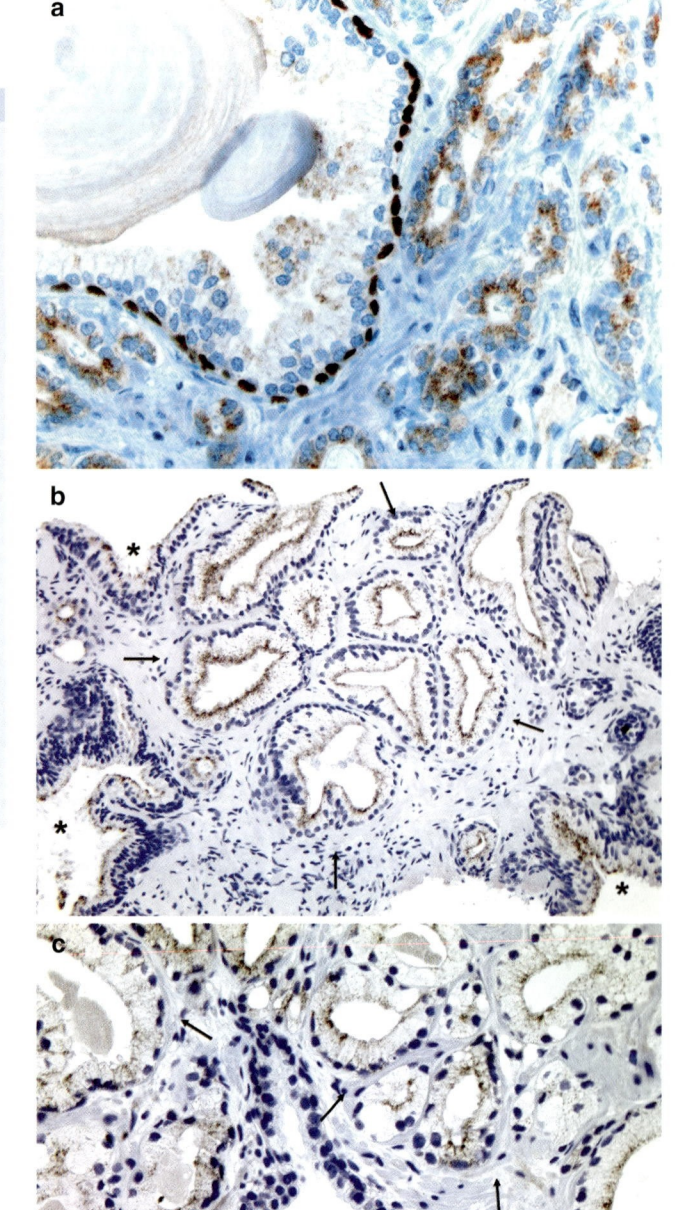

Fig. 4.6 Expression of AMACR appears as granular staining predominantly in the apical portion of cancer glands (**a**). An adjacent benign gland is also focally and weakly positive for AMACR (**a**). Benign glands are occasionally positive for AMACR staining, which is typically focal and weak and may represent field effect. However, this raises the question as to what should be considered as positive AMACR staining. Positive AMACR staining is defined as significantly stronger than that of adjacent benign glands [13]. For example, a prostate cancer (*arrows*) with strong and circumferential AMACR staining will be considered negative if adjacent benign glands (*asterisks*) have similar strong and circumferential staining (**b**). In contrast, a prostate cancer (*arrows*) with weak apical staining is considered positive for AMACR when the adjacent benign glands (*asterisks*) are completely negative (**c**)

4.3 α-Methylacyl-CoA-Racemase

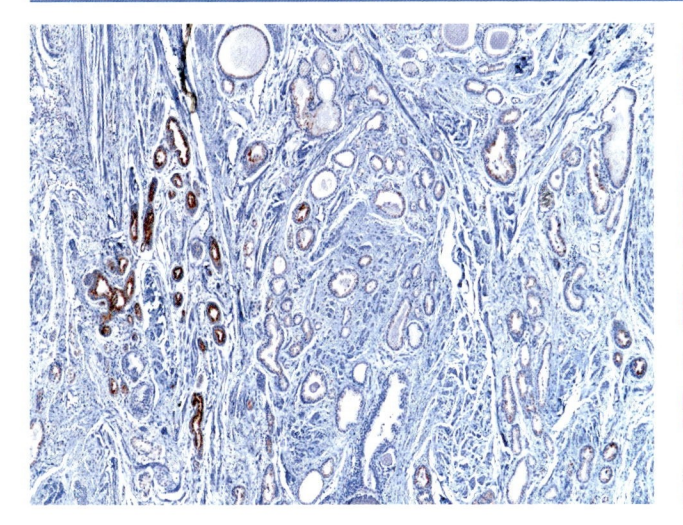

Fig. 4.7 Heterogeneous AMACR staining in cancer glands. The staining is strong in some cancer glands and weak or negative in others. This staining pattern is typical in prostate cancer and accounts for an 80% AMACR positive rate in prostate cancer detected on needle biopsy

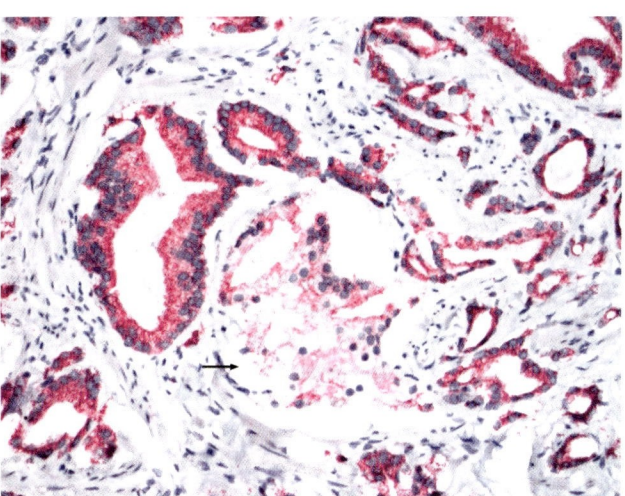

Fig. 4.9 Weak AMACR staining in foamy gland carcinoma. The typical acinar cancer glands are strongly positive for AMACR expression, while foamy gland cancer (*arrow*) is only weakly positive

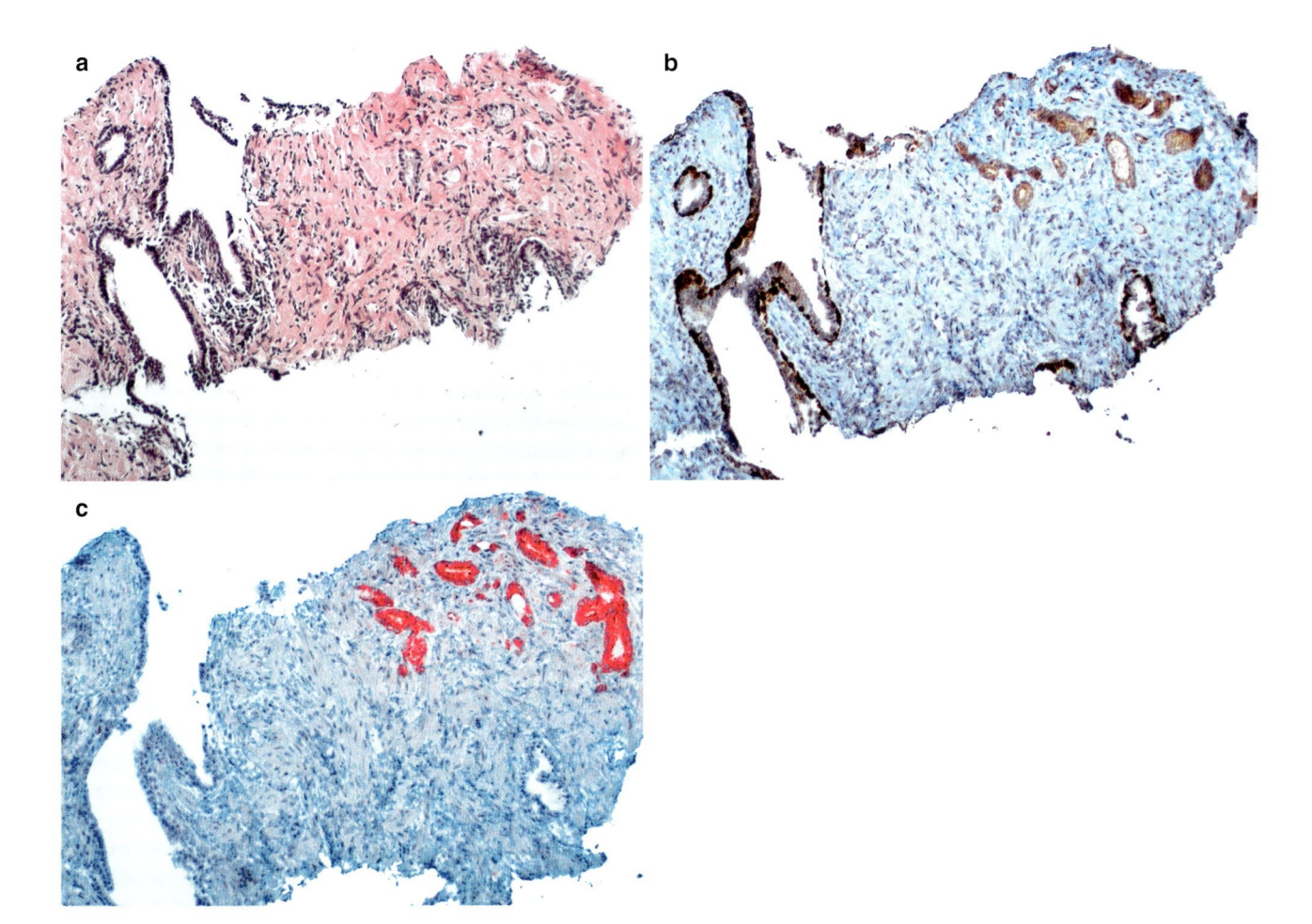

Fig. 4.8 Positive AMACR staining converts an ATYP to cancer diagnosis. A needle biopsy contains a small focus of atypical glands with architectural atypia but minimal cytological atypia (**a**). These glands are negative for basal cell marker K903 (**b**). These glands are highly suspicious for but not diagnostic of cancer due to lack of nuclear atypia. These glands are strongly positive for AMACR (**c**). A cancer diagnosis was established based on the morphological features, negative basal cell marker, and positive AMACR staining

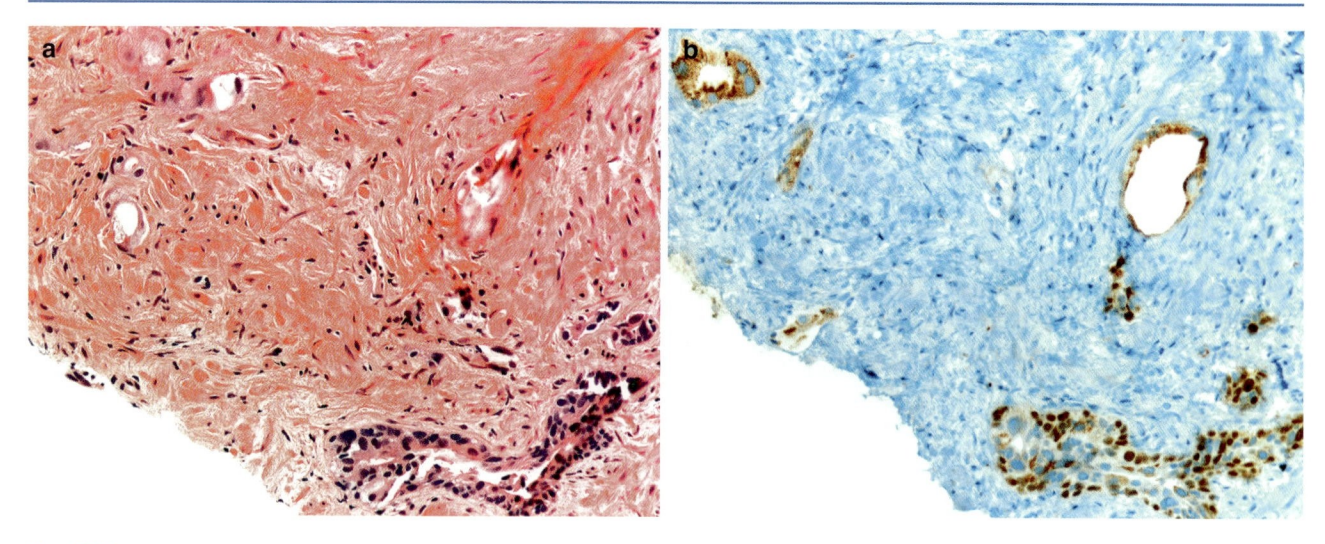

Fig. 4.10 Prostate cancer after radiation treatment. The cancer glands are small and atrophic with foamy cytoplasm after radiation (**a**). Also note the adjacent benign gland (*right lower corner*) is large and has irregular contour, stratified, and scattered hyperchromatic nuclei. The cancer glands are positive for AMACR but negative for basal cell marker p63 (**b**)

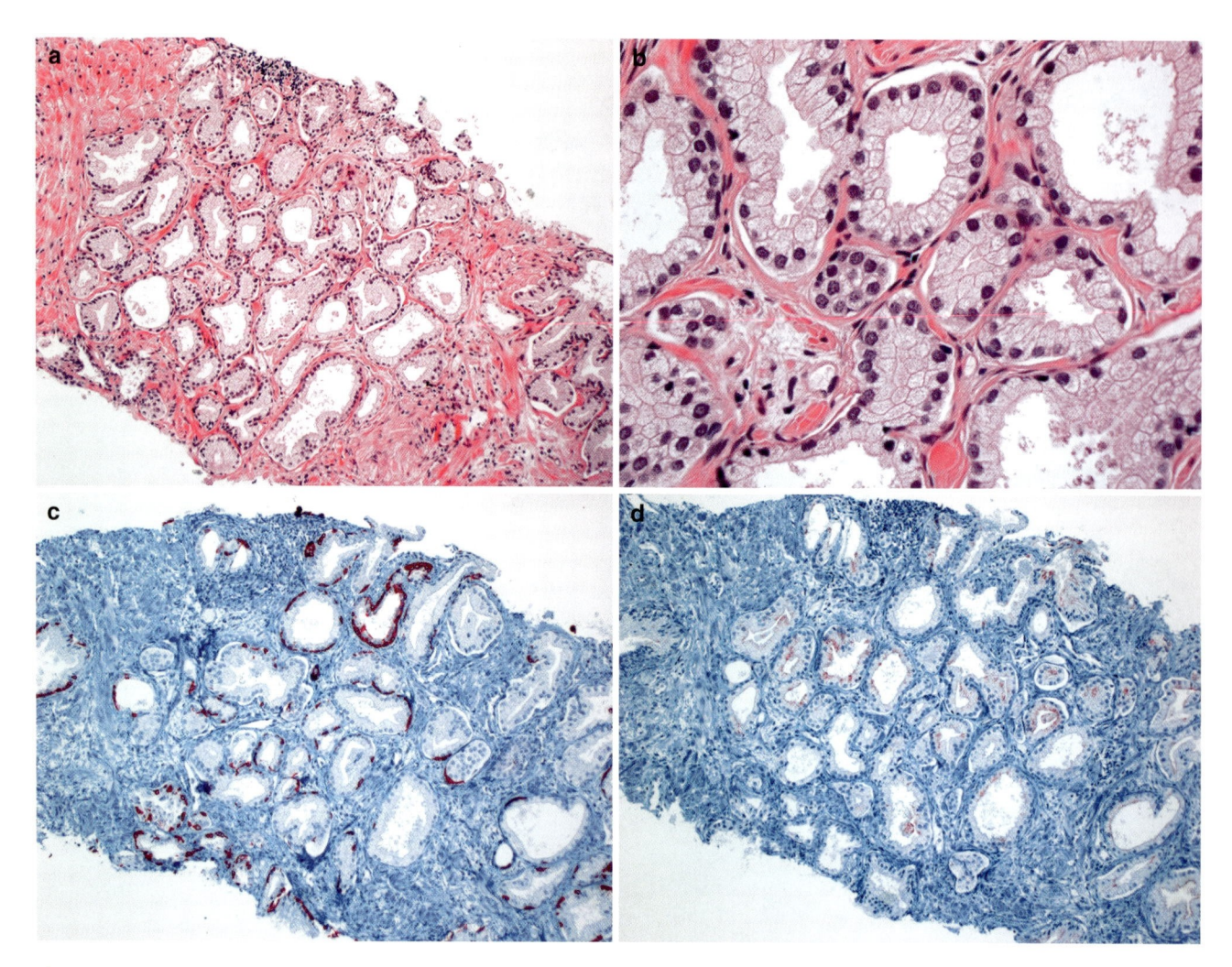

Fig. 4.11 AMACR expression in adenosis. The biopsy contains a well-circumscribed focus of closely packed small and large glands (**a**), whose cells have slight nuclear enlargement and inconspicuous nucleoli (**b**). The basal cell staining HMWCK is positive in a patchy fashion (**c**). These glands are focally positive for AMACR (**d**)

4.4 ERG Protein

Table 4.4 ERG protein

Genetics

ERG is a member of the *ETS* gene family, which is commonly involved by chromosomal translocation in prostate cancer [24, 25]

Staining pattern

Nuclear staining

ERG immunostaining correlates highly with *ERG* gene alteration [26, 27]

Endothelial cells are strongly positive for *ERG* and serve as the positive internal control

Diagnostic utility

Positive staining supports cancer diagnosis but lack of staining does not rule out cancer

Positive staining is exceedingly rare in noncancer glands distant from prostate carcinoma [26]

Pitfalls

Positive in 40–50% of prostate carcinomas

Positive in 20% of HGPIN that intermingles with prostate carcinoma (*see* Figs. 4.12 and 4.13) [24, 25, 28]

Fig. 4.12 Prostate biopsy with cancer stained with an antibody cocktail for both basal cell marker p63 (brown nuclear staining) and ERG (red nuclear staining). Cancer glands are positive for ERG and negative for p63, whereas benign glands are positive for p63 and negative for ERG

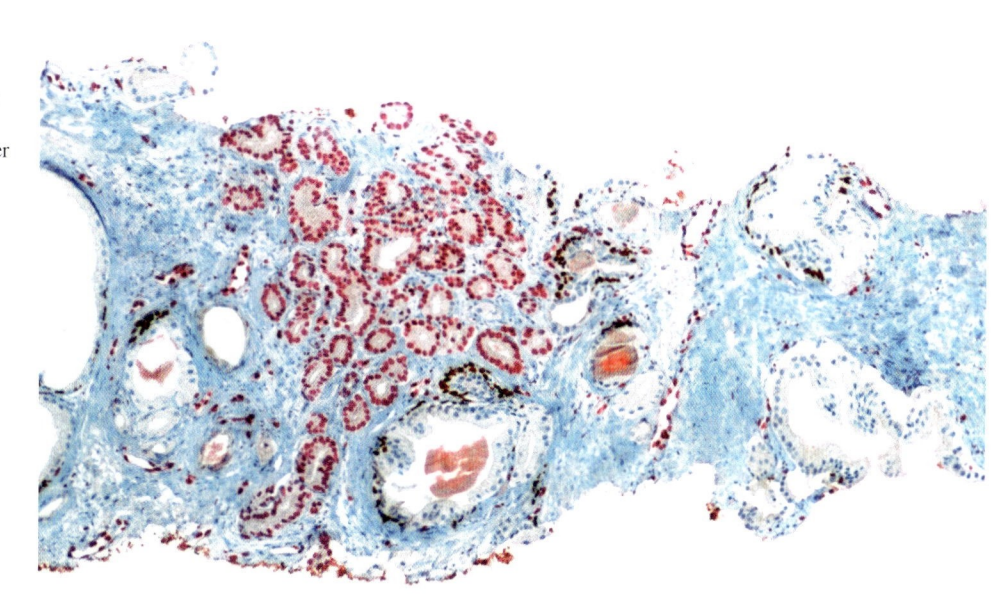

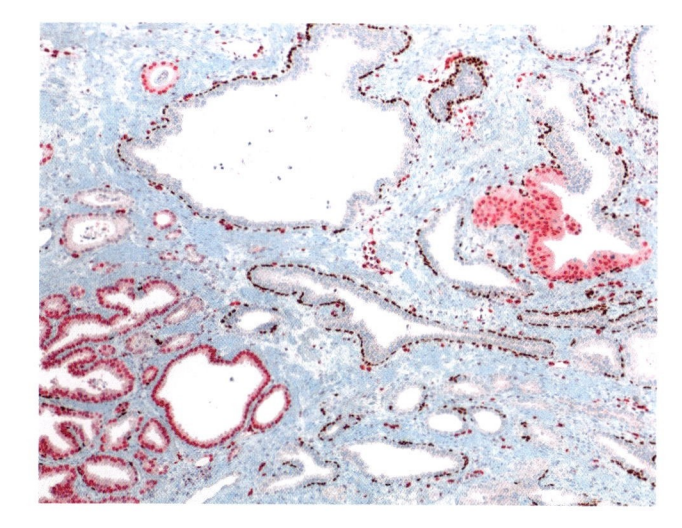

Fig. 4.13 ERG protein expression in prostate cancer and high-grade PIN. Prostate biopsy contains an HGPIN gland (*right upper corner*) that is adjacent to the cancer glands (*left lower corner*). The cancer glands and part of HGPIN glands are positive for ERG

4.5 Antibody Cocktails

Table 4.5 Combination of AMACR and basal cell markers

Types
Contains AMACR and basal cell marker (HMWCK and/or p63) antibodies in the same staining (see Fig. 4.14) [29, 30]

Staining pattern
Staining sensitivity and specificity similar to each antibody used separately

Diagnostic utility
Useful on prostate biopsy with limited amount of cancer

Allows simultaneous evaluation of basal cell marker and AMACR in the same small focus of cancer/atypical glands

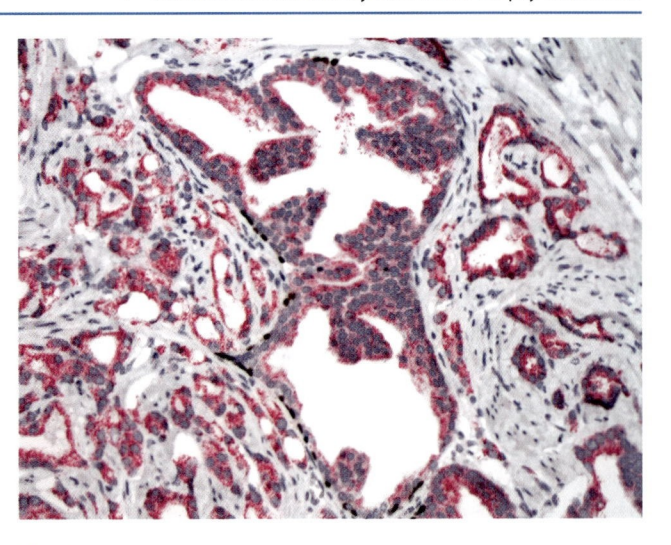

Fig. 4.14 Prostate biopsy containing cancer stained with a cocktail of AMACR and basal cell markers (HMWCK and p63). The cancer glands are positive for AMACR (*red signal*) and negative for basal cell markers (*brown signal*), whereas benign glands are negative for AMACR but positive for basal cell markers. Several different preparations with antibodies against basal cell markers (HMWCK, p63, or both) and AMACR are commercially available. Immunostains with such antibody cocktails allow simultaneous evaluation of basal cell markers and AMACR on the same tissue section and therefore provide an excellent definition of the nature of atypical glands. Antibody cocktails are extremely useful for prostate biopsies with minute focus of cancer that may be present on only one or two sections

4.6 Differential Diagnosis of Prostate Cancer by Immunohistochemistry

Table 4.6 Differential diagnosis of prostate cancer by immunohistochemistry

Diagnosis		Pancytokeratin	Basal cell marker	AMACR	Prostate-specific markers	Other marker(s)
Prostate carcinoma		+	–	+	+	
Prostate carcinoma with treatment effect		+	–	+ (may be reduced)	+ (may be reduced)	
Normal prostate/ nonprostatic structures	Seminal vesicle-ejaculatory duct epithelium	+	+	–	–	Pax 2 and Pax 6+, MUC6+
	Verumontanum mucosal gland hyperplasia	+	+	–	+	
	Cowper's glands	+	+	–	–, variable prostate-specific antigen staining	Mucicarmine, PAS-D, Alcian blue +
	Paraganglia	–	–	–	–	Neuroendocrine markers +
	Mesonephric remnants	+	Variable	–	–	
Benign prostatic lesion	Partial atrophy	+	Variable	Variable	+	
	Postatrophic hyperplasia	+	+	–	+	
	Urothelial metaplasia	+	+	–	–	
	Squamous metaplasia	+	+	–	–	
	Basal cell hyperplasia	+	+	–	Variable	
	Adenosis	+	Variable	Variable	+	
	Sclerosing adenosis	+	+	–	+	SMA and S100+
	Nonspecific granulomatous prostatitis	–	–	–	–	Cd68+
	Benign prostatic hyperplasia	+	+	–	+	
HGPIN		+	Variable	+	+	
Intraductal carcinoma of the prostate		+	+ in residual basal cells	+	+	

"+" indicates positive; "–" indicates negative

4.7 Practical Guideline for Using Immunohistochemistry in Workup of Prostate Biopsies

Table 4.7 Practical guideline for using immunohistochemistry in workup of prostate biopsies

Apply to selected cases in which the differential diagnosis includes prostatic carcinoma based on histologic evaluation

Immunostains must be interpreted in the context of hematoxylin–eosin (H&E) stain morphology
- Clearly define benign and atypical glands on H&E slide
- Define the nature of atypical glands: "favor cancer" vs "favor benign"
- Use immunostain results to corroborate the H&E impression
- Diagnosis should not be solely based on the immunostains
- If atypical glands are considered not diagnostic of cancer regardless of staining results, do not order immunostains

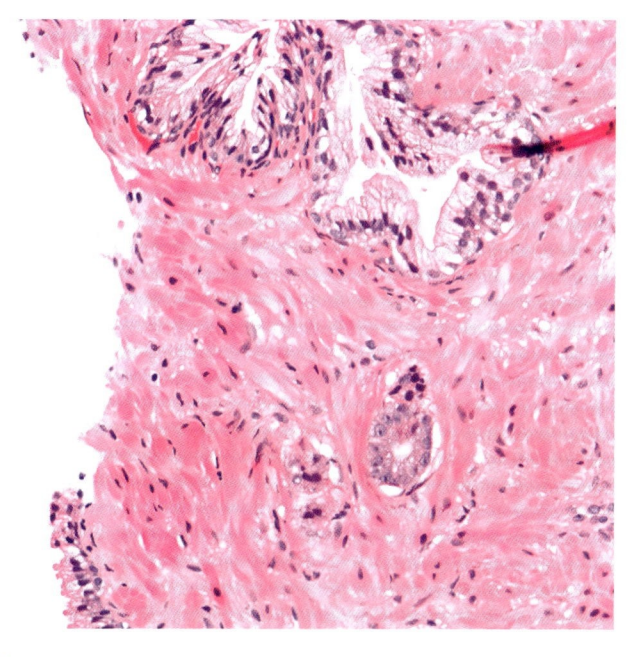

Fig. 4.15 A prostate biopsy containing two small atypical glands. A definitive cancer diagnosis cannot be established even if these atypical glands are negative for basal cell markers and positive for AMACR. It is therefore diagnosed as "atypical gland suspicious for cancer" without performing ancillary immunostains

References

1. Paner GP, Luthringer DJ, Amin MB (2008) Best practice in diagnostic immunohistochemistry: prostate carcinoma and its mimics in needle core biopsies. Arch Pathol Lab Med 132:1388–1396
2. Varma M, Jasani B (2005) Diagnostic utility of immunohistochemistry in morphologically difficult prostate cancer: review of current literature. Histopathology 47:1–16
3. Kahane H, Sharp JW, Shuman GB et al (1995) Utilization of high molecular weight cytokeratin on prostate needle biopsies in an independent laboratory. Urology 45:981–986
4. Wojno KJ, Epstein JI (1995) The utility of basal cell-specific anti-cytokeratin antibody (34 beta E12) in the diagnosis of prostate cancer. A review of 228 cases. Am J Surg Pathol 19:251–260
5. Zhou M, Aydin H, Kanane H, Epstein JI (2004) How often does alpha-methylacyl-CoA-racemase contribute to resolving an atypical diagnosis on prostate needle biopsy beyond that provided by basal cell markers? Am J Surg Pathol 28:239–243
6. Kunju LP, Mehra R, Snyder M, Shah RB (2006) Prostate-specific antigen, high-molecular-weight cytokeratin (clone 34betaE12), and/or p63: an optimal immunohistochemical panel to distinguish poorly differentiated prostate adenocarcinoma from urothelial carcinoma. Am J Clin Pathol 125:675–681
7. Shah RB, Kunju LP, Shen R et al (2004) Usefulness of basal cell cocktail (34betaE12 + p63) in the diagnosis of atypical prostate glandular proliferations. Am J Clin Pathol 122:517–523
8. Zhou M, Shah R, Shen R, Rubin MA (2003) Basal cell cocktail (34betaE12 + p63) improves the detection of prostate basal cells. Am J Surg Pathol 27:365–371
9. Shah RB, Zhou M, LeBlanc M et al (2002) Comparison of the basal cell-specific markers, 34betaE12 and p63, in the diagnosis of prostate cancer. Am J Surg Pathol 26:1161–1168
10. Varma M, Linden MD, Amin MB (1999) Effect of formalin fixation and epitope retrieval techniques on antibody 34betaE12 immunostaining of prostatic tissues. Mod Pathol 12:472–478
11. Osunkoya AO, Hansel DE, Sun X et al (2008) Aberrant diffuse expression of p63 in adenocarcinoma of the prostate on needle biopsy and radical prostatectomy: report of 21 cases. Am J Surg Pathol 32:461–467
12. Kunju LP, Chinnaiyan AM, Shah RB (2005) Comparison of monoclonal antibody (P504S) and polyclonal antibody to alpha methylacyl-CoA racemase (AMACR) in the work-up of prostate cancer. Histopathology 47:587–596
13. Zhou M, Jiang Z, Epstein JI (2003) Expression and diagnostic utility of alpha-methylacyl-CoA-racemase (P504S) in foamy gland and pseudohyperplastic prostate cancer. Am J Surg Pathol 27:772–778
14. Jiang Z, Wu CL, Woda BA et al (2002) P504S/alpha-methylacyl-CoA racemase: a useful marker for diagnosis of small foci of prostatic carcinoma on needle biopsy. Am J Surg Pathol 26:1169–1174
15. Magi-Galluzzi C, Luo J, Isaacs WB et al (2003) Alpha-methylacyl-CoA racemase: a variably sensitive immunohistochemical marker for the diagnosis of small prostate cancer foci on needle biopsy. Am J Surg Pathol 27:1128–1133
16. Kunju LP, Rubin MA, Chinnaiyan AM, Shah RB (2003) Diagnostic usefulness of monoclonal antibody P504S in the work-up of atypical prostatic glandular proliferations. Am J Clin Pathol 120:737–745
17. Yang XJ, Laven B, Tretiakova M et al (2003) Detection of alpha-methylacyl-coenzyme A racemase in postradiation prostatic adenocarcinoma. Urology 62:282–286
18. Tang X, Serizawa A, Tokunaga M et al (2006) Variation of alpha-methylacyl-CoA racemase expression in prostate adenocarcinoma cases receiving hormonal therapy. Hum Pathol 37:1186–1192
19. Zhou M, Chinnaiyan AM, Kleer CG et al (2002) Alpha-Methylacyl-CoA racemase: a novel tumor marker over-expressed in several human cancers and their precursor lesions. Am J Surg Pathol 26:926–931
20. Rubin MA, Zhou M, Dhanasekaran SM et al (2002) Alpha-Methylacyl coenzyme A racemase as a tissue biomarker for prostate cancer. JAMA 287:1662–1670
21. Skinnider BF, Oliva E, Young RH, Amin MB (2004) Expression of alpha-methylacyl-CoA racemase (P504S) in nephrogenic adenoma: a significant immunohistochemical pitfall compounding the

differential diagnosis with prostatic adenocarcinoma. Am J Surg Pathol 28:701–705
22. Wu CL, Yang XJ, Tretiakova M et al (2004) Analysis of alpha-methylacyl-CoA racemase (P504S) expression in high-grade prostatic intraepithelial neoplasia. Hum Pathol 35:1008–1013
23. Yang XJ, Wu CL, Woda BA et al (2002) Expression of alpha-methylacyl-CoA racemase (P504S) in atypical adenomatous hyperplasia of the prostate. Am J Surg Pathol 26:921–925
24. Clark JP, Cooper CS (2009) ETS gene fusions in prostate cancer. Nat Rev Urol 6:429–439
25. Shah RB, Chinnaiyan AM (2009) The discovery of common recurrent transmembrane protease serine 2 (TMPRSS2)-erythroblastosis virus E26 transforming sequence (ETS) gene fusions in prostate cancer: significance and clinical implications. Adv Anat Pathol 16:145–153
26. Furusato B, Tan SH, Young D et al (2010) ERG oncoprotein expression in prostate cancer: clonal progression of ERG-positive tumor cells and potential for ERG-based stratification. Prostate Cancer Prostatic Dis 13:228–237
27. Park K, Tomlins SA, Mudaliar KM et al (2010) Antibody-based detection of ERG rearrangement-positive prostate cancer. Neoplasia 12:590–598
28. Perner S, Mosquera JM, Demichelis F et al (2007) TMPRSS2-ERG fusion prostate cancer: an early molecular event associated with invasion. Am J Surg Pathol 31:882–888
29. Molinie V, Fromont G, Sibony M et al (2004) Diagnostic utility of a p63/alpha-methyl-CoA-racemase (p504s) cocktail in atypical foci in the prostate. Mod Pathol 17:1180–1190
30. Sanderson SO, Sebo TJ, Murphy LM et al (2004) An analysis of the p63/alpha-methylacyl coenzyme A racemase immunohistochemical cocktail stain in prostate needle biopsy specimens and tissue microarrays. Am J Clin Pathol 121:220–225

Contemporary Approach to Gleason Grading of Prostate Cancer

5

Since its inception in 1966 by Dr. Donald Gleason, the Gleason grading system has remained a cornerstone in the diagnosis and management of prostate cancer [1, 2]. With widespread utilization of prostate-specific antigen (PSA) screening, the diagnosis and management of prostate cancer have dramatically changed [3]. Clinical outcomes have also drastically changed over the past several decades. Furthermore, there is a better understanding of the morphological spectrum of prostate cancer. All these changes have prompted modification and refinement of the Gleason grading criteria and reporting for contemporary practice [4].

This chapter addresses several important changes to the original Gleason grading system in contemporary practice: rare utilization of Gleason patterns 1 and 2; the refinement of histological criteria for Gleason patterns 3 and 4; grading of unusual variant morphologies of prostate cancer; the significance of tertiary pattern 5; and recommendations for reporting in the setting of extended biopsy and multifocal prostate cancers. Finally, the impact of the 2005 International Society of Urologic Pathology (ISUP) consensus recommendations on current practice, its limitations and pitfalls and future trends, are also addressed.

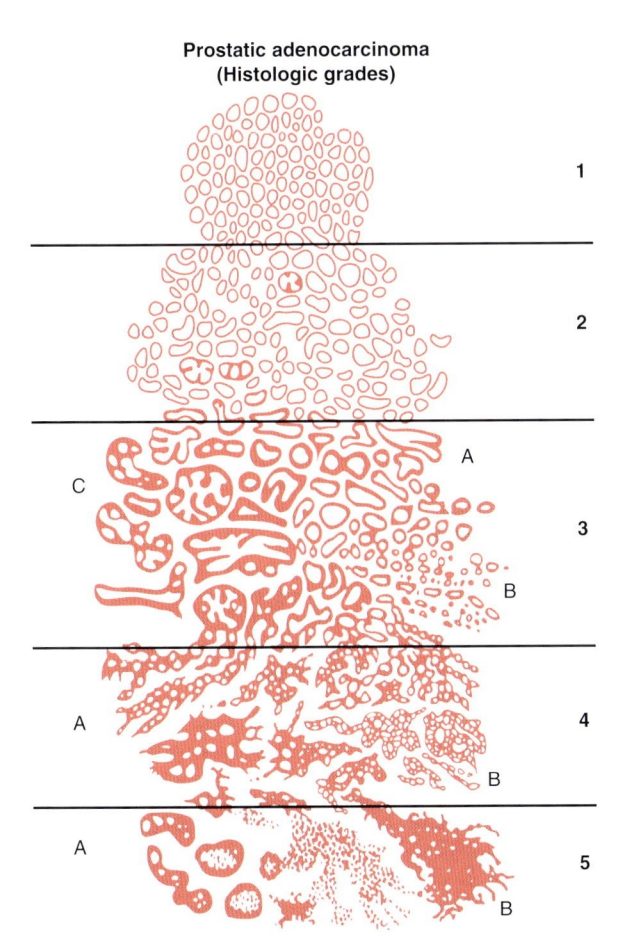

Fig. 5.1 Conventional Gleason grading system. In 1966, Donald F. Gleason created the Gleason grading system based on low-power architectural features of prostate cancer [1, 2]. This system was originally based on a study of 270 patients and later expanded to include 1032 men [5]. Dr. Gleason made further refinements to the system in 1974 and 1977. Using the architectural features, all tumors are put into one of the five patterns representing a continuum of progressively complex morphologies. Another unique aspect of the system is that, rather than assigning the worst grade, a sum of the most prevalent and second-most prevalent pattern (Gleason score = primary + secondary pattern) is assigned to the tumor. Of many grading systems for prostate cancer proposed over the years, the Gleason system is currently the most widely accepted and utilized system and has been endorsed by the World Health Organization [6]

R.B. Shah, M. Zhou, *Prostate Biopsy Interpretation: An Illustrated Guide*, DOI 10.1007/978-3-642-21369-4_5, © Springer-Verlag Berlin Heidelberg 2012

5.1 Significance of Gleason Grading in Prostate Cancer Management

Table 5.1 Significance of Gleason grading in prostate cancer management

Significance of Gleason grading in prognosis and therapy decisions
1. Predicts various outcome measures (PSA biochemical failure, pathologic stage, metastasis, and death) after various forms of treatment modalities (surveillance, radiation, and radical prostatectomy) [7–10]
2. Independent predictor of biochemical failure in patients receiving neo- or adjuvant hormonal therapy [11]
3. Patients with Gleason score of ≤6 are often candidates for active surveillance (watchful waiting)
4. Gleason score of 7 is a critical decision-making point; patients usually need some form of definitive therapy (e.g., lymph node sampling during radical prostatectomy and definitive therapy for patients on active surveillance)
5. Patients with Gleason score of 8–10 are often candidates for multimodality treatments, including adjuvant therapy or radiation treatment
6. An essential parameter in various multivariate prognosis and outcome models (nomograms) [12–14]

5.2 Prostate Cancer Nomograms Recurrence Categories and Prediction Models

Table 5.2 Prostate cancer nomograms and National Comprehensive Cancer Network (NCCN) recurrence categories and prediction models. The prediction of the natural history of prostate cancer remains challenging as we now increasingly detect it at an early stage with PSA screening. Specifically, it remains difficult to decide which localized cancers will progress and metastasize and which are innocuous or indolent and can be conservatively managed. Urologists use several multivariate systems to help answer some of these questions. The most popular multivariate systems are Partin and Han tables (urology.jhu.edu/prostate/partintables.php and urology.jhu.edu/prostate/hanTables.php) and Kattan nomograms (mskcc.org/applications/nomograms/Prostate). An example of a Partin table is shown for nonpalpable T1c prostate cancer detected by abnormal PSA, which uses biopsy Gleason score, serum PSA, and clinical stage to predict the definitive pathologic stage in radical prostatectomy. Partin tables help clinicians decide the primary treatment for localized prostate cancer based on the predicted extent of disease. The Han tables use pretreatment PSA, the biopsy Gleason score, and the clinical or pathologic stage to determine the likelihood of prostate cancer recurrence up to 10 years after surgery. These tables help clinicians determine which, if any, postoperative treatment should be prescribed. In the National Comprehensive Cancer Network (NCCN) recurrence risk-estimation model, Gleason score is utilized with other variables to place patients into various risk categories from very low to very high risk. Several other forms of nomograms have been proposed that utilize different clinical and pathologic information to predict specific outcome endpoints

Clinical State T1c (Nonpalpable, PSA Elevated)						
PSA range (ng/mL)	Pathologic stage	Gleason score				
		2–4	5–6	3+4=7	4+3=7	8–10
0–2.5	Organ confined	95 (89–99)	90 (88–93)	79 (74–85)	71 (62–79)	66 (54–76)
	Extraprostatic extension	5 (1–11)	9 (7–12)	17 (13–23)	25 (18–34)	28 (20–38)
	Seminal vesicle (+)	–	0 (0–1)	2 (1–5)	2 (1–5)	4 (1–10)
	Lymph node (+)	–	–	1 (0–2)	1 (0–4)	1 (0–4)
2.6–4	Organ confined	92 (82–98)	84 (81–86)	68 (62–74)	58 (48–67)	52 (41–63)
	Extraprostatic extension	8 (2–18)	15 (13–18)	27 (22–33)	37 (29–46)	40 (31–50)
	Seminal vesicle (+)	–	1 (0–1)	4 (2–7)	4 (1–7)	6 (3–12)
	Lymph node (+)	–	–	1 (0–2)	1 (0–3)	1 (0–4)
4.1–6	Organ confined	90 (78–98)	80 (8–83)	63 (58–68)	52 (43–60)	46 (36–56)
	Extraprostatic extension	10 (2–22)	19 (16–21)	32 (27–36)	42 (35–50)	45 (36–54)
	Seminal vesicle (+)	–	1 (0–1)	3 (2–5)	3 (1–6)	5 (3–9)
	Lymph node (+)	–	0 (0–1)	2 (1–3)	3 (1–5)	3 (1–6)
6.1–10	Organ confined	87 (72–97)	75 (72–77)	54 (49–59)	43 (35–51)	37 (28–46)
	Extraprostatic extension	13 (3–27)	23 (21–25)	36 (32–40)	47 (40–54)	48 (39–57)
	Seminal vesicle (+)	–	2 (2–3)	8 (6–11)	8 (4–12)	13 (8–19)
	Lymph node (+)	–	0 (0–1)	2 (1–3)	2 (1–4)	3 (1–5)
>10	Organ confined	80 (61–95)	62 (58–64)	37 (32–42)	27 (21–34)	22 (16–30)
	Extraprostatic extension	20 (5–39)	33 (30–36)	43 (38–48)	51 (44–59)	50 (42–59)
	Seminal vesicle (+)	–	4 (3–5)	12 (9–17)	11 (6–17)	17 (10–25)
	Lymph node (+)	–	2 (1–3)	8 (5–11)	10 (5–17)	11 (5–18)

PSA prostate-specific antigen, *T1c* nonpalpable cancer detected by elevated PSA

5.2 Prostate Cancer Nomograms Recurrence Categories and Prediction Models

Table 5.2 (continued)

NCCN recurrence risk categories	
Risk category	Definition
Very low	T1c plus Gleason score 2–6 plus PSA < 10 ng/mL
Low	T1-T2a plus Gleason score 2–6 plus PSA < 10 ng/mL (only 1 in 14 will die from prostate cancer)
Intermediate	T2b-T2c or Gleason score 7 or PSA 10–20 ng/mL (11% will die from prostate cancer within 15 y)
High	T3a or Gleason score 8–10 or PSA > 20 ng/mL
Very high	T3b-T4 (locally advanced) or metastasis present

NCCN National Comprehensive Cancer Network, *T1a* tumor incidental histologic finding in 5% or less of tissue resected, *T1b* tumor incidental histologic finding in more than 5% of tissue resected, *T1c* nonpalpable cancer detected by elevated PSA, *T2a* palpable cancer involving < 50% of one side of lobe, *T2b* palpable cancer involving more than 50% of one lobe, *T2c* involving bilateral lobe, *T3a* extraprostatic extension, *T3b* seminal vesicle invasion, *T4* invasion grossly into bladder or rectum or pelvic sidewalls

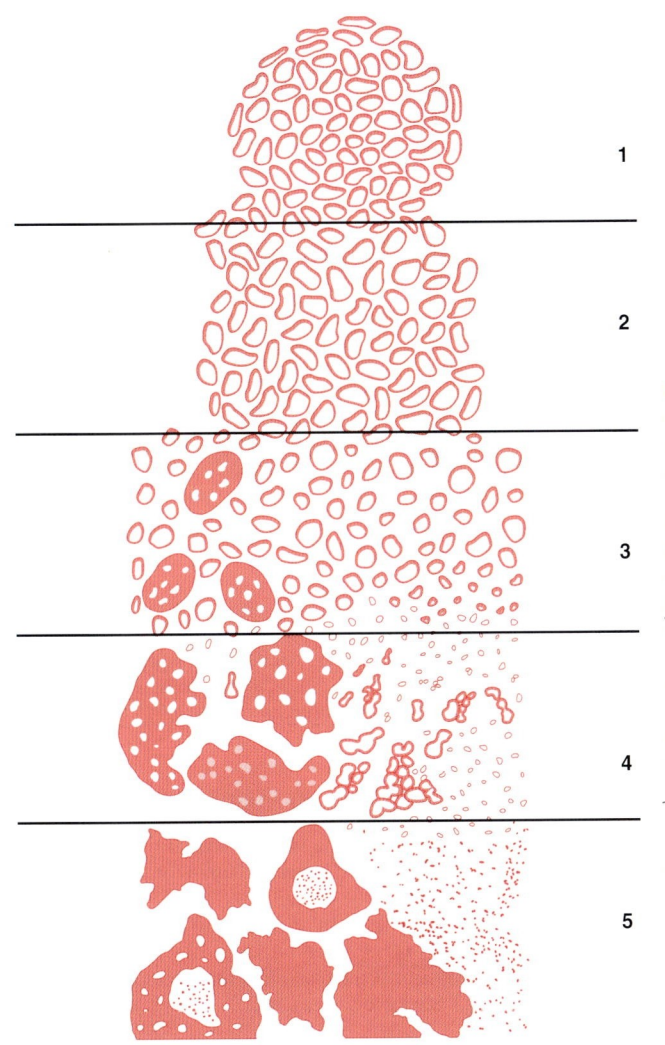

Fig. 5.2 Modified Gleason grading system proposed by ISUP in response to dramatic changes in the diagnosis and management of prostate cancer in the past 40 years. With widespread PSA screening, there is a remarkable shift toward low-volume, low-stage prostate cancers. Accordingly, extended biopsy templates, instead of limited targeted biopsies, are increasingly utilized to improve prostate cancer detection [15]. Surgical pathologists are increasingly grading prostate cancer in multiple cores from separate anatomic sites. Many atypical cribriform lesions are now recognized as cribriform high-grade prostatic intraepithelial neoplasia or intraductal carcinoma [16], and many of Gleason score 2–4 carcinomas are recognized as adenosis due to utilization of immunohistochemistry. Several prostate cancer histological variants were described recently and their grading was not discussed in the original Gleason grading system. A tertiary pattern, in addition to the primary and secondary patterns, is frequently present and it is controversial whether to include such a tertiary pattern in the final grade. The correlation between the biopsy and radical prostatectomy still remains poor; specifically, the undergrading of the biopsy is a significant problem [17–19]. These issues prompted the refinement of conventional grading criteria and reporting practices. The ISUP has proposed modification to the conventional Gleason grading system [4]. A schematic diagram of the modified Gleason grading system is shown here. Major changes from the previous version reflect a refinement of the criteria of Gleason patterns 3 and 4. (*Adapted from* Epstein et al. [4].)

5.3 Current Concepts of Gleason Grading

Table 5.3 Current concepts of Gleason grading of prostate cancer [3, 4, 13, 20–32]

1. Gleason pattern 1 or 2 should be rarely if ever applied in the biopsy setting
2. Gleason grade in the biopsy setting essentially starts with Gleason pattern 3
3. A few malignant glands located between benign glands indicate pattern 3 (small focus of cancer does not necessarily mean low-grade cancer)
4. Virtually all cribriform carcinomas represent pattern 4 or 5 if associated with necrosis
5. Clusters of glands with poorly formed glandular lumina where tangential sectioning is ruled out represent Gleason pattern 4
6. Percentage of pattern 4 in the setting of Gleason score 7 (3+4 versus 4+3) bears prognostic importance
7. Multiple cores with cancer of different Gleason grades, grade information of individual core(s) better correlates with Gleason grade of radical prostatectomy
8. Any amount of higher pattern in the needle biopsy should be reported
9. In the setting of high-grade tumor of large volume, a small amount (≤5%) of lower-grade pattern can be ignored and need not be reported
10. Tertiary pattern 5 in the biopsy should be reported as the secondary pattern in the needle biopsy due to its prognostic significance
11. Many "special" types of prostate cancers are considered examples of Gleason pattern 4 or 5

5.4 Contemporary Gleason Pattern 1

Table 5.4 Contemporary Gleason pattern 1

Definition
Circumscribed nodule of closely packed but separate, uniform, round-to-oval, medium-sized acini (glands larger than pattern 3)

Key differences from conventional grading system
None

Application in clinical practice
Most cases diagnosed as Gleason score 1+1=2 in the Gleason era would be diagnosed as *adenosis* (atypical adenomatous hyperplasia) today with basal cell immunohistochemistry. This pattern should not be diagnosed regardless of specimen type, with extremely rare exception

Key pitfalls
A smooth edge of an otherwise infiltrative tumor nodule may mimic pattern 1
Adenosis (AAH) may mimic as Gleason pattern 1 cancer

5.5 Contemporary Gleason Pattern 2

Table 5.5 Contemporary Gleason pattern 2

Definition
Like pattern 1, fairly circumscribed yet there may be minimal infiltration at the edge of tumor nodule
Glands are more loosely arranged and not quite as uniform as pattern 1

Key differences from conventional grading system
Cribriform glands are not allowed in contemporary Gleason pattern 2

Application in clinical practice
This pattern occasionally exists in transurethral resections and in multifocal low-grade tumors in the radical prostatectomy specimens
Due to poor reproducibility, lack of good correlation with prostatectomy grade, sampling issues, and potentially misleading clinical implications, Gleason score of 3–4 on needle biopsy should "rarely, if ever" be made when all the strict criteria are met and adenosis is excluded

Key pitfall
A smooth edge of an otherwise infiltrative tumor nodule may mimic pattern 2 in needle biopsy (*see* Fig. 5.3)

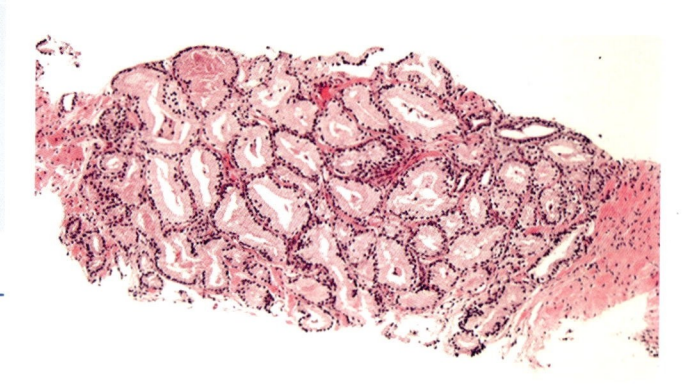

Fig. 5.3 Pitfalls of diagnosing Gleason patterns 1 and 2 in needle biopsy (NBX) samples. Although the definitions of patterns 1 and 2 are essentially the same as Gleason's original description, their application in contemporary biopsy practice is drastically different. Patterns 1 and 2 occasionally exist on prostate transurethral resection (TURP) and in multifocal low-grade tumors in radical prostatectomy specimens. Due to poor reproducibility, lack of good correlation with prostatectomy grade, sampling issues, and potentially misleading clinical implications, Gleason score of 3–4 on needle biopsy should "rarely, if ever" be made only when all strict criteria are met and adenosis is excluded. A major limitation of assigning a Gleason pattern 1 or 2 on a needle biopsy is that one may not see the border of the entire lesion as shown in this example. Therefore, most of such lesions in NBX should be assigned a score of 3+3=6. A score of 3+2=5 or 2+3=5 may be assigned with a comment that the Gleason score in radical prostatectomy is almost always higher in such a case

5.6 Contemporary Gleason Pattern 3

Table 5.6 Contemporary Gleason pattern 3

Definition

Discrete glandular units, typically smaller glands than those seen in Gleason pattern 1 or 2, infiltrate in and among nonneoplastic prostate acini (*see* Fig. 5.4a)

Glands typically have marked variation in size and shape (*see* Fig. 5.4a)

Only smooth circumscribed small cribriform nodules of same size as normal benign glands may qualify as cribriform carcinoma pattern 3 (*see* Fig. 5.4c)

Key differences from conventional grading system

Only smooth circumscribed small cribriform nodules the same size as normal glands should be diagnosed as Gleason pattern 3

"Individual cells" are not allowed in Gleason pattern 3

Application in clinical practice

The most common pattern encountered in needle biopsy specimens

Minute foci of individual, infiltrating tumor glands seen frequently in needle biopsy represent Gleason score 3 + 3 = 6 (*see* Fig. 5.4b)

The vast majority of cribriform cancer glands should be diagnosed as Gleason pattern 4 with only rare cribriform cancer glands assigned pattern 3

Some experts assign all cribriform carcinomas regardless of its architecture as pattern 4 or 5 if associated with necrosis

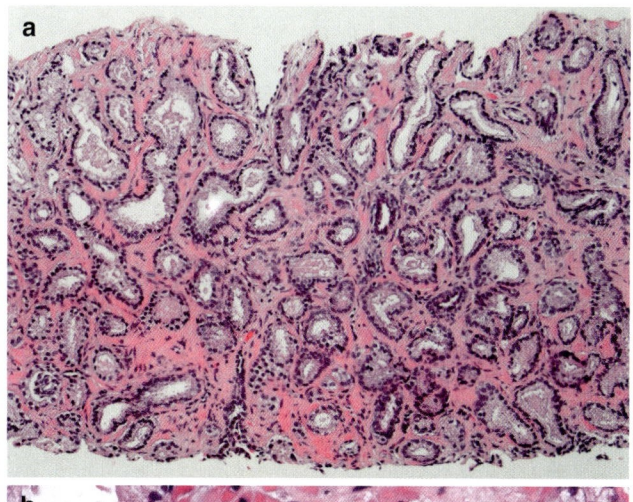

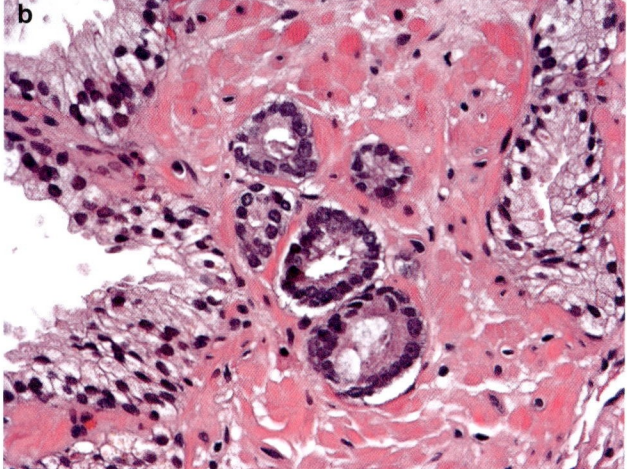

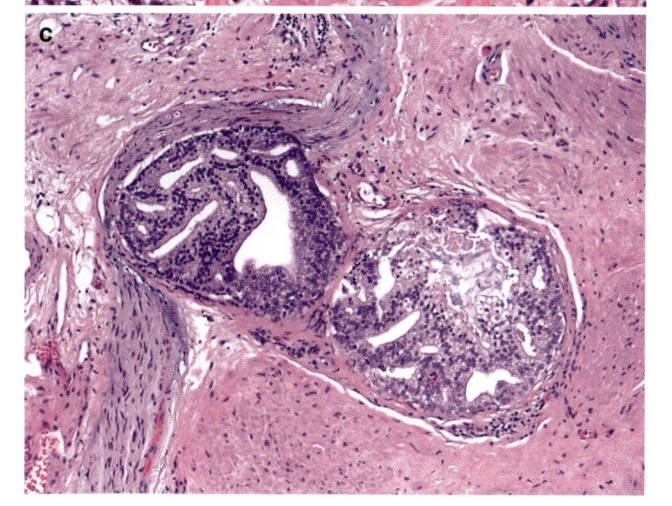

Key pitfalls

Tangentially sectioned pattern 3 glands may appear poorly formed and mimic pattern 4 (*see* Fig. 5.5a, b)

Cancer glands demonstrating complex branching such as "U" or "Y" shape or closely packed glands may be mistaken for Gleason pattern 4 (*see* Fig. 5.5c, d)

Fig. 5.4 Pattern 3 cancer glands in contemporary Gleason grading system. (**a**) From a practical standpoint, Gleason grading in contemporary practice begins with pattern 3. Gleason pattern 3 represents the most common pattern encountered in needle biopsy. Variably sized individual glands typically smaller than those seen in Gleason pattern 1 or 2, infiltrating between benign glands, represent the classic form of Gleason pattern 3. (**b**) A very small focus of cancer, as seen in this example, should still be graded as 3 + 3 = 6. (**c**) A cribriform lesion that may be graded as Gleason pattern 3. Such pattern 3 cribriform glands are small and have round and regular contour with regular lumina. They should be differentiated from cribriform PIN. Such distinction may rely on the presence of either a large number of glands negative for basal cell markers or the presence of specific features of cancer such as perineural invasion (as seen in this example), extraprostatic extension, or based on the presence of adjacent conventional carcinoma. In a recent study, when biopsies containing small invasive cribriform carcinomas were reviewed by expert urologic pathologists, overall interobserver reproducibility was poor and the majority of the lesions were considered to represent Gleason pattern 4 [24]. Therefore some experts assign all cribriform carcinomas regardless of its architecture as pattern 4 or 5 if associated with necrosis

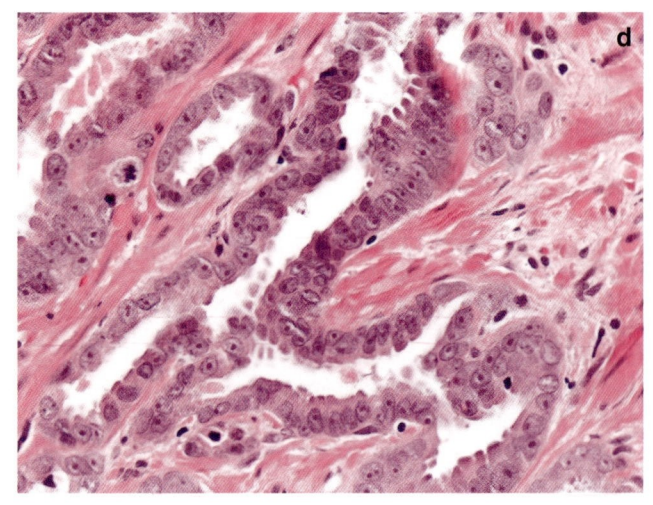

Fig. 5.5 (continued)

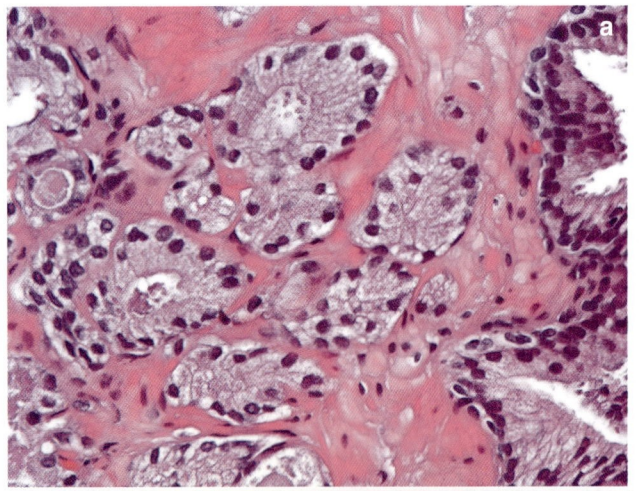

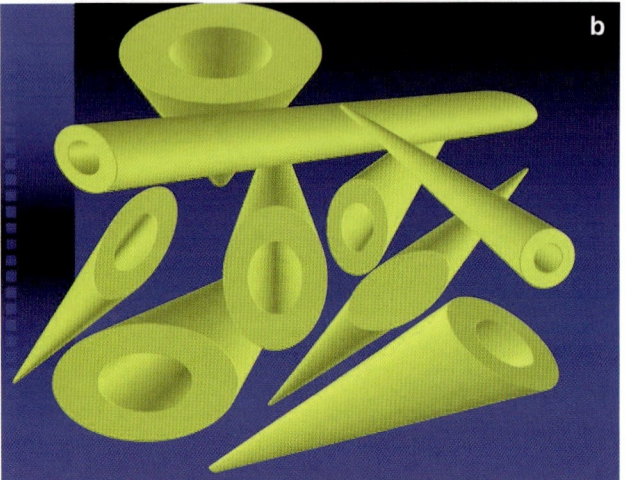

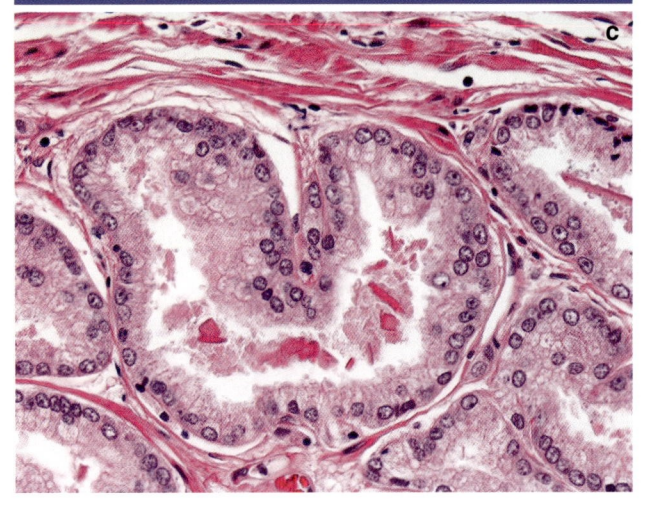

Fig. 5.5 Common pitfalls of interpretation of Gleason pattern 3 prostate cancers. (**a**) Tangentially sectioned cancer glands at the periphery of a tumor nodule mimic poorly formed pattern 4 glands. (**b**) This diagram illustrates how a group of cancer glands, sectioned at different angles, may give rise to seemingly poorly formed glands. Therefore, only a group or entire cluster of glands with poorly formed lumina should be considered as pattern 4. It is also a good practice to examine multiple levels of biopsy. (**c, d**) Large pattern 3 cancer glands may show complex branching and appear as "V" or "Y" shaped

5.7 Contemporary Gleason Pattern 4

Table 5.7 Contemporary Gleason pattern 4

Definition

Fused glands (*see* Fig. 5.6a)

Hypernephroid morphology (*see* Fig. 5.6b)

Large or irregular cribriform glands (*see* Fig. 5.6c, d)

Ill-defined glands or cluster with poorly formed glandular lumina where tangential sectioning is ruled out (*see* Fig. 5.6f)

Key differences from conventional grading system

The majority (>95%) of cribriform carcinomas are Gleason pattern 4

Ill-defined glands with poorly formed glandular lumina where tangential sectioning is ruled out are pattern 4

Application in clinical practice

Gleason pattern 4 constitutes an important clinical decision-making point. Presence of any Gleason pattern 4 typically is considered clinically significant prostate cancer and usually necessitates some form of definitive therapy

In the most recent Partin tables, Gleason score 7 (3+4) and Gleason score 7 (4+3) are considered separately. This emphasizes the importance of determining the quantity of Gleason pattern 4

Key pitfalls

A few poorly formed glands seen randomly within a focus or only at the edge likely represent tangential sectioning of pattern 3 glands (*see* Fig. 5.5a).

On needle biopsy, cribriform pattern 4 tumor often manifests as a fragment of cribriform glands as there is little supporting stroma

5.7 Contemporary Gleason Pattern 4

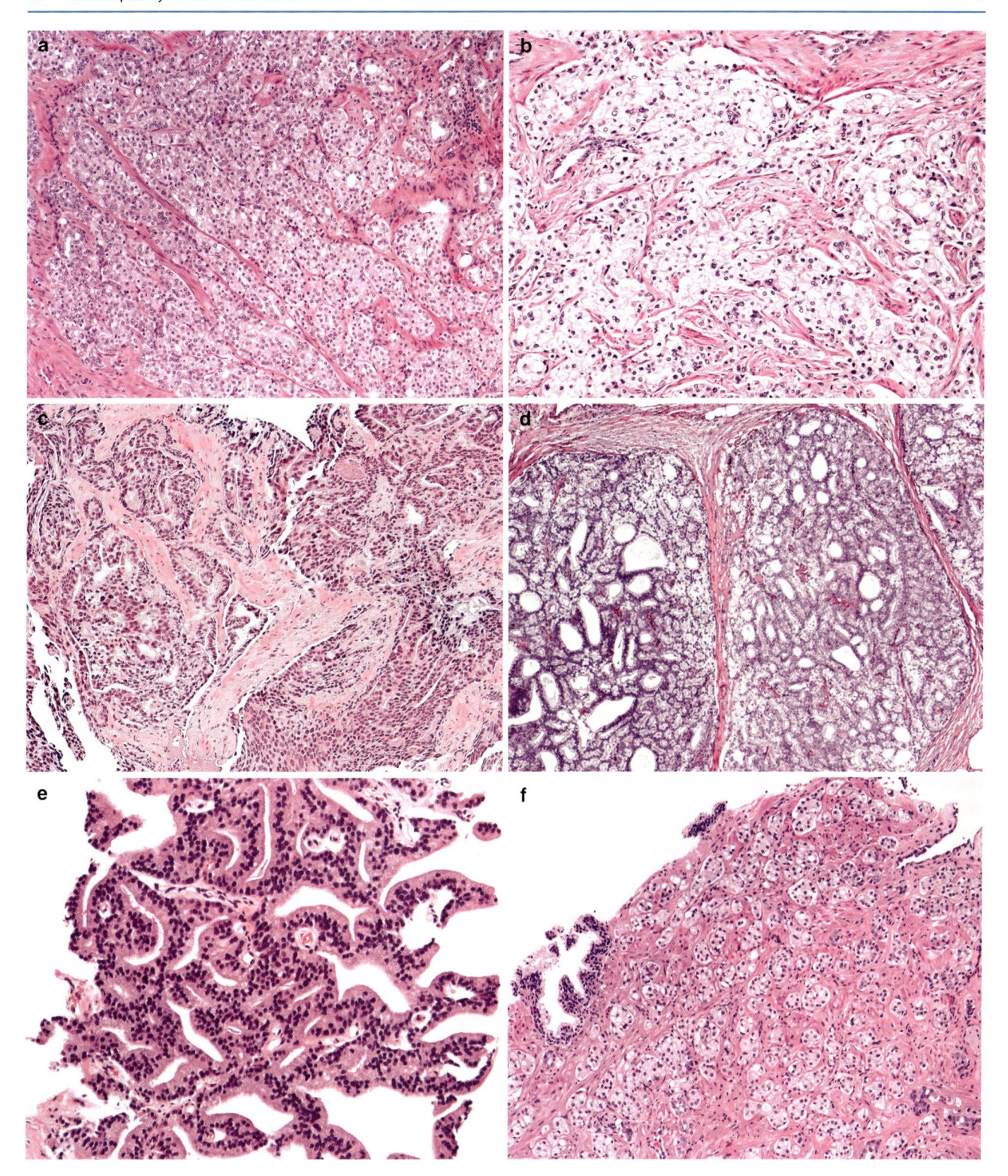

Fig. 5.6 Morphological spectrum of pattern 4 cancer in contemporary practice. (**a**) Ragged and fused cancer glands representing Gleason pattern 4. (**b**) Hypernephroid pattern may mimic foamy gland differentiation. Hypernephroid morphology usually has clear vacuolated cytoplasm rather than bubbly xanthomatous cytoplasm seen in the latter. Distinction between the two is of little clinical significance. Most importantly, grading should be based on the underlying architecture of the tumor rather than the hypernephroid or foamy appearance. (**c–e**) Gleason pattern 4 cribriform carcinoma spectrum includes small but irregular cribriforming glands (**c**); round and regular uniform cribriform cancers much larger than normal prostate glands (**d**); and adenocarcinoma with ductal differentiation characterized by confluent cribriform glands lined by tall columnar cells and demonstrating slit-like pattern and papillary differentiation (**e**). (**f**) A cluster of poorly formed or ill-defined glands where tangential sectioning is ruled out warrants the diagnosis of Gleason pattern 4. Although glands are discrete and not fused, they are poorly formed with barely recognizable lumina. Strict criteria should be applied as tangential sectioning of pattern 3 cancer glands may result in several seemingly poorly formed glands

5.8 Gleason Grading of Cribriform Carcinomas

Table 5.8 Gleason grading of cribriform carcinomas

Histologic pattern[a]	Gleason pattern
1. Rounded, well-circumscribed cribriform glands the same size of normal glands	3
2. Large cribriform glands	4
3. Cribriform glands with irregular borders	4
4. Cribriform carcinoma with ductal/papillary/PIN-like differentiation	4

[a]The vast majority of cribriform carcinoma patterns (>95%) fall into Gleason pattern 4, with only rare cribriform lesions satisfying criteria for pattern 3 (See histological pattern #1); Some experts assign all cribriform carcinomas regardless of its architecture as pattern 4 or 5 if associated with necrosis

5.9 Contemporary Gleason Pattern 5

Table 5.9 Contemporary Gleason pattern 5

Definition

Essentially no glandular differentiation, composed of solid sheets, cords, or single cells (*see* Fig. 5.7a, b)

Comedonecrosis characterized by dirty necrosis with karyorrhectic debris surrounded by papillary, cribriform, solid masses (*see* Fig. 5.7c)

Key differences from conventional grading system

No major difference

Application in clinical practice

Any amount of pattern 5 is clinically significant and puts the patient in the high-risk group category

In needle biopsy, pattern 5 should be included in the final Gleason score even present in an amount less than the secondary pattern

Some studies recommend reporting volume or percentage pattern of 4/5 in needle biopsy as it is of independent prognostic significance. However, percent pattern 4/5 in biopsy is usually predictive of radical prostatectomy percent 4/5 only when present at extreme percentages

Key pitfalls

Recognition of pattern 5 in needle biopsy could be challenging and is prone to both over- and under-interpretation

Tangentially sectioned or poorly formed glands may mimic single cells or cords

Amorphous intraluminal eosinophilic secretions or intraluminal inflammatory debris may mimic comedonecrosis

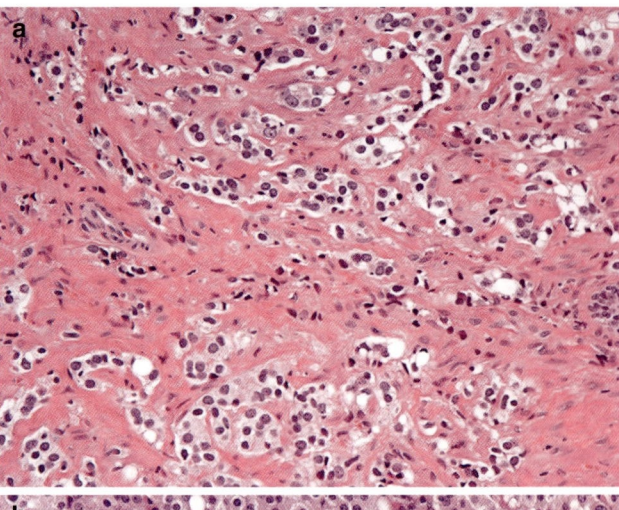

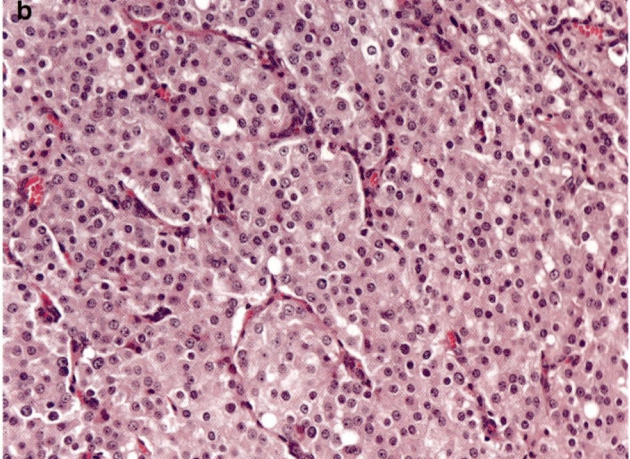

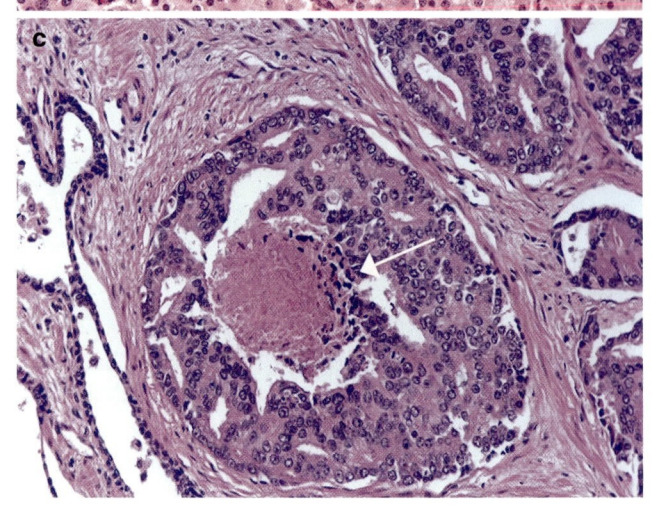

Fig. 5.7 Morphologic spectrum of Gleason pattern 5. Pattern 5 is the most consistently reproduced pattern, including tumor with single rows and cords of cells (**a**), solid nests (**b**), and solid/cribriform/papillary tumor with comedonecrosis (**c**). In general, this pattern should be recognizable at low power to be considered significant (*see* Fig. 5.12). Occasional random or peripherally distributed single cells or cord-like tumor cells may represent tangential sectioning. Sometimes abundant intraluminal amorphous secretions may mimic comedonecrosis. Only dirty necrosis with karyorrhectic debris represents comedonecrosis (*arrow*)

5.10 Gleason Grading of Unusual "Variant" Histology Types and Patterns

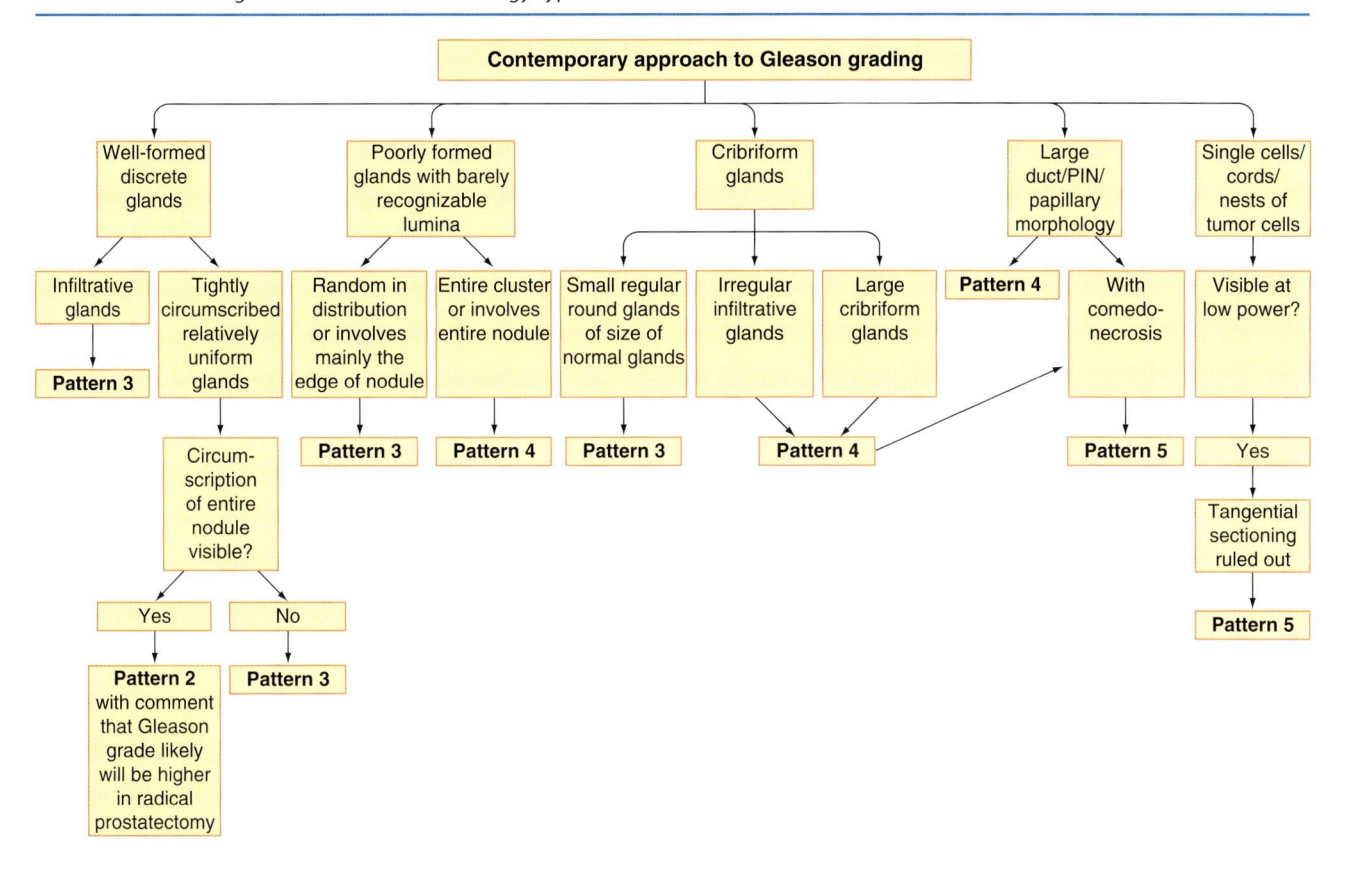

Fig. 5.8 Contemporary Gleason grading based on major architectural features

5.10 Gleason Grading of Unusual "Variant" Histology Types and Patterns

Table 5.10 Gleason grading of unusual "variant" histology types and patterns

Gleason grading of unusual "variant" histology types and patterns	
Histologic type or pattern	Gleason pattern
Foamy gland pattern	Grade based on underlying architecture
Pseudohyperplastic	Pattern 3
Atrophic	Pattern 3
Intracytoplasmic clear vacuoles	Grade based on underlying architecture
Ductal adenocarcinoma	Pattern 4, pattern 5 with necrosis
Signet-ring cell carcinoma	Pattern 5
Small cell carcinoma	Not graded
Adenosquamous and squamous carcinoma	Not graded
Sarcomatoid carcinoma	Not graded
Glomeruloid pattern	3 or 4; recent data suggest pattern 4
Collagenous micronodules	Grade based on underlying architecture
Mucinous (colloid) carcinoma	Grade based on underlying architecture (3 or 4)

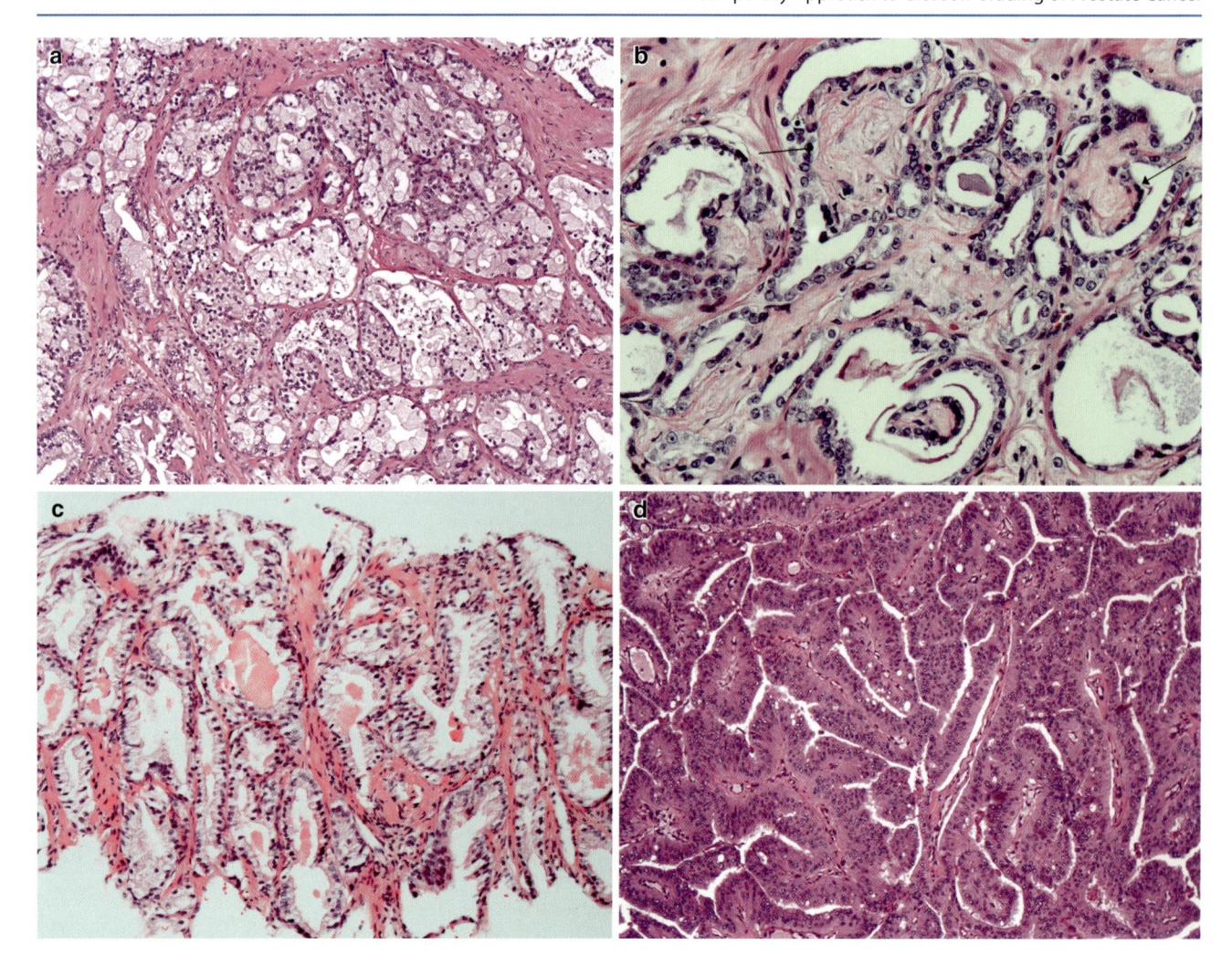

Fig. 5.9 Prostate cancer morphological variants and their Gleason grading in contemporary practice [4]. (**a**) Moderately differentiated foamy gland cancer, Gleason score 4+3=7. Although foamy gland cancers appear morphologically bland, their biological behavior is wide ranging. The majority represents intermediate-grade tumors, containing a Gleason pattern 4 component. From a grading perspective, these tumors should be graded on overall architecture rather than foamy appearance. (**b**) When grading cancer with collagenous micronodules, one should try to subtract this feature from analysis and grade based on the underlying architecture of the tumor. Although the epithelium often assumes a complex architecture, most of these cases represent Gleason pattern 3 (*arrows*). (**c**) Pseudohyperplastic carcinoma with large undulating and branching contour should be graded as Gleason pattern 3. (**d**) Confluent cancer glands with papillary architecture lined by tall columnar epithelium represent large-duct morphology and should be graded as Gleason pattern 4. With intraluminal necrosis, it is graded as Gleason pattern 5. Other large-duct morphologies include endometrioid growth pattern with cribriform/papillary morphology and PIN-like large discrete glands, demonstrating tall columnar lining epithelium. (**e**) Small cell neuroendocrine carcinoma should not be graded due to its unique tumor biology and therapeutic significance. Any amount of such differentiation is significant and should be reported. (**f**) Intraluminal cribriform proliferation representing glomeruloid differentiation (*arrows*). Grading of such differentiation remains controversial. Although some experts consider it either pattern 3 or pattern 4, recent data suggest that intraluminal cribriform architecture should be regarded as pattern 4 [25]. (**g**) Grading of colloid carcinoma consisting of tumor cells in pools of extravasated mucin is controversial. Previously, such tumors were considered high grade, Gleason score 4+4=8 tumors. New data suggest that they are not uniformly aggressive [33]. Again, one should use the architecture as a major feature to grade these tumors. If there are discrete glands floating within the pools of mucin, it should be considered pattern 3; however, if cribriform glands are present it should be considered pattern 4. In this example, the primary pattern is 3, with a small component of secondary pattern 4 (*lower right*). (**h**) Intracytoplasmic vacuoles can be seen in many prostate cancers of different patterns and do not equate to signet-ring differentiation or pattern 5. In this example, cytoplasmic vacuoles are seen in Gleason pattern 3 cancer. Such cases should be graded based on underlying architecture rather than the presence of intracytoplasmic vacuoles (*Image courtesy of* Dr. Kirk Wojno; Royal Oak, MI)

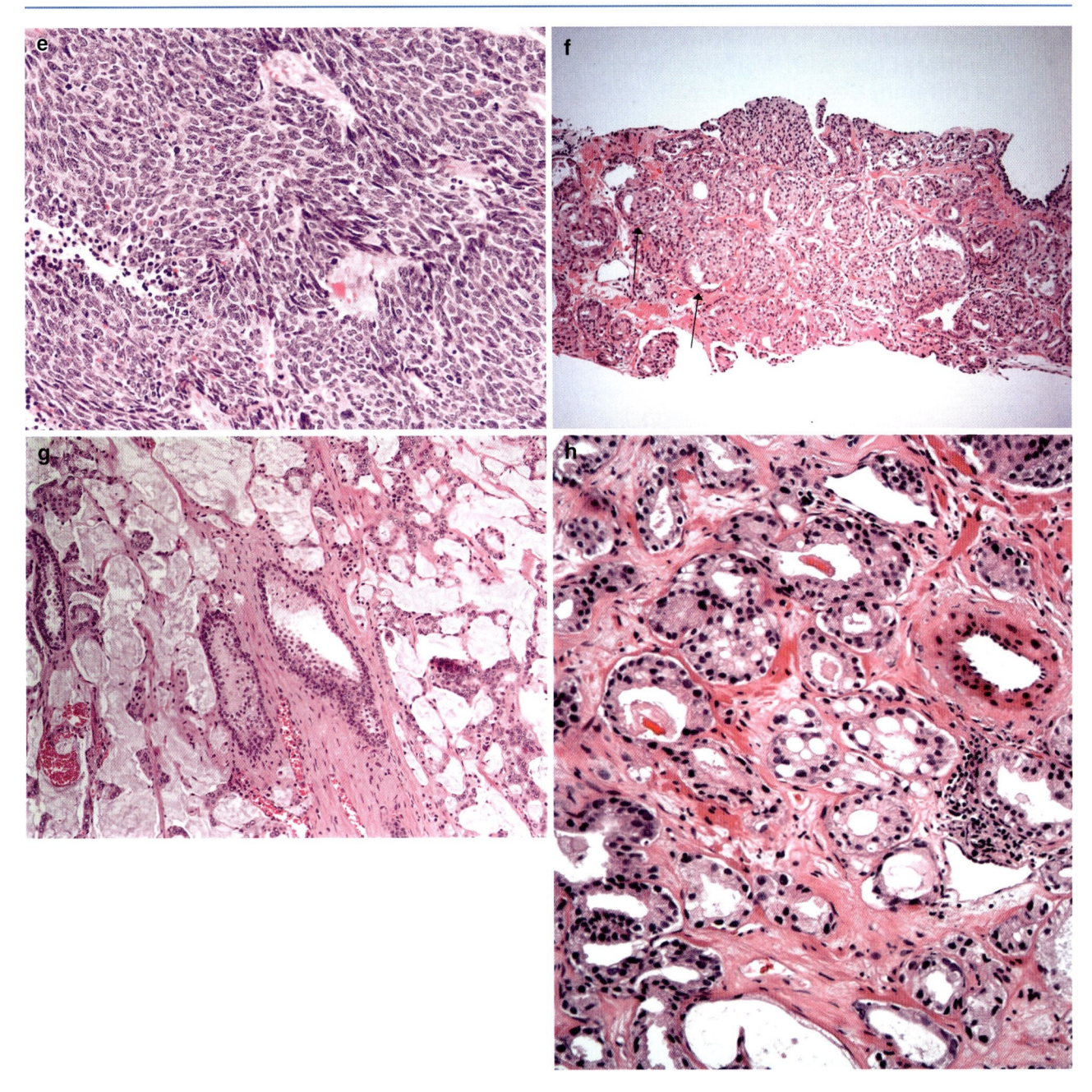

5.10 Gleason Grading of Unusual "Variant" Histology Types and Patterns 51

Fig. 5.9 (continued)

5.11 Gleason Grading in the Setting of Multiple Cores with Prostate Cancer of Different Gleason Patterns

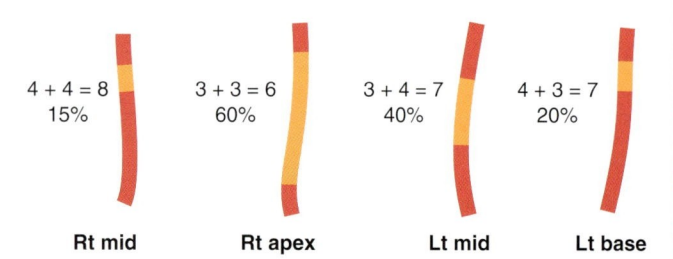

Fig. 5.10 Gleason grading in the setting of multiple cores with prostate cancer of different Gleason patterns. In contemporary practice of extended biopsy, it is common to see different cores containing cancers of different Gleason patterns. In this setting, should only a global Gleason score or worst score be assigned? Emerging data suggest that one should assign Gleason score to individual cores as long as the cores were submitted in the separate containers or their anatomic sites are specified by urologists if they are submitted in the same container [4, 23, 28, 32, 34]. Assigning an overall Gleason score is optional. In our experience, overall worst Gleason score demonstrates the best correlation between biopsy and prostatectomy Gleason grade and, more importantly, the likelihood of upgrading at prostatectomy remains lowest [32]. This is especially true when the radical prostatectomy has multifocal cancer. In another study, one core has a Gleason score of 4+4=8 and other cores have pattern 3+3=6, the pathological stage at radical prostatectomy is comparable to cases with all cores having Gleason score 4+4=8 [23]. In a recent survey, urological surgeons typically use the highest grade of all cores for clinical management [28]

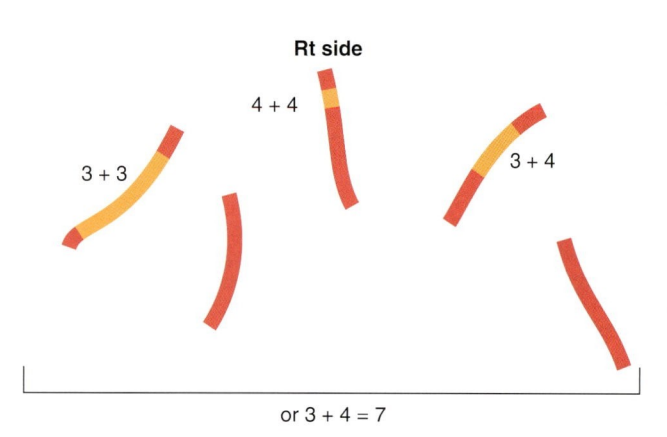

Fig. 5.11 Gleason grading in the setting of multiple cores with different Gleason grades in the same containers without specific site designation. Multiple cores placed in the same container without individual core specification – or only as "left" or "right" – are a relatively common practice. Currently, no clear guidelines address this issue. Recently, we simulated this scenario in our practice by artificially lumping the cores as if they were put in "right" or "left" side only and then determined a global score (average Gleason score of the entire case), worst Gleason score, and Gleason score of the largest cancer focus [22]. Overall correlation was best with the worst Gleason score, and chances of significant upgrading in radical prostatectomy were least when this parameter was used. These results suggest that when multiple intact cores are submitted in a container without specific site identifiers, the Gleason score of an individual core or worst Gleason score provide better information of the underlying Gleason grade. This approach is not recommended if cores are fragmented as there are potential chances of artificially upgrading the tumor

5.12 Tertiary Pattern 5 in Prostate Biopsy

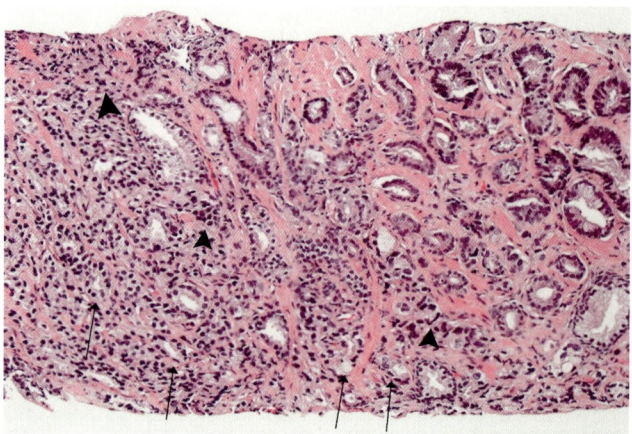

Fig. 5.12 Tertiary pattern 5. A prostate needle biopsy demonstrating primary pattern 3 (well-formed discrete glands, *upper right*), secondary pattern 4 (poorly formed fused glands, *arrows*), and tertiary pattern 5 (cords and individual single cells, *arrowheads*); such a case should be graded 3+5. It is important to document the tertiary pattern if it is higher than the secondary pattern. A typical scenario is the biopsy contains cancer of patterns 3, 4, and 5 in various proportions. Emerging data suggest that such tumors should be classified high grade [4, 30, 31]. This recommendation is critical for clinical management. The majority of clinicians use Partin tables or nomograms to predict outcomes such as pathological stage or prognosis after radical prostatectomy or radiation therapy. These algorithms typically use only primary and secondary pattern reported in the NBX and therefore tertiary pattern of higher grade would be dropped unless reported as secondary pattern. In our experience, the radical prostatectomy pathologic outcomes of biopsy Gleason score 3+4 or 4+3 with tertiary pattern 5 is comparable to the radical prostatectomy pathologic outcomes of biopsy Gleason score 8–10 [30]. Similarly, other investigators have demonstrated that PSA biochemical failure is higher for patients with Gleason 7 containing a tertiary pattern 5 compared with Gleason score 7 cancers without a tertiary pattern 5 [31]

5.13 Recommendations for Gleason Grading in the Post-therapy Setting

Table 5.11 Recommendations for Gleason grading in the post-therapy setting

Gleason grading after radiation and/or hormonal therapy
Do not grade when there is morphologic evidence of treatment effect
Treatment effect produces morphological changes mimicking high-grade cancer (*see* Fig. 5.13)
Grading may be appropriate if there is no morphological evidence of treatment effect

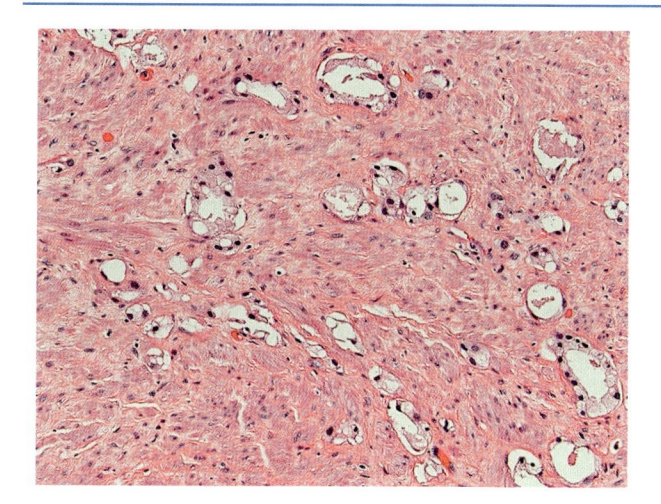

Fig. 5.13 Treatment produces histological changes mimicking high-grade cancer [35, 36]. A prostate needle biopsy post-radiation treatment demonstrating single cells and poorly formed glands, simulating a high-grade cancer. Both radiation and hormone therapy cause glandular breakdown, loss of glandular architecture with either poorly formed/compressed glands or single cells, cytoplasmic vacuolization, nuclear shrinkage, nuclear hyperchromasia and pyknosis, and mucinous degeneration. These morphological features simulate and may be mistaken for a high-grade cancer if the treatment is not suspected. Gleason grading should not be applied in this setting

5.14 Impact of ISUP-modified Gleason Grading System

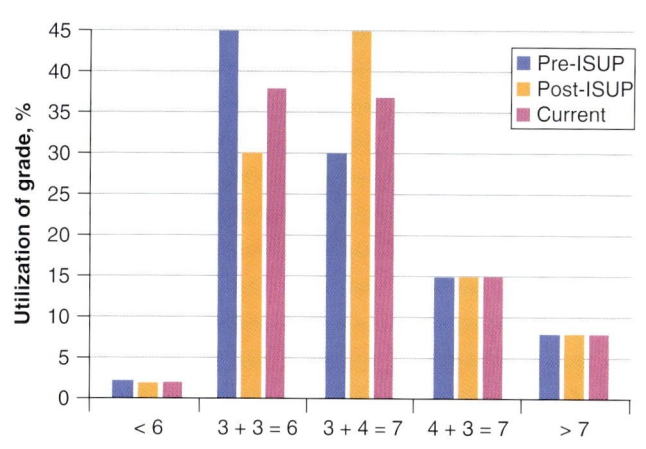

Fig. 5.15 Impact of ISUP-modified Gleason grading system. Before the ISUP Gleason grading recommendations, Gleason score 6 cancer was the most common grade. After ISUP recommendations, there was a significant decrease in Gleason score 6 diagnosis and an upward shift toward Gleason score 7 (3+4). With increasing experience and understanding, utilization of Gleason score 7 (3+4) has slightly shifted back and is now almost parallel to Gleason score 6 diagnosis. Overall, increased utilization of secondary Gleason pattern 4 is the most noticeable impact of ISUP grading recommendations in practice [39]. However, overall significance of this shift for patient management and prognosis remains to be validated. Billis et al. [40] found that modified but not conventional Gleason score better predicted PSA failure after radical prostatectomy. This study is one of the first to provide important evidence-based validation on the clinical impact of the 2005 revised Gleason grading system (*Image courtesy of* Dr. Kirk Wojno; Royal Oak, MI)

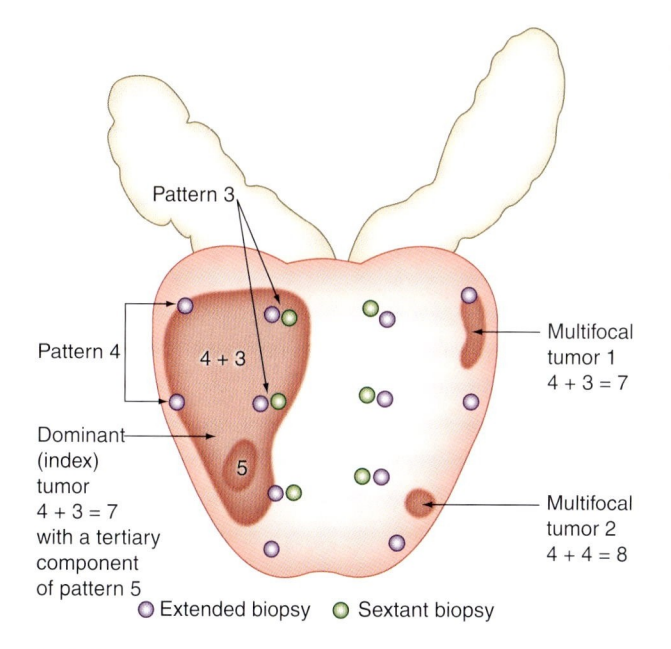

Fig. 5.14 Effect of tumor multifocality and biopsy sampling techniques on biopsy/radical prostatectomy Gleason score correlation. Correlation between biopsy and radical prostatectomy Gleason score remains poor in Gleason grading; specifically, biopsy undergrading remains a significant concern [17–19]. Recent studies suggest that this discrepancy is reduced when extended biopsy protocols are used [37, 38]. Various factors affect this correlation, most notably tumor multifocality and biopsy-sampling techniques. Most prostate cancers are multifocal, represented by a dominant or index tumor and other separate multifocal tumors. In this example, areas of Gleason pattern 4 tumor are primarily identified by laterally directed extended biopsy cores, whereas sextant biopsy cores undersample these areas. Areas of tertiary pattern 5 within the index tumor and nondominant multifocal tumor 2 with Gleason score 4+4 remains unsampled by both sextant and extended biopsy cores

5.15 Problem Areas in Gleason Grading and Future Trends

Table 5.12 Problem areas in Gleason grading and future trends [41–45]

Problem areas in Gleason grading	Future trends
Concordance between biopsy and radical prostatectomy grade	Three-dimensional (3D) extended and saturation biopsy protocols to reduce tissue sampling error and better sample the tumor with grade heterogeneity in the setting of multifocal prostate cancer
Predictability of "clinically insignificant" Gleason ≤6 cancer and its grade progression at individual patient level	Site-specific labeling and 3D extended and saturation biopsy protocols to better sample underlying high-grade tumor
	Utilization of morphometric parameters to improve predictive value of Gleason grading
	Utilization of gene-expression studies and molecular correlates and markers that predict clinically significant and/or higher-grade tumor
Inter- and intraobserver variability	Utilization of advanced computational, digital, and morphometric techniques

References

1. Gleason DF (1966) Classification of prostatic carcinomas. Cancer Chemother Rep 50:125–128
2. Bailar JC III (1966) Mellinger GT, Gleason DF: Survival rates of patients with prostatic cancer, tumor stage, and differentiation – preliminary report. Cancer Chemother Rep 50:129–136
3. Shah RB (2009) Current perspectives on the Gleason grading of prostate cancer. Arch Pathol Lab Med 133:1810–1816
4. Epstein JI, Allsbrook WC Jr, Amin MB et al (2005) The 2005 International Society of Urological Pathology (ISUP) consensus conference on Gleason grading of prostatic carcinoma. Am J Surg Pathol 29:1228–1242
5. Gleason DF, Mellinger GT (1974) Prediction of prognosis for prostatic adenocarcinoma by combined histological grading and clinical staging. J Urol 111:58–64
6. Eble JN, Sauter G, Epstein JI, Sesterhenn IA (eds) (2004) World Health Organization Classification of tumors: pathology and genetics of tumours of the urinary system and male genital organs, 1 edn. International Agency for Research on Cancer (IARC) Press, Lyons
7. Ennis RD, Malyszko BK, Rescigno J et al (1998) Biologic classification as an alternative to anatomic staging for clinically localized prostate cancer: a proposal based on patients treated with external beam radiotherapy. Urology 51:265–270
8. Roehl KA, Han M, Ramos CG et al (2004) Cancer progression and survival rates following anatomical radical retropubic prostatectomy in 3,478 consecutive patients: long-term results. J Urol 172:910–914
9. Schwartz E, Albertsen P (2002) Nomograms for clinically localized disease Part III: watchful waiting. Semin Urol Oncol 20:140–145
10. Zagars GK, Pollack A, von Eschenbach AC (1997) Prognostic factors for clinically localized prostate carcinoma: analysis of 938 patients irradiated in the prostate specific antigen era. Cancer 79: 1370–1380
11. Bentley G, Dey J, Sakr WA et al (2000) Significance of the Gleason scoring system after neoadjuvant hormonal therapy. Mol Urol 4:125; discussion 131
12. Partin AW, Yoo J, Carter HB et al (1997) Combination of prostate-specific antigen, clinical stage, and Gleason score to predict pathological stage of localized prostate cancer. A multi-institutional update. JAMA 277:1445–1451
13. Partin AW, Mangold LA, Lamm DM et al (2001) Contemporary update of prostate cancer staging nomograms (Partin Tables) for the new millennium. Urology 58:843–848
14. Pisansky TM, Kahn MJ, Rasp GM et al (1997) A multiple prognostic index predictive of disease outcome after irradiation for clinically localized prostate carcinoma. Cancer 79:337–344
15. Siu W, Dunn RL, Shah RB, Wei JT (2005) Use of extended pattern technique for initial prostate biopsy. J Urol 174:505–509
16. Amin MB, Schultz DS, Zarbo RJ (1994) Analysis of cribriform morphology in prostatic neoplasia using antibody to high-molecular-weight cytokeratins. Arch Pathol Lab Med 118:260–264
17. Bostwick DG (1994) Gleason grading of prostatic needle biopsies. Correlation with grade in 316 matched prostatectomies. Am J Surg Pathol 18:796–803
18. Cookson MS, Fleshner NE, Soloway SM, Fair WR (1997) Correlation between Gleason score of needle biopsy and radical prostatectomy specimen: accuracy and clinical implications. J Urol 157:559–562
19. Steinberg DM, Sauvageot J, Piantadosi S, Epstein JI (1997) Correlation of prostate needle biopsy and radical prostatectomy Gleason grade in academic and community settings. Am J Surg Pathol 21:566–576
20. Brinker DA, Potter SR, Epstein JI (1999) Ductal adenocarcinoma of the prostate diagnosed on needle biopsy: correlation with clinical and radical prostatectomy findings and progression. Am J Surg Pathol 23:1471–1479
21. Epstein JI (2000) Gleason score 2–4 adenocarcinoma of the prostate on needle biopsy: a diagnosis that should not be made. Am J Surg Pathol 24:477–478
22. Kunju LP, Daignault S, Wei JT, Shah RB (2009) Multiple prostate cancer cores with different Gleason grades submitted in the same specimen container without specific site designation: should each core be assigned an individual Gleason score? Hum Pathol 40:558–564
23. Kunz GM Jr, Epstein JI (2003) Should each core with prostate cancer be assigned a separate Gleason score? Hum Pathol 34: 911–914
24. Latour M, Amin MB, Billis A et al (2008) Grading of invasive cribriform carcinoma on prostate needle biopsy: an interobserver study among experts in genitourinary pathology. Am J Surg Pathol 32:1532–1539
25. Lotan TL, Epstein JI (2009) Gleason grading of prostatic adenocarcinoma with glomeruloid features on needle biopsy. Hum Pathol 40:471–477
26. Mosse CA, Magi-Galluzzi C, Tsuzuki T, Epstein JI (2004) The prognostic significance of tertiary Gleason pattern 5 in radical prostatectomy specimens. Am J Surg Pathol 28:394–398
27. Pan CC, Potter SR, Partin AW, Epstein JI (2000) The prognostic significance of tertiary Gleason patterns of higher grade in radical prostatectomy specimens: a proposal to modify the Gleason grading system. Am J Surg Pathol 24:563–569
28. Rubin MA, Bismar TA, Curtis S, Montie JE (2004) Prostate needle biopsy reporting: how are the surgical members of the Society of Urologic Oncology using pathology reports to guide treatment of prostate cancer patients? Am J Surg Pathol 28:946–952
29. Rubin MA, Dunn R, Kambham N et al (2000) Should a Gleason score be assigned to a minute focus of carcinoma on prostate biopsy? Am J Surg Pathol 24:1634–1640

References

30. Shah R, Daignault S, Kunju LP et al (2009) Significance of tertiary pattern 5 in prostate needle biopsies with Gleason score of 3+4 or 4+3 prostate cancer: pathologic correlation following radical prostatectomy. Mod Pathol 22:193A
31. Trpkov K, Zhang J, Chan M et al (2009) Prostate cancer with tertiary Gleason pattern 5 in prostate needle biopsy: clinicopathologic findings and disease progression. Am J Surg Pathol 33:233–240
32. Wu AJ, Daignault S, Wasco MJ et al (2008) Correlation of biopsy and radical prostatectomy Gleason score in contemporary extended ≥ 12 core biopsy practice: improved correlation with biopsy worst Gleason score. Mod Pathol 21:190A
33. Lane BR, Magi-Galluzzi C, Reuther AM et al (2006) Mucinous adenocarcinoma of the prostate does not confer poor prognosis. Urology 68:825–830
34. Dunn R, Shah R, Zhou M (2002) Global Gleason score, highest Gleason score, or weighted Gleason score: what Gleason score should be reported in prostate needle biopsies? Mod Pathol 15:161A/669
35. Gaudin PB, Zelefsky MJ, Leibel SA et al (1999) Histopathologic effects of three-dimensional conformal external beam radiation therapy on benign and malignant prostate tissues. Am J Surg Pathol 23:1021–1031
36. Montironi R, Schulman CC (1998) Pathological changes in prostate lesions after androgen manipulation. J Clin Pathol 51:5–12
37. Emiliozzi P, Maymone S, Paterno A et al (2004) Increased accuracy of biopsy Gleason score obtained by extended needle biopsy. J Urol 172:2224–2226
38. King CR, McNeal JE, Gill H, Presti JC Jr (2004) Extended prostate biopsy scheme improves reliability of Gleason grading: implications for radiotherapy patients. Int J Radiat Oncol Biol Phys 59:386–391
39. Zareba P, Zhang J, Yilmaz A, Trpkov K (2009) The impact of the 2005 International Society of Urological Pathology (ISUP) consensus on Gleason grading in contemporary practice. Histopathology 55:384–391
40. Billis A, Guimaraes MS, Freitas LL et al (2008) The impact of the 2005 international society of urological pathology consensus conference on standard Gleason grading of prostatic carcinoma in needle biopsies. J Urol 180:548–552; discussion 552–553
41. Burke HB, Goodman PH, Rosen DB et al (1997) Artificial neural networks improve the accuracy of cancer survival prediction. Cancer 79:857–862
42. Cordon-Cardo C, Kotsianti A, Verbel DA et al (2007) Improved prediction of prostate cancer recurrence through systems pathology. J Clin Invest 117:1876–1883
43. Piert M, Park H, Khan A et al (2009) Detection of aggressive primary prostate cancer with 11C-choline PET/CT using multimodality fusion techniques. J Nucl Med 50:1585–1593
44. Schulte RT, Wood DP, Daignault S et al (2008) Utility of extended pattern prostate biopsies for tumor localization: pathologic correlations after radical prostatectomy. Cancer 113:1559–1565
45. Shah RB, Chinnaiyan AM (2009) The discovery of common recurrent transmembrane protease serine 2 (TMPRSS2)-erythroblastosis virus E26 transforming sequence (ETS) gene fusions in prostate cancer: significance and clinical implications. Adv Anat Pathol 16:145–153

Histologic Variants of Prostate Carcinoma

Histologic variants and variations of prostate adenocarcinoma account for 5–10% of prostate carcinomas and typically are associated with ordinary acinar prostate adenocarcinoma. The morphologic spectrum of histologic variants ranges from tumors often resembling benign conditions, such as foamy and pseudohyperplastic carcinoma, to highly aggressive forms, such as small cell neuroendocrine carcinoma. These histologic variants often differ from acinar carcinoma in clinical, immunophenotypic, ultrastructural, and genetic features [1]. Some of these histologic variants also differ in prognosis and may necessitate a different therapeutic approach. This chapter outlines important clinical and pathologic characteristics of histologic variants and variations.

6.1 Histological Variants of Prostate Carcinoma

Table 6.1 Histological variants of prostate carcinoma

Foamy gland carcinoma
Pseudohyperplastic carcinoma
Adenocarcinoma with atrophic features
Adenocarcinoma with glomeruloid features
Ductal adenocarcinoma
Mucinous (colloid) carcinoma
Small cell neuroendocrine carcinoma
Sarcomatoid carcinoma (carcinosarcoma)
Signet ring cell carcinoma
Squamous and adenosquamous carcinoma
Adenoid cystic basal cell carcinoma
Urothelial carcinoma

6.2 Histologic Variants of Prostate Carcinoma Mimicking Benign Lesions

Table 6.2 Histologic variants of prostate carcinoma mimicking benign lesions

Histological pattern of cancer	Benign condition they may mimic
Foamy gland carcinoma	Cowper's glands
	Mucinous metaplasia
	Xanthomatous inflammation
Atrophic carcinoma	Benign atrophy
Pseudohyperplastic carcinoma	Benign prostatic hyperplasia (BPH)
	Prostatic intraepithelial neoplasia (PIN)

6.3 Foamy Gland Carcinoma

Table 6.3 Foamy gland carcinoma [1–5]

Microscopical features

Low-power architecture

Crowded and/or infiltrative glands with abundant foamy/xanthomatous cytoplasm (*see* Fig. 6.1a–b)

Nucleus-to-cytoplasm (N:C) ratio is very low due to abundant foamy cytoplasm, resembling histiocytes

Amorphous eosinophilic luminal secretions are common

Majority of foamy gland carcinomas also contain conventional acinar differentiation

High-power cytology

Nuclei are typically small and dense; nuclear enlargement, hyperchromasia, and prominent nucleoli are usually not conspicuous

Nuclei are typically rounder than oval nuclei of benign glands

The cytoplasm has bubbly empty vacuoles

Immunohistochemical and molecular features

Basal cell markers are negative

α-Methylacyl-CoA racemase (AMACR) is variably expressed with overall low sensitivity (68–70%)

ETS gene fusions demonstrate lower frequency (~30%) [1]

Differential diagnosis

Cowper's gland and mucinous metaplasia. Cowper's glands and mucinous metaplasia contain intracytoplasmic mucin, whereas foamy carcinoma contains luminal mucin but lack intracytoplasmic mucin and demonstrate variable degree of cytological atypia

Xanthomatous inflammation. The lack of nuclear atypia, lack of glandular differentiation, and conventional acinar cancer favors xanthomatous inflammation (*see* Fig. 7.30). In small needle biopsy samples, immunohistochemical markers for CD-68, prostate-specific antigen (PSA), and cytokeratin help confirm the diagnosis.

Gleason grading and clinical significance

Graded based on its underlying architecture and not based on foamy appearance

Some foamy gland carcinomas behave as an intermediate-to-aggressive cancers. Majority represent Gleason score 6–7 tumors.

R.B. Shah, M. Zhou, *Prostate Biopsy Interpretation: An Illustrated Guide*,
DOI 10.1007/978-3-642-21369-4_6, © Springer-Verlag Berlin Heidelberg 2012

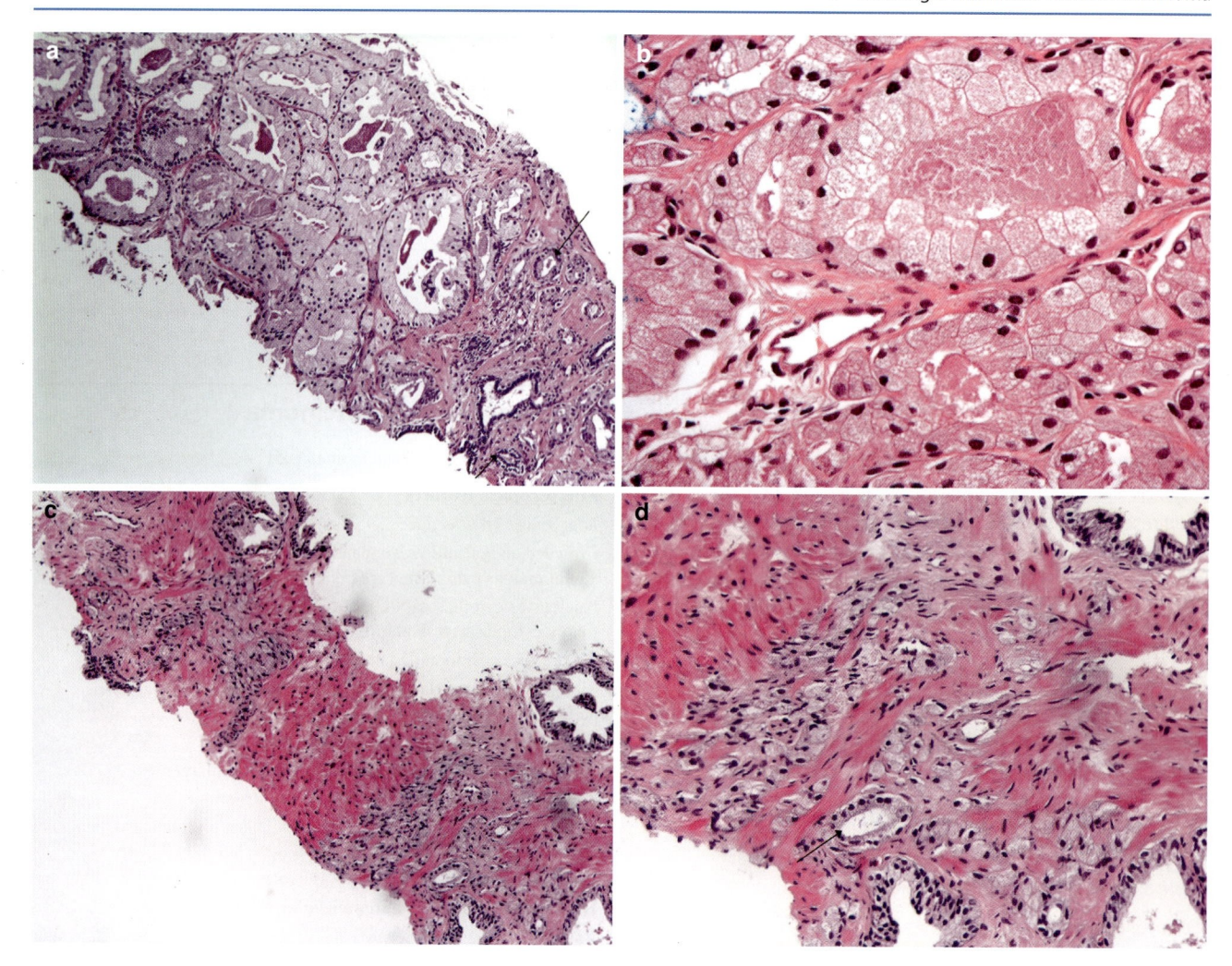

Fig. 6.1 Morphological spectrum of foamy gland carcinoma. (**a**, **b**) At low power, a foamy gland carcinoma is characterized by abundant xanthomatous cytoplasm with low N:C ratio, simulating a benign process. Intraluminal, dense, pink, acellular secretions are common. Conventional acinar differentiation (*arrow*) is also common in foamy carcinoma (**a**). The nuclei are small and dense; typical malignant nuclear features of prostate cancer are only variably present, making recognition of cancer difficult. Occasional prominent nucleoli and nuclear enlargement are also present (**b**). (**c**, **d**) A poorly differentiated foamy gland carcinoma simulating xanthomatous inflammation in needle biopsy. Presence of cytological atypia and/or any glandular differentiation (*arrow*) supports the diagnosis of foamy gland carcinoma (**d**). An immunohistochemical panel consisting of histiocytic markers and pancytokeratin may be needed to arrive at a definitive diagnosis in such cases, particularly in small needle biopsy samples. Gleason grading should be based on architecture rather than foamy appearance [2]

6.4 Pseudohyperplastic Carcinoma

Table 6.4 Pseudohyperplastic carcinoma [2, 5–7]

Microscopical features

Low-power architecture

Many closely packed glands of varying size with complex and undulating architecture and frequent papillary infolding. Large glands with undulating architecture are a prominent feature (*see* Fig. 6.2).

The cytoplasm is amphophilic with frequent amorphous secretions and blue mucin

High-power cytology

Nuclear enlargement, hyperchromasia, and prominent nucleoli are present and required for making a cancer diagnosis in needle biopsy

Immunohistochemical features

Basal cell markers are negative and are required in most cases

AMACR is variably expressed with overall low sensitivity (68–70%)

Differential diagnosis

High-grade PIN (HGPIN) and BPH

The diagnosis of pseudohyperplastic carcinoma should be made with caution in needle biopsy samples when the focus of concern is small, as the diagnosis of HGPIN or BPH cannot be excluded with certainty. Immunohistochemical markers are not always helpful in this situation (*see* Fig. 6.3). When present, conventional acinar differentiations aid in this differential diagnoses.

Gleason grading and clinical significance

Usually considered to be Gleason score 3 + 3 = 6 carcinoma

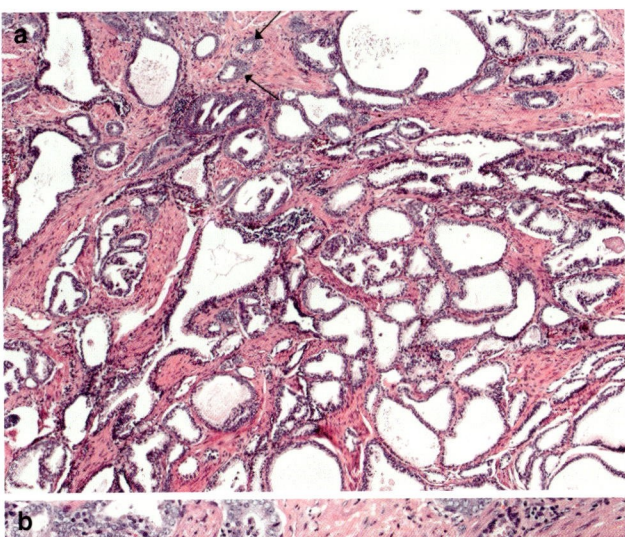

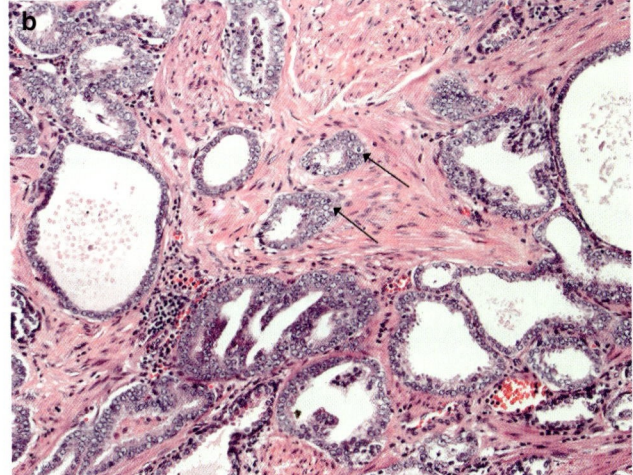

Fig. 6.2 Pseudohyperplastic prostate carcinoma. (**a**, **b**) At low magnification, pseudohyperplastic carcinoma demonstrates crowded proliferation of large dilated glands with branching and papillary infoldings and luminal secretions. These glands are deceptively bland at low power and mimic BPH. Also note the presence of small conventional acinar cancer glands (*arrow*, **a**). At high magnification, both large and small glands display cytoplasmic amphophilia and nuclear atypia suggestive of cancer (**b**). (**c–f**) Another pseudohyperplastic carcinoma in needle biopsy. Note relatively deceptive, bland appearance of large glands at low power. Crowding, admixture with some small glands and differences in cytoplasmic characteristics bring attention to these glands at low power (**c**). At higher magnification, single layer of nuclei, with nuclear enlargement and prominent nucleoli, is visible (**d–e**). The lack of basal cell markers (HMWCK and p63) and strong AMACR expression (**f**) support the diagnosis of pseudohyperplastic prostate carcinoma

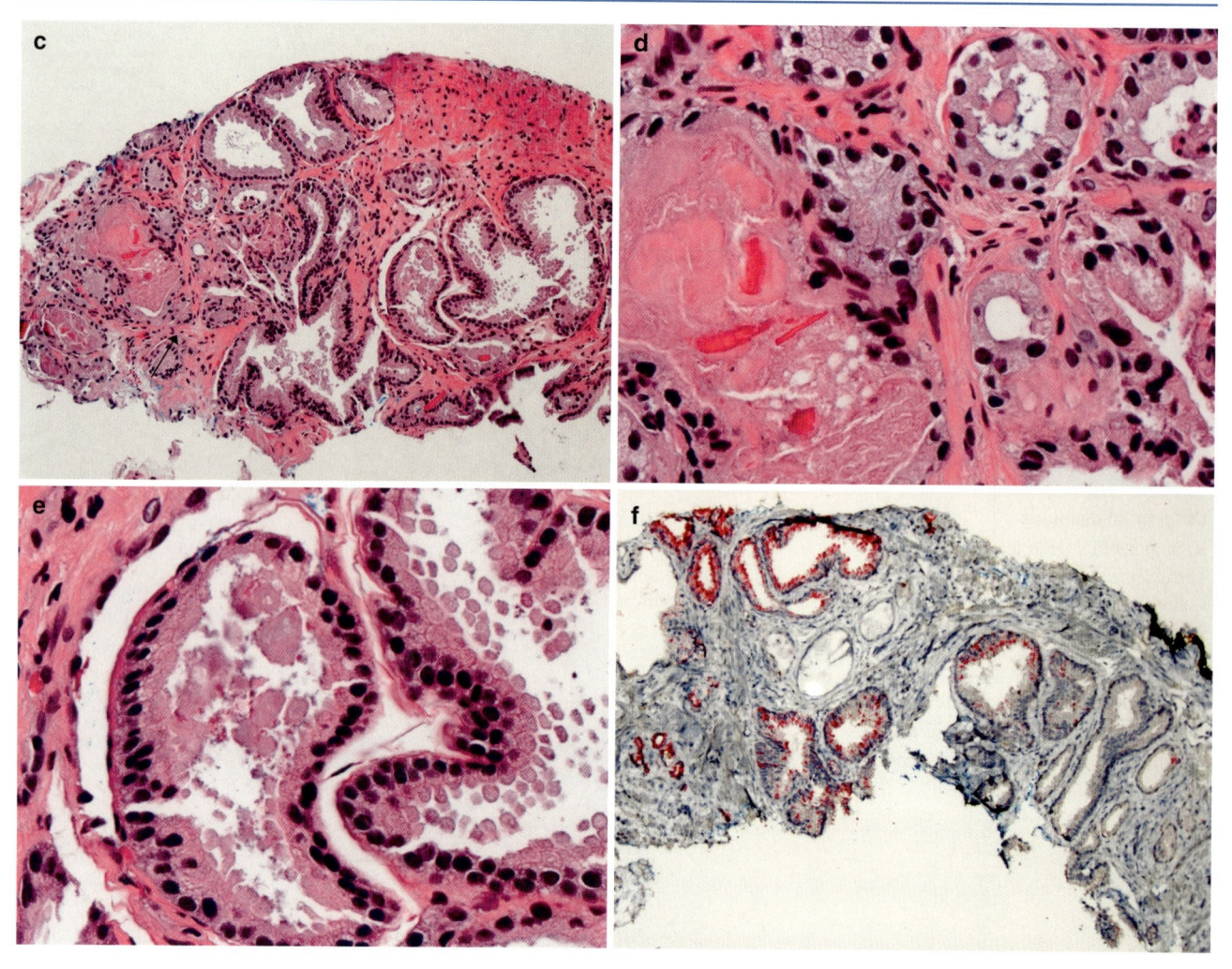

Fig. 6.2 (continued)

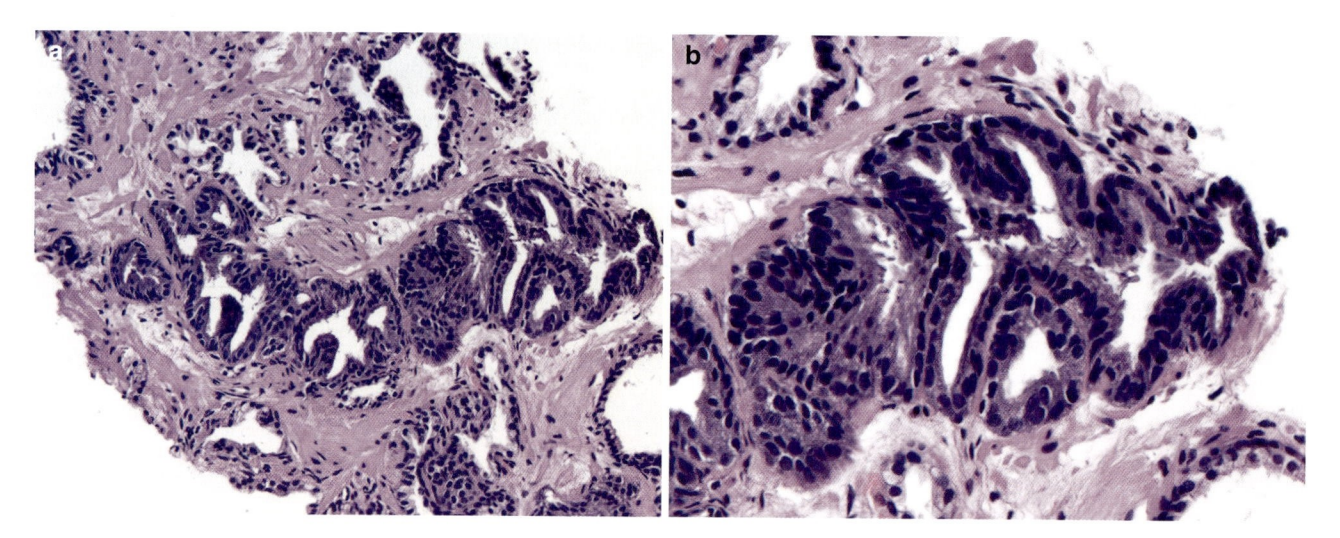

Fig. 6.3 Atypical glands suspicious for pseudohyperplastic carcinoma. Diagnosis of a small focus of pseudohyperplastic prostate carcinoma in needle biopsy should be made with extreme caution. (**a–d**) In this example, there is a small focus of crowded large- to mid-size glands with undulated architecture, papillation and nuclear stratification, and dense cytoplasmic eosinophilia, suspicious for pseudohyperplastic carcinoma (**a**). High-power view demonstrates marked cytological atypia (**b**). Immunostains show these glands demonstrating rare basal cells (**c**) and are strongly positive for AMACR (**d**). Note here that the focus of concern is very small and a diagnosis of HGPIN cannot be excluded based on morphology or immunoprofile. In this circumstance, a diagnosis of atypical prostate glands suspicious for but not diagnostic of carcinoma (AYTP) would be appropriate

6.5 Prostate Adenocarcinoma with Atrophic Features

Table 6.5 Prostate adenocarcinoma with atrophic features [2, 5, 8, 9]

Microscopical features

Low-power architecture

Infiltrative and/or crowded glands with scant yet basophilic/amphophilic cytoplasm (*see* Fig. 6.4)

Intraluminal secretions including amorphous eosinophilic concretions and blue mucin are often present

Usually intermixed with nonatrophic conventional acinar adenocarcinoma

In cases after treatment, other features of androgen deprivation or radiation are usually evident

High-power cytology

Significant nuclear enlargement, hyperchromasia, and prominent nucleoli are usually present and are required for making the diagnosis

(*see* Fig. 6.4b–e)

Immunohistochemical features

Basal cell markers are negative

AMACR is variably expressed with overall low sensitivity (68–70%)

Differential diagnosis

Simple lobular atrophy, postatrophic hyperplasia, and partial atrophy

Atrophic carcinoma despite scant cytoplasm usually displays an infiltrative growth pattern, with atrophic glands intermingling with larger benign glands. In contrast, benign atrophy conditions are characterized by lobulated or circumscribed proliferation. Atrophic carcinoma appears less dark or basophilic compared to postatrophic hyperplasia or complete atrophy, as the cytoplasm is relatively decreased but is appreciable in the former.

Atrophic carcinoma demonstrates significantly more cytological atypia compared to benign atrophy

Atrophic prostate carcinoma is often intermixed with nonatrophic conventional prostate carcinoma

Gleason grading and clinical significance

Atrophic carcinomas not associated with therapy typically behave as conventional Gleason score 3 + 3 = 6 prostate carcinoma

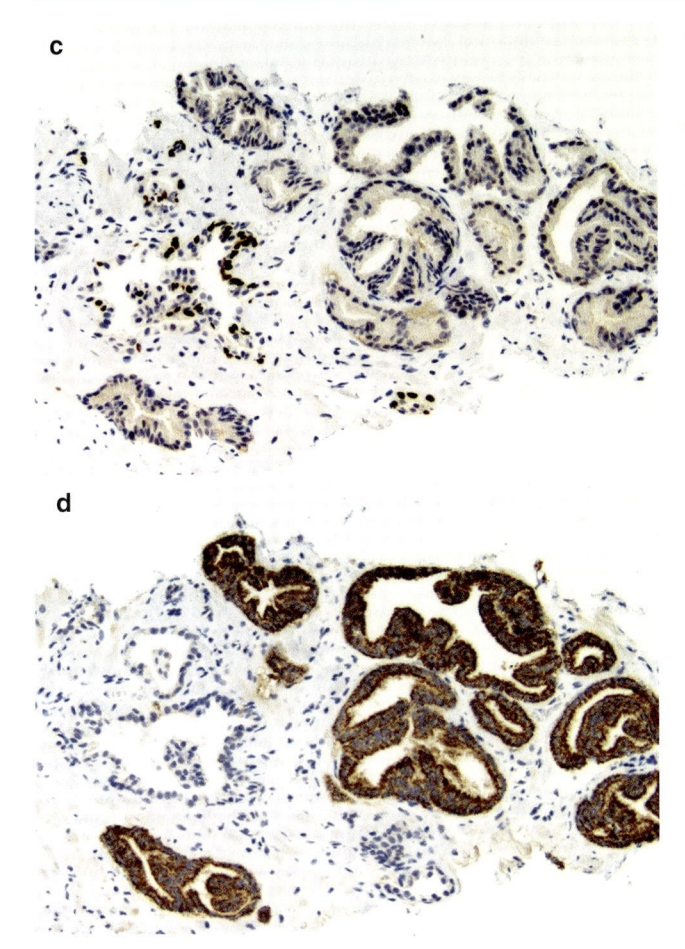

Fig. 6.3 (continued)

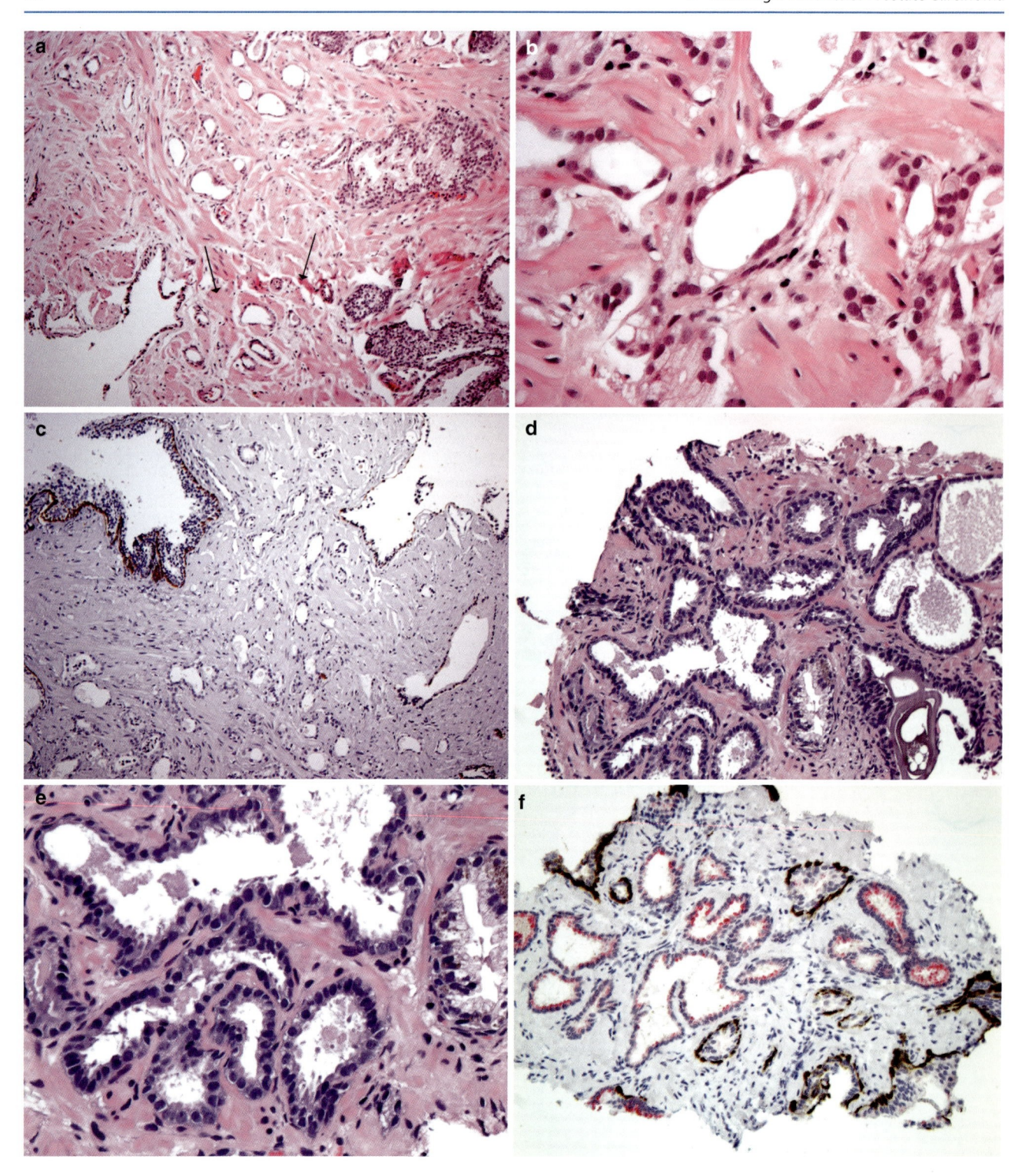

Fig. 6.4 Prostate adenocarcinoma with atrophic features. (**a–c**) At low-power examination, the cancer glands demonstrate scant amphopilic cytoplasm mimicking partially atrophic benign glands. However, infiltrative growth is obvious (*arrows*, **a**). At higher magnification, the cancer glands are not completely atrophic and still retain a small amount of cytoplasm. Also note that the cancer glands display unequivocal malignant histologic features (**b**). Cancer glands lack immunohistochemical markers for basal cells; benign glands demonstrate strong staining (**c**). (**d–f**) Another example in biopsy. Cancer glands impart a basophilic appearance at low power due to marked reduction in cytoplasm mimicking completely atrophic glands (**d**). Significant cytological atypia argues against the diagnosis of benign atrophy (**e**). PIN-4 cocktail antibodies demonstrate lack of basal cell expression and strong expression of AMACR, supporting the diagnosis of cancer (**f**). Significant cytological atypia and/or presence of admixed conventional acinar cancer is required to make a definitive diagnosis of atrophic adenocarcinoma

6.6 Prostate Adenocarcinoma with Glomeruloid Features

Table 6.6 Prostate adenocarcinoma with glomeruloid features [2, 10]

Microscopical features

Low-power architecture

Tufts or balls of cancer cells projecting into the cancer lumina, superficially resembling renal glomeruli (*see* Fig. 6.5)

The central portion typically has cribriform architecture; a prominent central fibrovascular core may be present

Conventional acinar component is usually present

High-power cytology

Nuclear enlargement, hyperchromasia, and prominent nucleoli are usually present

Immunohistochemical features

Identical to conventional acinar prostate cancer

Differential diagnosis

Invasive cribriform carcinoma of the prostate

Glomeruloid body represents an intraluminal cribriform proliferation with a dominant cellular bridge connecting the central mass to the periphery of the acini (*see* Fig. 6.5), whereas in true cribriform carcinoma, the cellular bridges are transluminal and relatively evenly spaced and similar in size. Fibrovascular cores are less common in cribriform carcinoma.

Gleason grading and clinical significance

No consensus in assigning a Gleason grade to this histologic variant. A recent study suggests grading as pattern 4. Adjacent carcinoma frequently demonstrates Gleason pattern 4 cribriform glands.

A specific feature of prostate cancer that can be used to diagnose prostate cancer in challenging cases. It is typically observed in <3% of prostate needle biopsies and <5% of radical prostatectomy specimens.

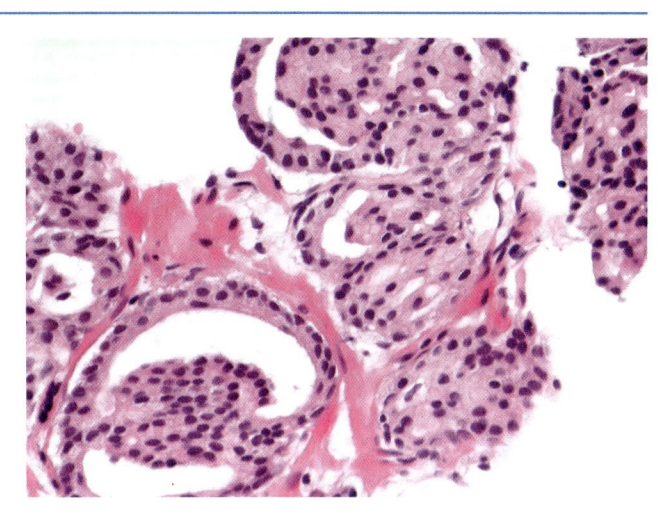

Fig. 6.5 Prostate adenocarcinoma with glomeruloid differentiation. There is cribriform proliferation spanning the lumen, mimicking renal glomeruli. Although Gleason grading for glomerulation is controversial and no consensus has been reached by the International Society of Urological Pathology, some data suggest it should be graded as Gleason pattern 4 [10]. Importantly, glomerulation is usually a focal phenomenon; conventional acinar or cribriform carcinoma is usually present (*not shown*) and helps define the tumor grade

6.7 Ductal Adenocarcinoma

Table 6.7 Ductal adenocarcinoma [2, 11–15]

Microscopical features

Low-power architecture

Ductal adenocarcinoma grows within and expands the prostatic urethra and periurethral ducts, or more commonly involves prostatic ducts and acini

A variety of architectural patterns often intermingle, including confluent papillary, cribriform, "PIN-like," single large gland duct-type morphology, "endometroid" and solid (*see* Fig. 6.6)

Cancer glands are lined by pseudostratified tall columnar cells with abundant amphophilic cytoplasm

In papillary pattern, true fibrovascular cores are seen

In cribriform and endometroid patterns, lumina are often compressed with slit-like architecture

Ductal adenocarcinoma commonly demonstrates intraductal spread into preexisting ducts with preservation of basal cell layers (*see* Fig. 6.6e)

High-power cytology

Cytological atypia is minimal in some cases, but most cases demonstrate nuclear atypia, including nuclear pleomorphism and mitoses and necrosis

Immunohistochemical features

Positive for PSA, prostatic acid phosphatase (PSAP), prostate-specific membrane antigen (PSMA), and AMACR, and usually negative for HMWCK and p63, although residual basal cell layer is common with intraductal spread

Differential diagnosis

Centrally located tumors often present with papillary or solid morphology and may be confused with high-grade, poorly differentiated urothelial carcinoma (*see* Fig. 6.13). Urothelial adenocarcinoma often has prominent cytological pleomorphism, nested morphology, and lack acinar differentiation. A panel of PSA, PSMA, HMWCK 903, p63, and thrombomodulin is helpful and typically required in this differential.

Secondary involvement by colonic adenocarcinoma. Presence of more typical ductal and/or acinar morphology, along with an immunohistochemical panel of PSA, PSMA, β-catenin, CDX-2, and villin can be helpful. Colorectal tumors often demonstrate luminal dirty necrosis and are negative for PSA and PSMA, whereas often positive for B-catenin, CDX-2, and villin.

In needle biopsies, large gland, papillary, or PIN-like morphology of ductal carcinoma is often confused for HGPIN (*see* Fig. 6.6b). Presence of numerous crowded glands, confluence, and true fibrovascular cores or necrosis are helpful to separate from PIN. Basal cell markers also may help in this differentiation, but lack of basal cell staining in small focus does not rule out HGPIN diagnosis. Definitive distinction may not be feasible in small needle biopsy samples, and possibility of ductal carcinoma should be raised.

Centrally located tumors in small biopsy samples may mimic prostatic urethral polyp. Prostatic urethral polyps are polypoid nodules consisting entirely of benign-appearing prostatic acini lined by prostatic glandular epithelium and urothelium.

Gleason grading and clinical significance

Ductal adenocarcinomas are more aggressive than acinar carcinoma, present at more advanced stages (non-organ-confined disease), and are now regarded as Gleason pattern 4 or pattern 5 with necrosis

Known previously as endometrial or endometrioid carcinoma of the prostate, this tumor is currently recognized as a variant of acinar prostate adenocarcinoma

Pure ductal adenocarcinoma is rare (1.3%); majority has mixed ductal and acinar morphology (incidence of ~5%)

Periurethral or centrally located tumor may manifest with urinary obstruction and hematuria

Ductal adenocarcinoma seen only in small transurethral biopsies may require transrectal ultrasound-guided prostate needle biopsy sampling to document true extent of disease, as this disease is usually associated with large volume tumor with frequent acinar adenocarcinoma component

6.7 Ductal Adenocarcinoma

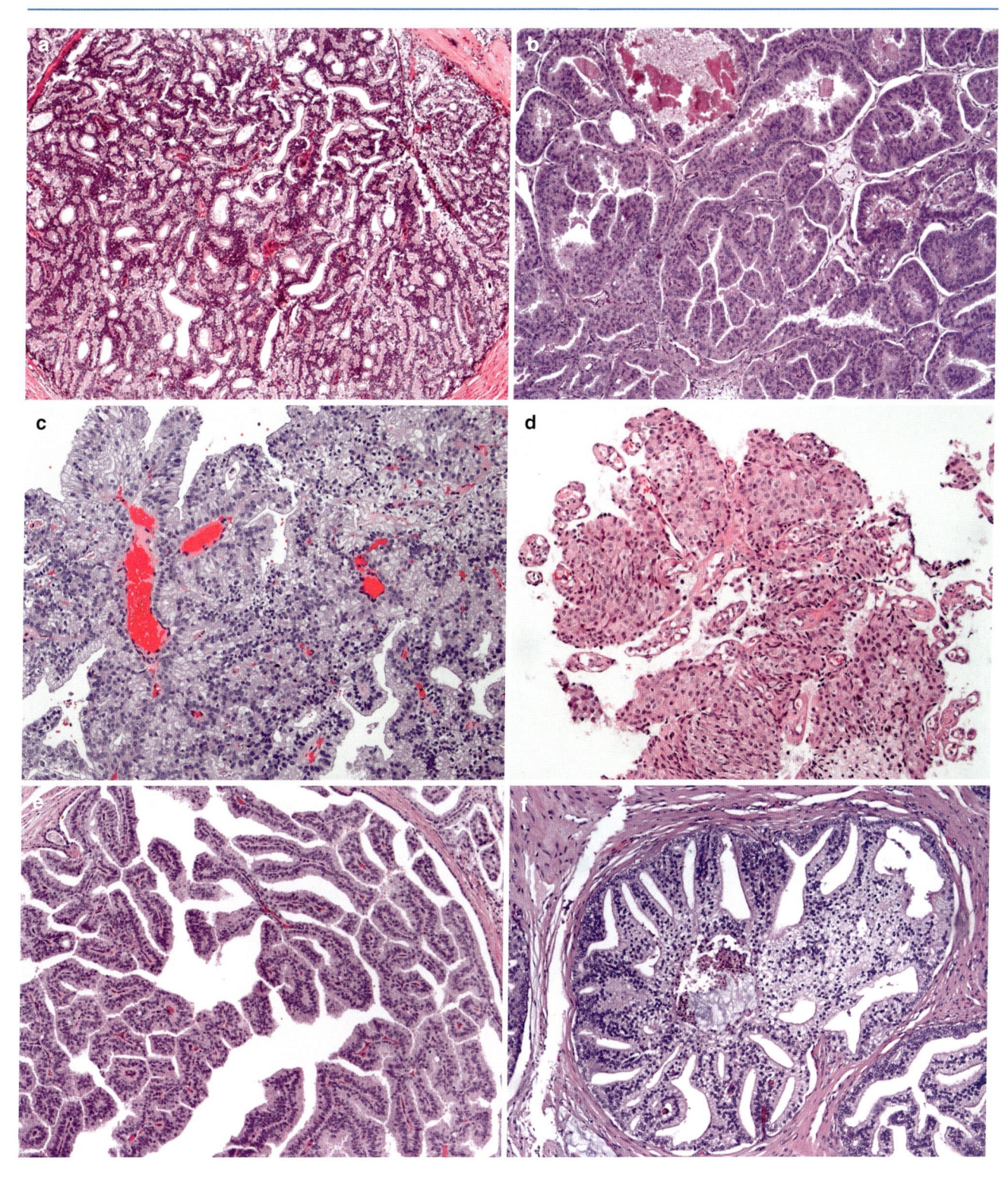

Fig. 6.6 Morphological spectrum of ductal prostate adenocarcinoma. (**a**) Large nodule of ductal adenocarcinoma showing endometrioid growth pattern with admixture of confluent cribriform and papillary patterns with irregular slit-like lumina and glands lined by tall columnar lining epithelium. (**b**) PIN-like ductal adenocarcinoma often has large well-formed glands lined by pseudostratified tall columnar cells, mimicking HGPIN. Large glandular architecture and tall columnar cell-lining distinguishes PIN-like ductal adenocarcinoma from conventional acinar cancer. Marked glandular crowding distinguishes it from HGPIN. Lack of basal cells by immunohistochemistry may further aid in difficult cases. In small needle biopsy cases, diagnosis may not be possible, and possibility of ductal carcinoma should be raised. (**c–d**) Ductal adenocarcinoma with papillary and solid-papillary growth patterns. Ductal adenocarcinoma often grows within the urethra as a papillary or polypoid mass. The tumor often has prominent papillary or solid architecture that is typically encountered in transurethral resection specimens where the distinction from urothelial carcinoma could be problematic. An immunohistochemical panel of p63, high-molecular weight cytokeratin (HMWCK) 903 (34βE12), PSA, PSMA, and thrombomodulin should be performed to rule out high-grade urothelial carcinoma [16]. (**e**) Ductal carcinoma often demonstrates intraductal spread. (**f**) Ductal adenocarcinoma is graded as pattern 4; cases with intraluminal necrosis (*shown*) or with solid architecture are graded as pattern 5

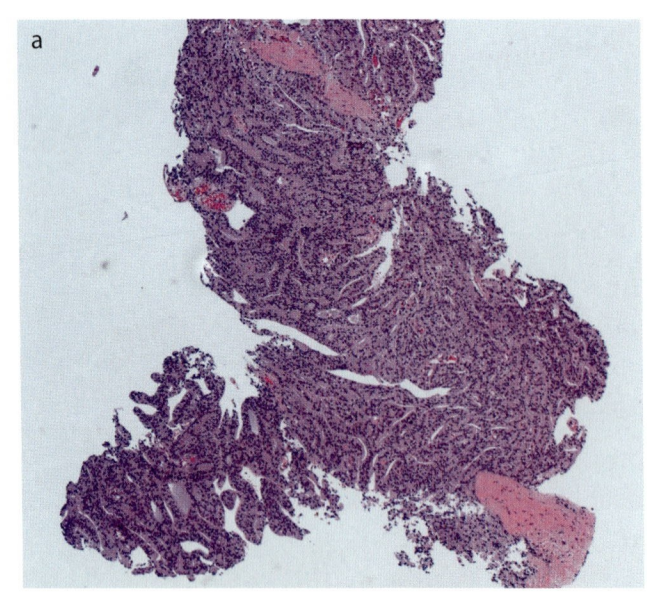

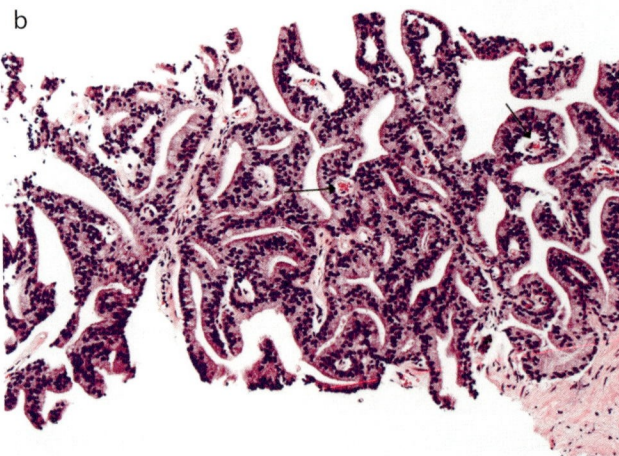

Fig. 6.7 Ductal carcinoma in needle biopsy often is fragmented. Note confluent proliferation of cribriform glands (**a**) with slit-like lumina and pseudostratified tall columnar epithelium (**b**). Also note the presence of fibrovascular cores in some glands suggesting a papillary architecture (*arrow*, **b**)

6.8 Mucinous (Colloid) Carcinoma

Table 6.8 Mucinous (colloid) carcinoma [2, 17–20]

Microscopical features

Low-power architecture

Tumor cells floating within the mucin pool sharply demarcated from the stroma (*see* Fig. 6.8); mucin accounts for >25% of the tumor volume

Tumor cells are arranged in cribriform configurations, individual acinar architecture, tubules, cords, or strands

Collagenous micronodules representing hyalinization of extravasated mucin, one of three specific features of prostate cancer (*see* Fig. 6.8d)

High-power cytology

Tumor cells are often monotonous, bland-looking, with frequent prominent nucleoli

Immunohistochemical and molecular features

Identical to conventional acinar prostate cancer: positive for PSA and PSAP; negative for basal cell markers. AMACR is variably expressed

Highest frequency of *ETS* gene fusions (~80%) in this morphologic subtype [1]

Differential diagnosis

Diagnosis of mucinous carcinoma is restricted to tumors showing ≥25% of the tumor with lakes of extracellular mucin

Prostate carcinoma with <25% mucinous component should be classified as having mucinous features, whereas prostate acinar carcinoma demonstrating intraluminal prominent mucin is not considered colloid carcinoma

Colloid carcinoma of the prostate mimics colorectal colloid carcinoma in small biopsy samples (*see* Fig. 6.8a–c). PSA, PSAP, and PSMA positivity suggest the prostate origin. Presence of conventional acinar cancer is a helpful feature. CDX-2 marker not entirely reliable in the differential diagnosis, as prostate carcinoma may express CDX-2 [21]

Gleason grading and clinical significance

Gleason grading should be based on overall architecture of the tumor, ignoring mucinous differentiation (*see* Fig. 6.8d)

Pure colloid carcinoma are rare; the majority demonstrate concomitant conventional acinar carcinoma

Average age at presentation similar to conventional acinar adenocarcinoma

The clinical stage of mucinous carcinoma is often advanced, with locally advanced or metastatic disease

6.8 Mucinous (Colloid) Carcinoma

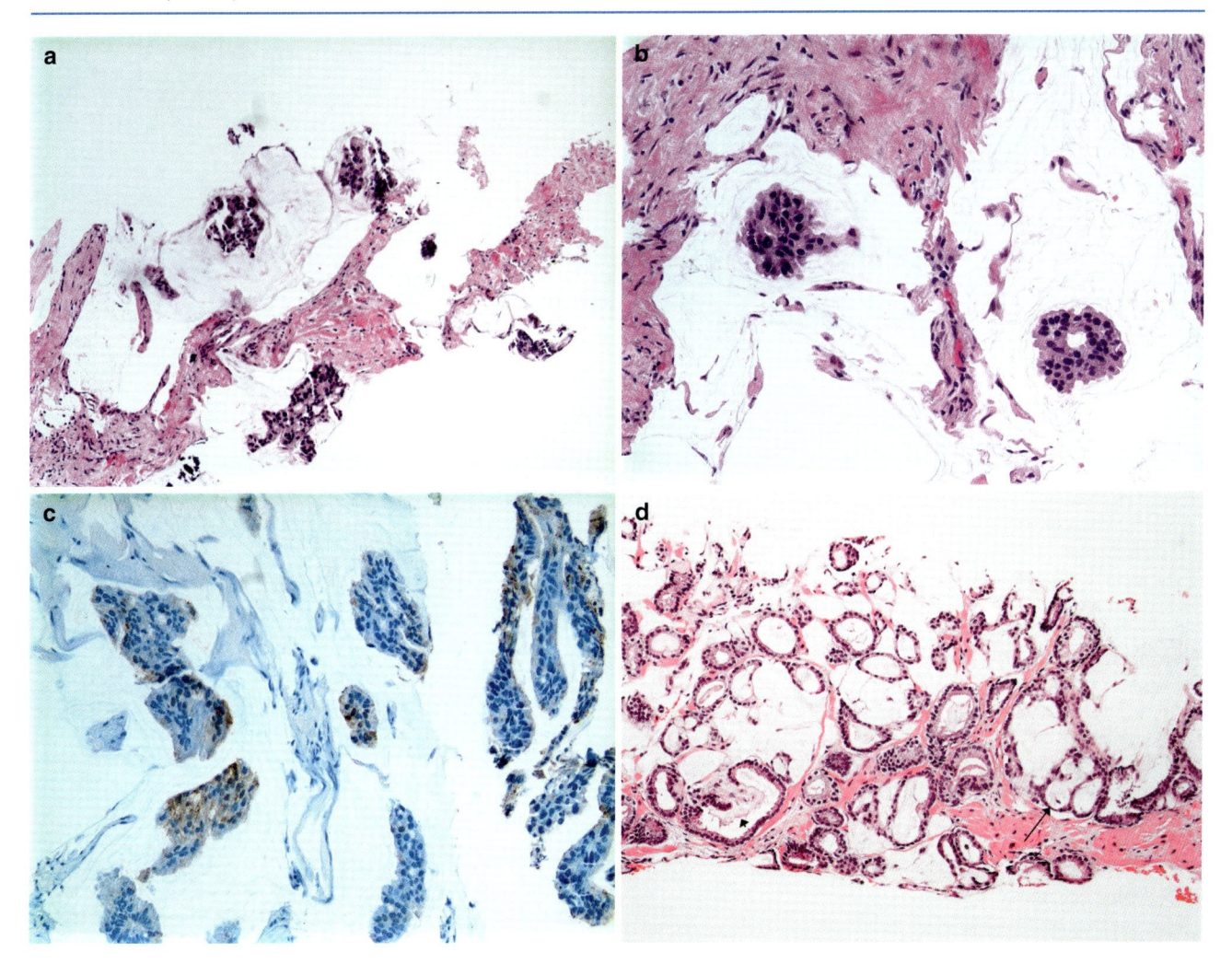

Fig. 6.8 Mucinous (colloid) carcinoma. (**a–d**) Cancer cells float in lakes of extracellular mucin (**a**) and are arranged in acini and cribriform growth pattern. This is distinct from the intraluminal mucin seen in conventional prostate acinar carcinoma. Cytologically, they usually appear bland (**b**). When this finding is seen exclusively in biopsy without a component of acinar carcinoma, immunohistochemical staining for prostate markers should be utilized to rule out colorectal primary. Tumor cells in this case demonstrated strong PSA reactivity supporting the diagnosis of primary prostate cancer (**c**). Example of prostate carcinoma with mucinous features demonstrating well-formed discrete glands with occasional cribriform gland (*arrow*), floating within the mucin pool. Also note the presence of intraluminal collagenous nodule in some glands (*arrowheads*), which is common in this variant morphology. Previously, all colloid carcinomas were designated as aggressive Gleason pattern 4+4=8 carcinoma but recent data suggest that they are not uniformly aggressive and grade should be applied based on the underlying architecture (3+4=7 in **d**)

6.9 Small Cell Neuroendocrine Carcinoma

Table 6.9 Small cell neuroendocrine (NE) carcinoma [2, 22–35]

Microscopical features

Low-power architecture

Relatively uniform population of small-to-intermediate-sized blue cells with scant cytoplasm and hyperchromatic nuclei arranged in diffuse sheets or broad organoid nests (*see* Fig. 6.9b–c)

Small cell component may be intimately mixed with acinar component

High-power cytology

Nuclei demonstrate molding, fine, powdery chromatin, and inconspicuous nucleoli

Apoptotic bodies and mitoses are numerous

Necrosis is usually conspicuous

Immunohistochemical and molecular features

Cancer cells positive for one or more NE markers, including synaptophysin, chromogranin A, and CD56. CD56 is the most sensitive marker

Evidence of hormone production, including adrenocorticotropic hormone, calcitonin, serotonin, and antidiuretic hormone, can be demonstrated by immunostaining

PSA and PSAP are typically negative (~80%) or very focal positive in the small cell component

~20–30% cases demonstrate expression of basal cell markers p63 and CK 903

TTF1 expression may be positive; therefore, does not discriminate between a small cell carcinoma arising in the prostate and metastasis from the lung

Higher frequency of *ETS* gene fusions predominately (~70%) through interstitial deletion mechanism [1]

Differential diagnosis

Poorly differentiated prostate adenocarcinoma; small cell carcinoma from other sites; other blue cell tumors (lymphoma, primitive neuroectodermal tumor [PNET], and rhabdomyosarcoma); and rarely primary carcinoid tumor

Careful analysis of patient's age, clinical findings, morphology, and a panel of immunohistochemical markers usually leads to a definitive diagnosis (*see* Fig. 6.11)

Gleason grading and clinical significance

Small cell carcinoma should not be graded

The prognostic significance of neuroendocrine differentiation (presence of cytoplasmic neuroendocrine granules or cells positive for neuroendocrine markers; *see* Fig. 6.9a) in an ordinary acinar prostate carcinoma is uncertain and usually inconsequential

The clinical outcome for both pure small cell carcinoma and mixed small cell and acinar forms is extremely poor

The emergence of a small cell component during the course of acinar prostate carcinoma signals an aggressive terminal phase of the disease. The average median survival time after the diagnosis is 7–17 months.

Treatment typically consists of platinum-based chemotherapy

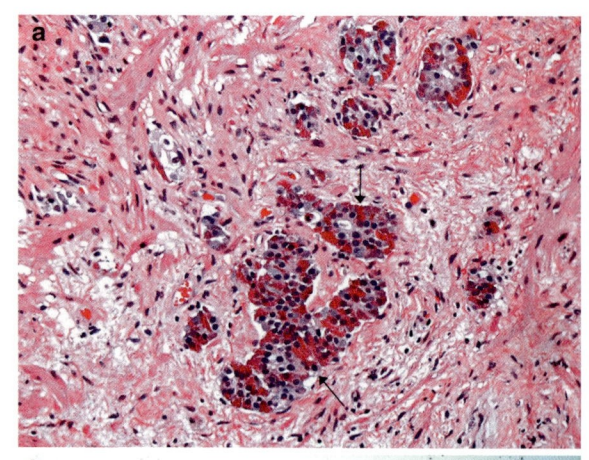

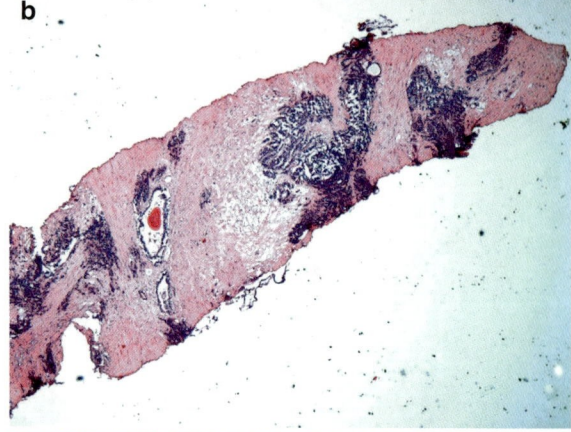

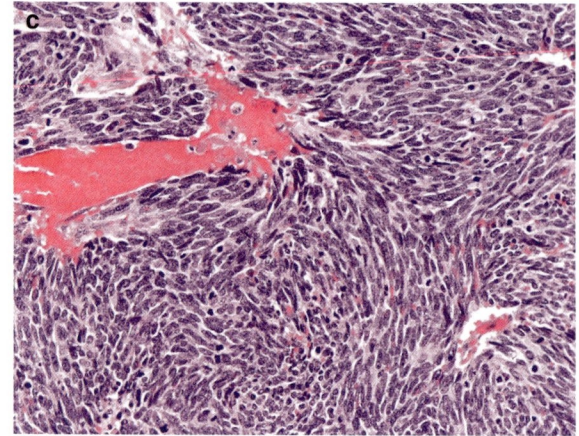

Fig. 6.9 Spectrum of NE differentiation in prostate adenocarcinoma. (**a**) Conventional prostate adenocarcinoma demonstrates Paneth cell–like differentiation, characterized by occasional cells with bright eosinophilic cytoplasmic granules resembling Paneth cells (*arrows*) of the gastrointestinal tract. The significance of such NE differentiation is controversial but overall data do not indicate an adverse prognosis [31–34]. (**b**) Small cell carcinoma involving the prostate shows basophilic tumor cells arranged in haphazard nests and trabeculae with infiltration between benign glands. (**c**) At higher magnification, small cell carcinoma of the prostate is identical to its pulmonary counterpart with scant cytoplasm, spindling of nuclei with salt-and-pepper chromatin, indistinct nucleoli, increased mitosis, and apoptosis. Presence of acinar differentiation is a very useful feature to suggest the prostate origin. Small cell carcinoma, regardless of its amount in prostate biopsy, should be reported due to its prognostic and therapeutic significance

6.9 Small Cell Neuroendocrine Carcinoma

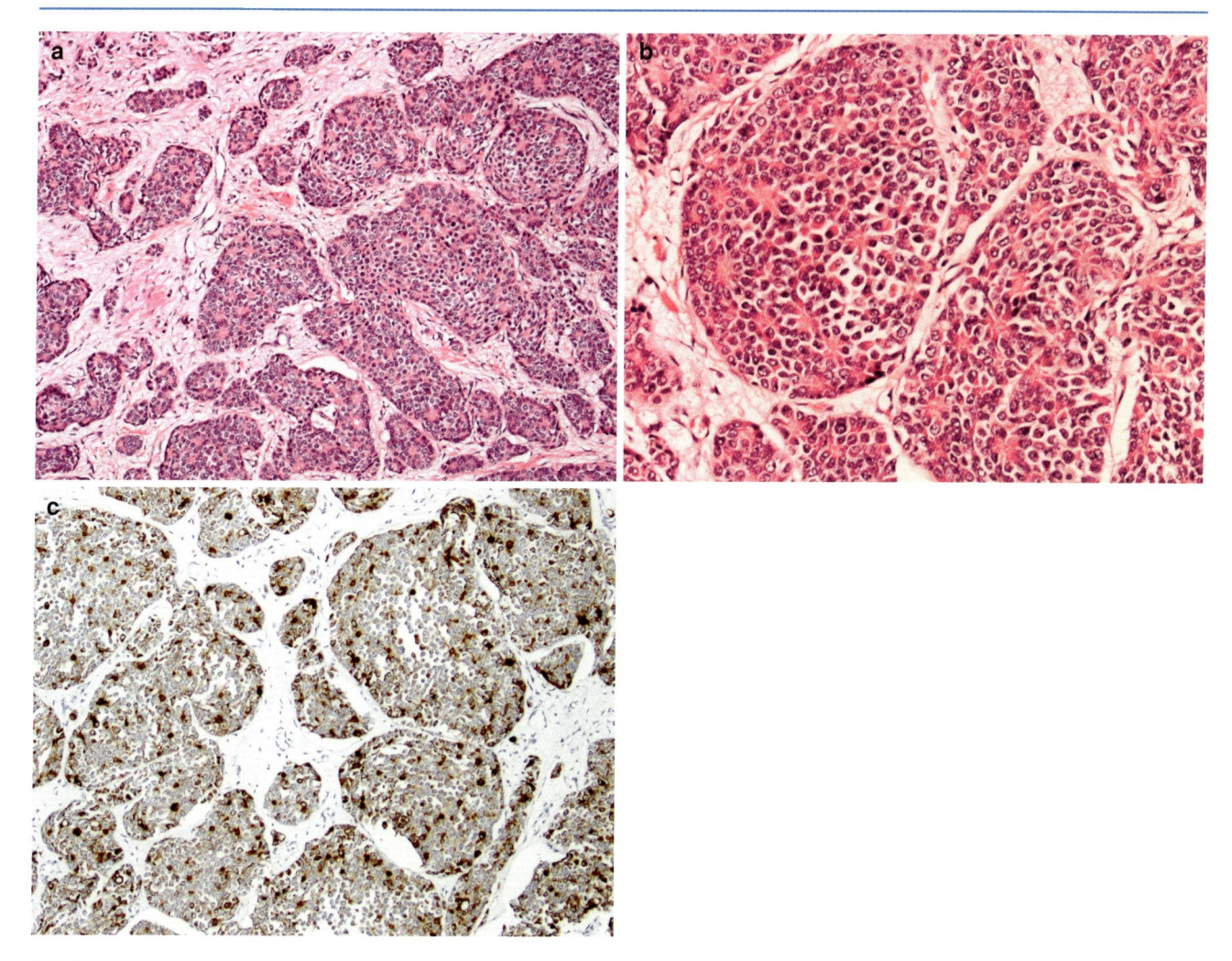

Fig. 6.10 (**a–c**) Carcinoid-like differentiation in acinar prostate adenocarcinoma [36]. Prostate adenocarcinoma is occasionally composed of uniform cells forming acini and organoid nests that superficially resemble carcinoid tumor (**a**). Cells may occasionally express NE markers. But note here that nuclear features are more typical of prostatic adenocarcinoma, with open chromatin and nucleolar prominence, rather than the granular chromatin and inconspicuous nucleoli of a carcinoid tumor (**b**). Lack of diffuse NE marker reactivity (*not shown*) and strong reactivity for PSA (**c**) suggest that this is not a true carcinoid tumor but an unusual carcinoid-like morphology of prostate adenocarcinoma (**c**)

6.10 Approach to Neuroendocrine Differentiation in Prostate Cancer

Approach to neuroendocrine differentiation in prostate cancer

- Conventional acinar prostate cancer with Paneth cell-like change
  → A form of focal NE differentiation
  → Prognostic significance controversial; overall no significance; do not need to report; grade and treat as a conventional acinar prostate cancer

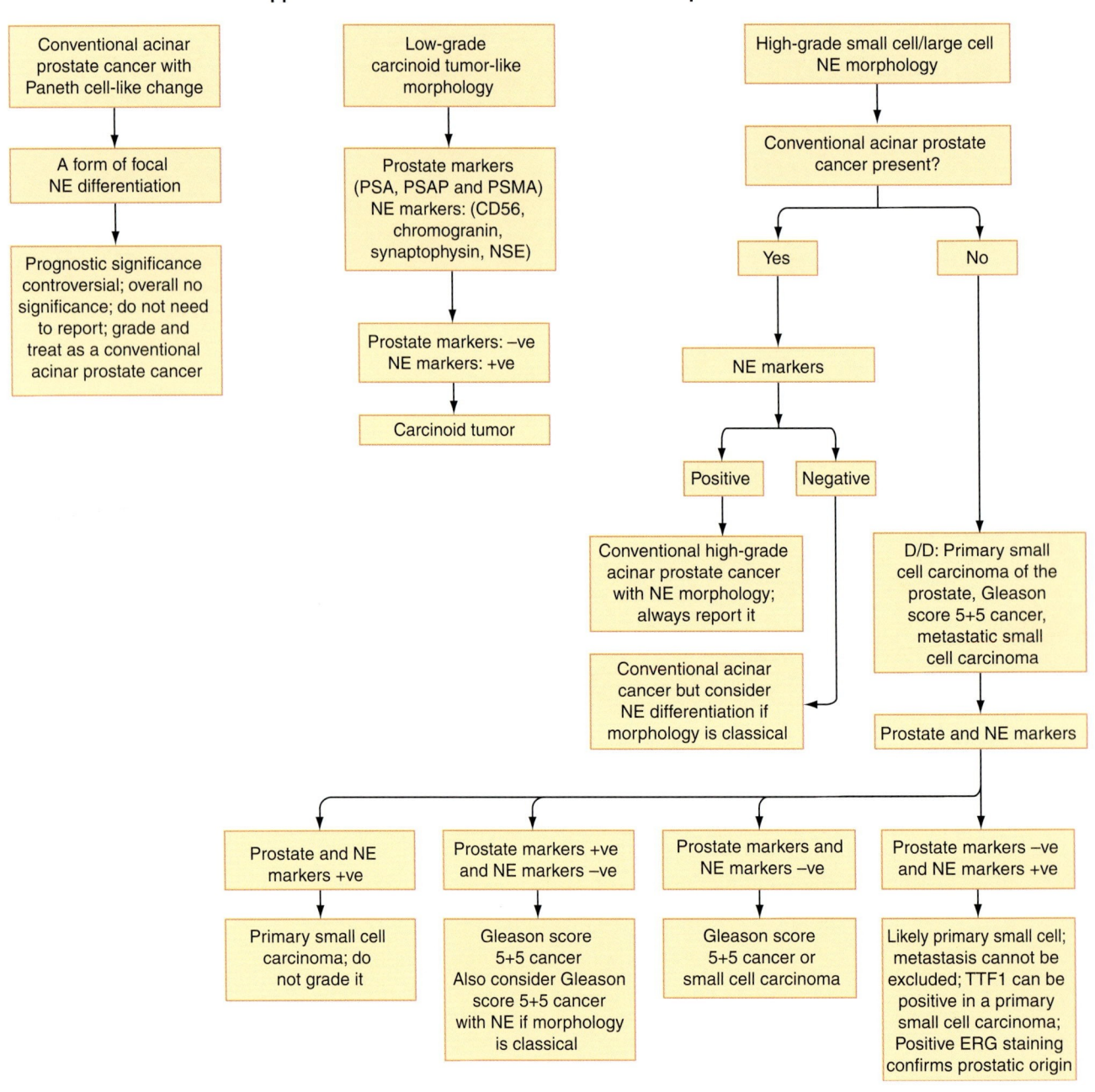

- Low-grade carcinoid tumor-like morphology
  → Prostate markers (PSA, PSAP and PSMA) NE markers: (CD56, chromogranin, synaptophysin, NSE)
  → Prostate markers: –ve NE markers: +ve
  → Carcinoid tumor

- High-grade small cell/large cell NE morphology
  → Conventional acinar prostate cancer present?
    - Yes → NE markers
      - Positive → Conventional high-grade acinar prostate cancer with NE morphology; always report it
      - Negative → Conventional acinar cancer but consider NE differentiation if morphology is classical
    - No → D/D: Primary small cell carcinoma of the prostate, Gleason score 5+5 cancer, metastatic small cell carcinoma
      → Prostate and NE markers
        - Prostate and NE markers +ve → Primary small cell carcinoma; do not grade it
        - Prostate markers +ve and NE markers –ve → Gleason score 5+5 cancer Also consider Gleason score 5+5 cancer with NE if morphology is classical
        - Prostate markers and NE markers –ve → Gleason score 5+5 cancer or small cell carcinoma
        - Prostate markers –ve and NE markers +ve → Likely primary small cell; metastasis cannot be excluded; TTF1 can be positive in a primary small cell carcinoma; Positive ERG staining confirms prostatic origin

Fig. 6.11 Approach to differential diagnosis of NE differentiation in prostate cancer. *D/D* differential diagnosis NE Neuroendocrine differentiation

6.11 Sarcomatoid Carcinoma (Carcinosarcoma)

Table 6.10 Sarcomatoid carcinoma (carcinosarcoma) [37–41]

Microscopical features

Low-power architecture

Usually a biphasic tumor, with epithelial/glandular component showing variable Gleason patterns or epithelial differentiation and sarcomatoid component often exhibiting nondescript malignant spindle cell proliferation (*see* Fig. 6.12)

In some cases, pure mesenchymal differentiation may be present

Heterologous mesenchymal differentiation can also be present, including osteosarcoma, leiomyosarcoma, chondrosarcoma, and rhabdomyosarcoma

High-power cytology

Marked nuclear crowding, nuclear pleomorphism, atypical mitoses, and necrosis are commonly present

Immunohistochemical features

The epithelial elements are variably positive for PSA and/or pancytokeratins, whereas the sarcomatoid elements react with markers of corresponding mesenchymal differentiation and variably express cytokeratins, and PSA is frequently undetectable

Broad-spectrum cytokeratins including HMWCK should be used

Aberrant reactivity for keratins can occur in some leiomyosarcomas, this finding alone is usually insufficient to identify a tumor as of epithelial origin (*see* Fig. 11.5). A panel of keratins and mesenchymal markers should be utilized

Differential diagnosis (*see* Fig. 11.7)

Tumors of specialized prostatic stroma, primary sarcoma, and sarcomatoid carcinoma of the urinary bladder

History of previous prostate cancer and treatment, presence of variable epithelial differentiation, and immunohistochemistry help in the differential diagnosis

Differentiation from primary sarcoma can be especially difficult but is often clinically unimportant

Gleason grading and clinical significance

Sarcomatoid carcinoma should not be graded

Patients tend to be older men who often present with symptoms of urinary obstruction

Sarcomatoid carcinoma may be a de novo diagnosis but patients usually have a previous history of prostate carcinoma treated with radiation and/or hormonal therapy

Serum PSA can be normal or undetectable, despite the frequent presence of nodal and distant metastases

The 5-year survival rate is less than 40%

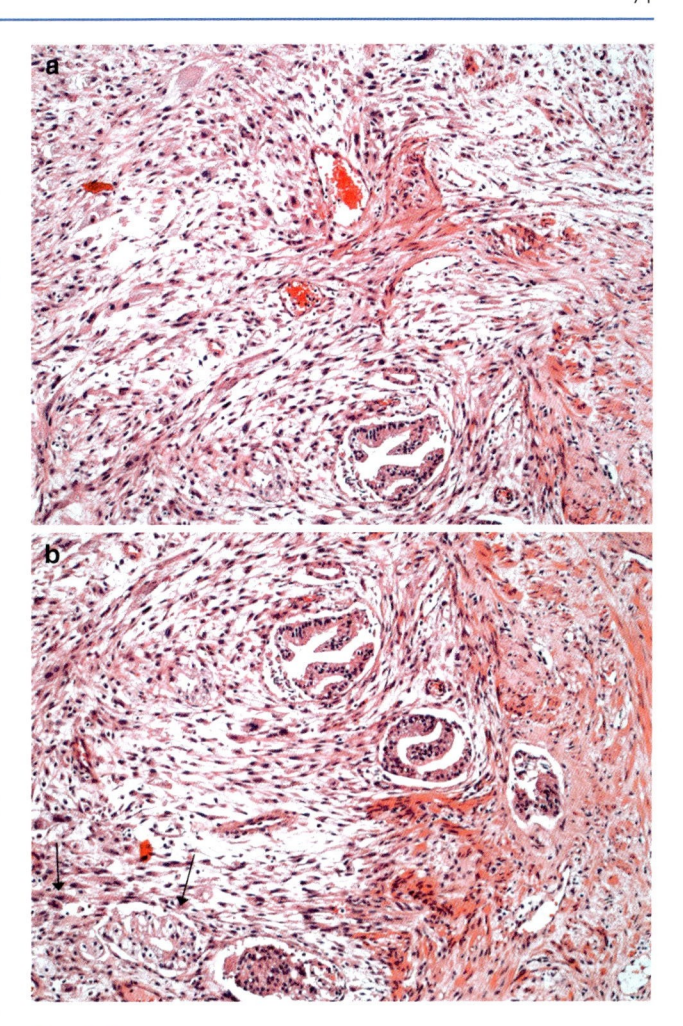

Fig. 6.12 Sarcomatoid carcinoma (carcinosarcoma). Sarcomatoid carcinoma has high-grade undifferentiated spindle cell sarcoma with a myxoid background (**a**). Acinar carcinoma is present (*arrow*) and is intimately admixed with the sarcomaotid component (**b**). In contrast to prostate stromal sarcoma, epithelial component in sarcomatoid carcinoma is malignant. Extensive sampling is usually required to document the presence of the epithelial component. History of previous prostate carcinoma is also very useful to diagnose a sarcomatoid carcinoma and rule out primary sarcoma

6.12 Urothelial Carcinoma

Table 6.11 Urothelial carcinoma [16, 42–48]

Microscopical features

Low-power architecture

Urothelial carcinoma involving the prostate is of two types:

1. The most common form is bladder urothelial carcinoma spreading into and expanding the preexisting prostate ducts and acini (*see* Fig. 6.13a–b)

Prostatic stroma invasion is characterized by small, irregular nests, cords, or single cells with stromal retraction or desmoplastic and inflamed stroma (*see* Fig. 6.13c)

2. Rarely, urothelial carcinoma arises within the prostate without concomitant bladder carcinoma

High-power cytology

Nuclei are high grade and pleomorphic with frequent central necrosis

Squamous and/or glandular differentiation may be present

Immunohistochemical features

Prostate urothelial carcinoma cells are negative for prostate-specific markers

Majority express CK7, CK20, basal cell markers p63 and HMWCK, and thrombomodulin

Differential diagnosis

Urothelial carcinoma involving prostatic ducts and acini often mimic intraductal spread of high-grade prostate adenocarcinoma or invasive, poorly differentiated prostate adenocarcinoma (*see* Fig. 8.3)

Presence of conventional acinar differentiation suggests prostate adenocarcinoma

Prostate adenocarcinoma often has relatively monotonous cytological atypia

A panel of PSA, PSMA, basal cell markers HMWCK K903 and p63, and thrombomodulin can be used for this differential diagnosis

Urothelial carcinomas are variably positive for basal cell markers and negative for prostate-specific markers. Preexisting peripheral basal cells may also be highlighted by basal cell markers

Urothelial metaplasia typically do not fill and expand the ducts and are characterized by cytologically benign urothelial cells

Clinical significance

Primary prostate urothelial carcinoma is rare, with the majority representing secondary involvement by urothelial carcinoma cells from the bladder or urethra

Biopsies of bladder should be performed to rule out primary bladder disease

Prostate involvement, with stromal invasion, indicates stage IV disease with significantly worse prognosis: 5-year survival 45% versus 100% urothelial carcinoma in situ after cystoprostatectomy

Differentiation from prostate adenocarcinoma is crucial as these tumors do not respond to androgen deprivation therapy and should be treated by radical cystoprostatectomy with lymph node dissection

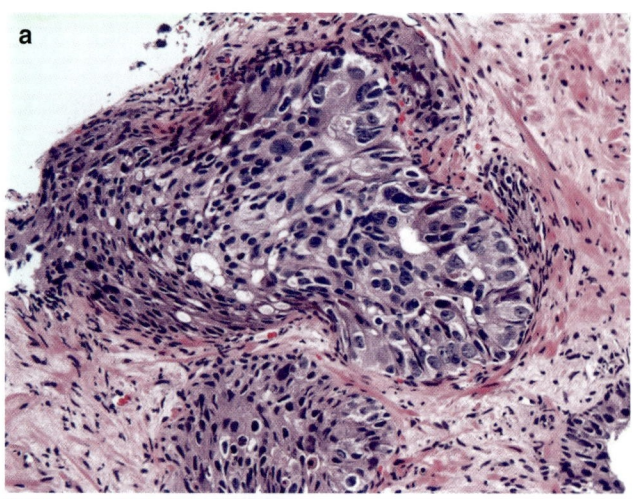

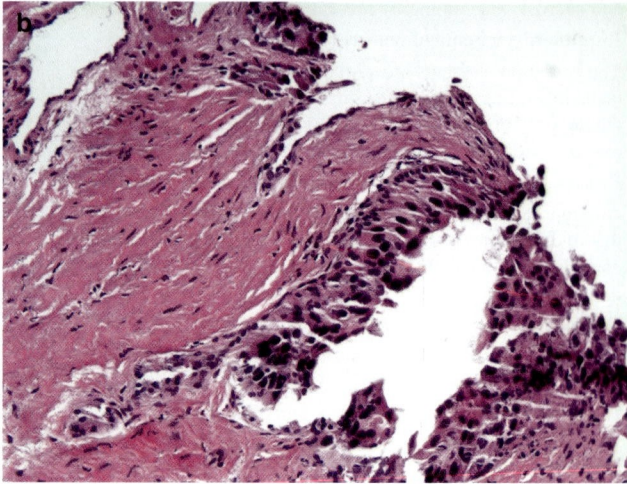

Fig. 6.13 High-grade urothelial carcinoma involving the prostate. (**a–d**) In urothelial carcinoma of the prostate, preexisting acini/ducts are expanded by high-grade pleomorphic cells without evidence of stromal invasion (**a**). At higher magnification, cytological pleomorphism of tumor cells and scattered peripheral basal cells are visible (**b**). This presentation mimics intraductal spread of high-grade prostate cancer. Stromal invasion is characterized by small irregular nests or single cells with stromal retraction artifacts and desmoplastic stroma (**c**). Invasion of stroma should be recognized using strict criteria as it indicates stage IV disease. Strong reactivity for p63 in tumor cells supports the diagnosis of urothelial carcinoma; benign prostate glands demonstrate a peripheral layer of basal cells (**d**)

6.13 Squamous and Adenosquamous Cell Carcinoma

Table 6.12 Squamous and adenosquamous cell carcinoma (SCC) [49–52]

Microscopical features

Low-power architecture

Identical to SCC of other anatomic sites

Pure SCC does not contain any malignant glandular component

Adenosquamous carcinoma harbors both malignant glandular and squamous components that can be distinct or exhibit direct transition from one pattern to another

High-power cytology

Depending on the degree of squamous differentiation, variable degree of keratin pearls or cytoplasmic keratinization is present

Immunohistochemical features

The malignant squamous component is in most cases negative for PSA and PSAP but positive for HMWCK and p63

Malignant glandular component variably expresses PSA and PSAP

Differential diagnosis

Prostate carcinoma after radiation or hormonal ablation treatment may exhibit prominent squamous differentiation, but the conventional acinar component is usually present

SCC should be differentiated from squamous metaplasia secondary to prostate infarcts or hormonal and radiation therapy (*see* Fig. 6.15). Squamous metaplasia adjacent to infarcts may demonstrate atypia but is associated with inflammation are reactive in nature

Radiation-induced atypia is degenerative in nature and the process is not infiltrative, and lacks the architecture disarray, destructive stromal reaction, and neoplastic nuclear atypia seen in the squamous or adenosquamous cell carcinoma

Secondary involvement of the prostate by a carcinoma with squamous differentiation from the bladder or other sites should be ruled out on clinical grounds

Gleason grading and clinical significance

SCC and adenosquamous carcinoma should not be graded

SCC account for less than 0.5% of all prostate cancers

An association between schistosomiasis and SCC of the bladder and prostate has been documented

Adenosquamous carcinoma is even rarer and may arise in patients with prostrate carcinoma after hormonal and radiation therapy

Squamous and adenosquamous carcinoma without such predisposing factors have been also documented

Clinically, patients present with symptoms of advanced stage prostate carcinoma, including urinary obstruction, hematuria, bone pain, and markedly abnormal digital rectal examination. The PSA level is usually normal

Prostate squamous and adenosquamous cell carcinoma are extremely aggressive diseases and are resistant to androgen deprivation, radiation therapy, and chemotherapy

In rare cases of organ-confined disease, patients may benefit from locally aggressive radical surgery

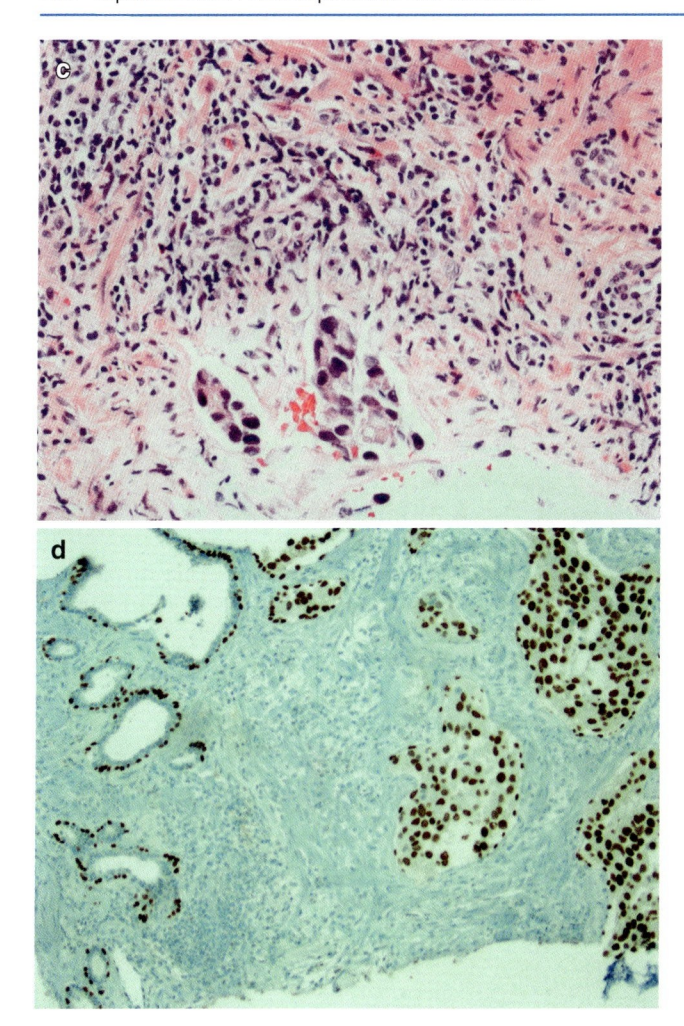

Fig. 6.13 (continued)

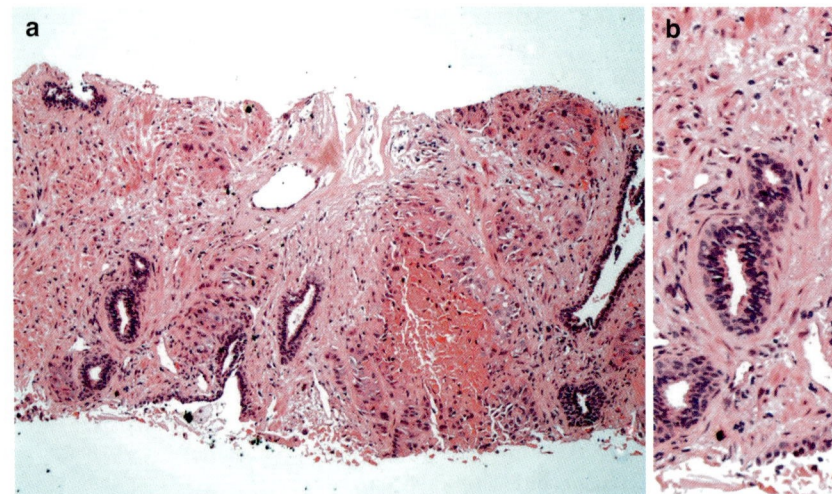

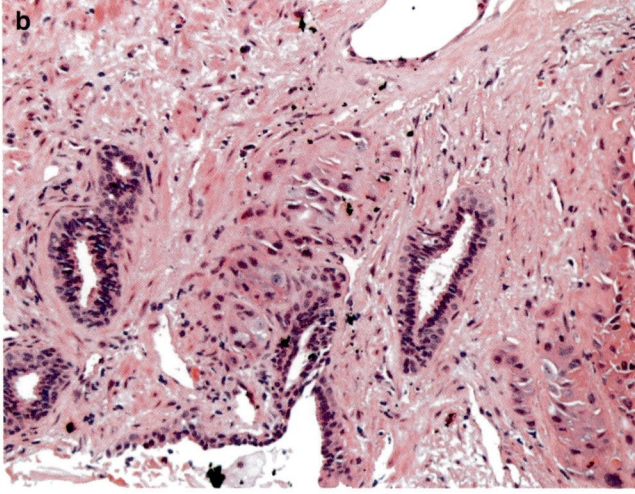

Fig. 6.14 Squamous cell carcinoma of the prostate. Pure SCC of the prostate, consisting of infiltrating nests of partially necrotic malignant cells between benign glands and a desmoplastic stroma (**a**). At higher magnification, evidence of squamous differentiation in the form of cytoplasmic eosinophilia is noted in some cells (**b**). Before a diagnosis of pure SCC is considered, extensive sampling is required to rule out a conventional prostate carcinoma or urothelial carcinoma. Lack of history of previous prostate cancer may also help establish the diagnosis of pure SCC

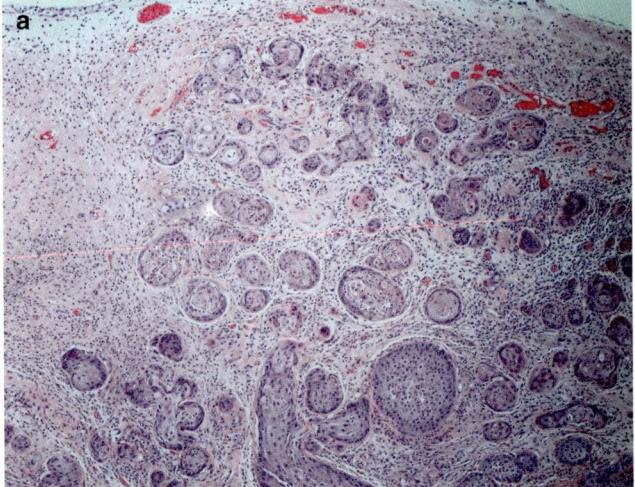

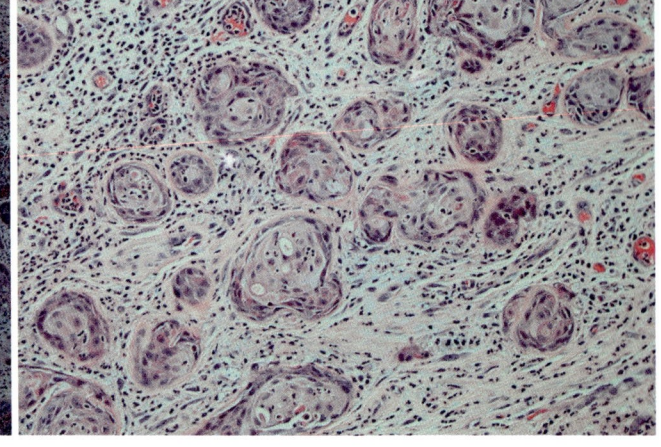

Fig. 6.15 Necrotizing squamous metaplasia of prostate, mimicking SCC. This transurethral resection of the prostate after ablative therapy shows necrotizing squamous metaplasia within the hyperplastic prostate glands mimicking SCC. At low power, lobulated appearance of the lesion (**a**) and, at high power (**b**), lack of definitive infiltrative features suggest the diagnosis of squamous metaplasia. Knowledge of previous therapy is also helpful in difficult cases

6.14 Signet Ring Cell Carcinoma

Table 6.13 Signet ring cell carcinoma [2, 53]

Microscopical features

Low-power architecture

Poorly differentiated tumor grows in sheets, small clusters, and as single cells (*see* Fig. 6.16)

Frequently admixed with ordinary acinar carcinoma

High-power cytology

Tumor cells demonstrate signet ring cell–like features, characterized by nuclear displacement and indentation by clear cytoplasmic vacuoles

The vacuoles does not contain mucin

The signet ring cell component should be ≥25% of the tumor mass to be considered as a signet ring variant

Immunohistochemical features

Variably positive for prostate-specific markers PSA and PSMA

Negative stains for CK7, CK20, HMWCK, and mucin

Differential diagnosis

Before establishing a diagnosis of prostate signet ring carcinoma, a metastasis from other anatomic sites, including stomach, lung, colon, and pancreaticobiliary system should be excluded

On the other hand, prostatic origin signet ring cell carcinoma should be considered when signet ring cell carcinoma of unknown primary is encountered, especially if mucin stains are negative

Pseudo signet ring features may be seen in lymphocytes, and focally within other benign mimics, sclerosing adenosis, and nephrogenic metaplasia

Gleason grading and clinical significance

Graded as Gleason pattern 5

The signet ring cell carcinoma is a rare histologic variant of prostate carcinoma with an aggressive clinical outcome

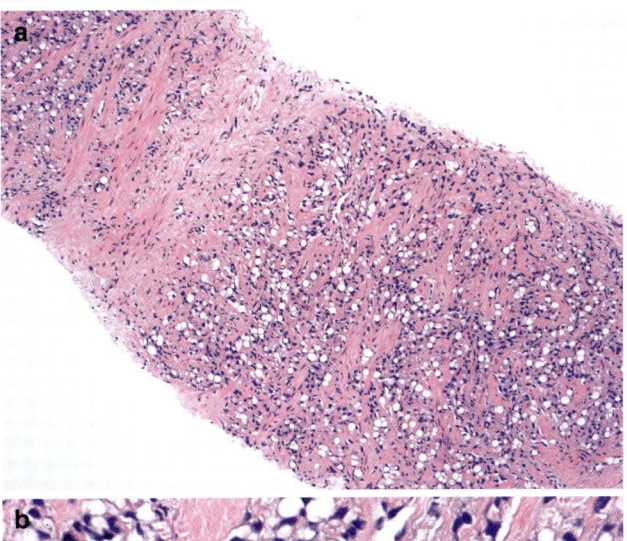

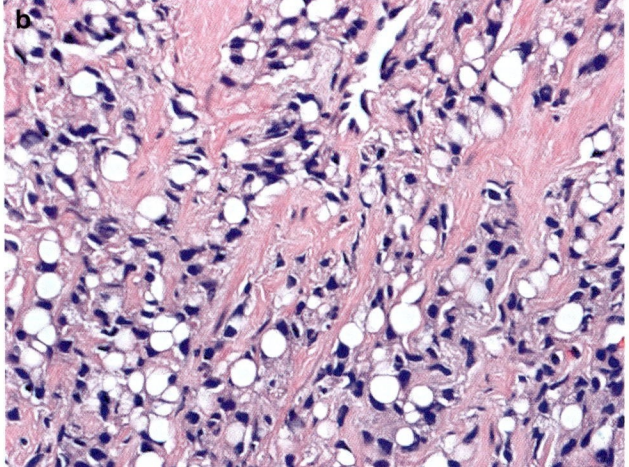

Fig. 6.16 Signet ring cell prostate carcinoma is composed of sheets of infiltrative discohesive cells with cytoplasmic vacuoles displacing the nuclei peripherally (**a**). At higher magnification, vacuoles are optically clear and cytological atypia is present (**b**). In most cases, the cytoplasmic vacuoles lack staining for mucin. The signet ring cell carcinoma is graded as Gleason pattern 5. Presence of vacuoles in cancer glands should not be viewed as signet ring cell differentiation and grading should be based on underlying architecture

6.15 Adenoid Cystic Basal Cell Carcinoma

Table 6.14 Adenoid cystic basal cell carcinoma (BCC) [54–58]

Microscopical features

Low-power architecture

Infiltrating nests, cords, trabeculae, and sheets or cribriform proliferation of basaloid cells that may exhibit peripheral palisading (*see* Fig. 6.17)

May demonstrate prominent luminal formation with cribriform architecture similar to "adenoid cystic carcinoma" of salivary glands

Infiltrative growth pattern is often characterized by desmoplastic stroma, invasion into preexisting structures, extraprostatic extension, perineural invasion, and tumor necrosis may be present

High-power cytology

Nuclear features are similar to basal cell hyperplasia characterized by high N:C ratio, hyperchromatic ovoid coffee bean-type nuclei, and nuclear stratification

Immunohistochemical features

BCC is positive for basal cell markers p63 and HMWCK 903

Prostate-specific markers PSA, PSAP, and PSMA are negative

High Ki-67 proliferative activity (>20%) compared to adenoid cystic basal cell hyperplasia (<5%)

Differential diagnosis

Differentiation from basal cell hyperplasia depends on identifying unequivocal features of malignancy, including infiltrative growth pattern, stromal desmoplasia, perineural and lymphovascular invasion, necrosis, and extraprostatic extension. Immunohistochemical features are not reliable in this separation

Prostate adenocarcinoma may rarely demonstrate basaloid features characterized by diffuse p63 positivity, but tumor is typically negative for HMWCK and positive for PSA

Extension of anal basaloid carcinoma and adenoid cystic carcinoma of the Cowper's glands should also be excluded. The distinction relies on history and determining the epicenter of the tumor

Clinical significance

BCC of the prostate is extremely rare and often manifests with symptoms of urinary obstruction

Serum PSA is often not elevated

The clinical outcome of BCC is uncertain due to insufficient data, although tumors usually present with locally advanced disease including extraprostatic extension. Distant metastasis has been reported

High Ki-67 staining in BCC is correlated with tumor aggressiveness

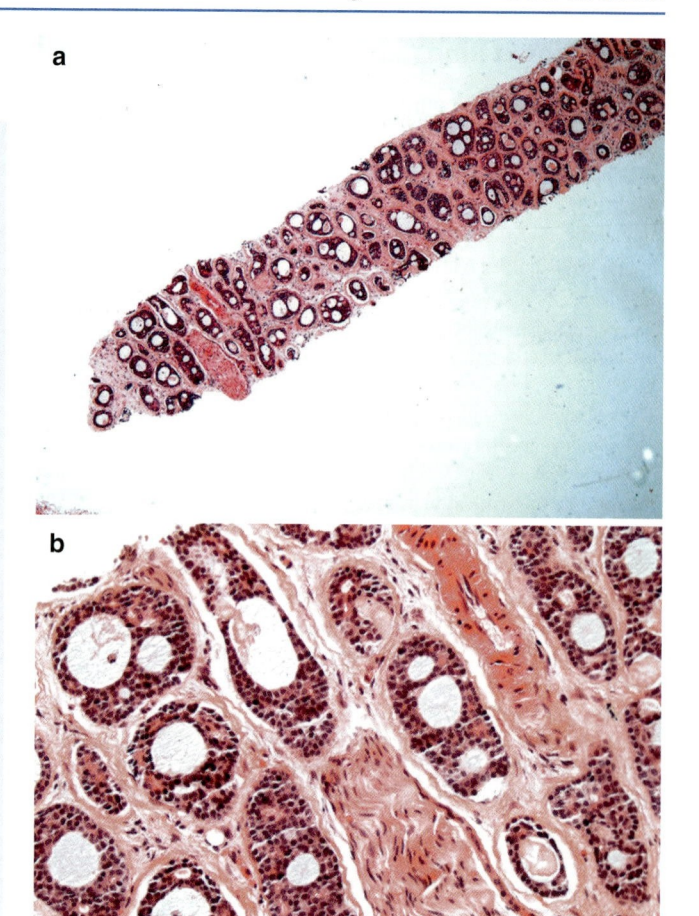

Fig. 6.17 Adenoid cystic BCC. (**a**, **b**) Adenoid cystic BCC with a solid and cribriform architecture, mimicking basal cell hyperplasia (**a**). The distinction from basal cell hyperplasia is especially difficult in needle biopsy samples, as cells can be relatively bland and infiltrative features may not be easily appreciated. In contrast to basal cell hyperplasia, tumor cells in BCC are dense, haphazardly arranged with infiltrative features characterized by edematous desmoplastic stroma, destruction of smooth muscle, and perineural invasion (**b**). Infiltrative growth is the hallmark of BCC and is required to differentiate from florid basal cell hyperplasia

References

1. Han B, Mehra R, Suleman K et al (2009) Characterization of ETS gene aberrations in select histologic variants of prostate carcinoma. Mod Pathol 22:1176–1185
2. Epstein JI, Allsbrook WC Jr, Amin MB et al (2005) The 2005 international society of urological pathology (ISUP) consensus conference on Gleason grading of prostatic carcinoma. Am J Surg Pathol 29:1228–1242
3. Nelson RS, Epstein JI (1996) Prostatic carcinoma with abundant xanthomatous cytoplasm. Foamy gland carcinoma. Am J Surg Pathol 20:419–426
4. Tran TT, Sengupta E, Yang XJ (2001) Prostatic foamy gland carcinoma with aggressive behavior: clinicopathologic, immunohistochemical, and ultrastructural analysis. Am J Surg Pathol 25:618–623
5. Zhou M, Jiang Z, Epstein JI (2003) Expression and diagnostic utility of alpha-methylacyl-CoA-racemase (P504S) in foamy gland and pseudohyperplastic prostate cancer. Am J Surg Pathol 27:772–778
6. Humphrey PA, Kaleem Z, Swanson PE, Vollmer RT (1998) Pseudohyperplastic prostatic adenocarcinoma. Am J Surg Pathol 22:1239–1246
7. Levi AW, Epstein JI (2000) Pseudohyperplastic prostatic adenocarcinoma on needle biopsy and simple prostatectomy. Am J Surg Pathol 24:1039–1046
8. Cina CJ, Epstein JI (1997) Adenocarcinoma of the prostate with atrophic features. Am J Surg Pathol 21:289–295
9. Egan AJ, Lopez-Beltran A, Bostwick DG (1997) Prostatic adenocarcinoma with atrophic features: malignancy mimicking a benign process. Am J Surg Pathol 21:931–935
10. Lotan TL, Epstein JI (2009) Gleason grading of prostatic adenocarcinoma with glomeruloid features on needle biopsy. Hum Pathol 40:471–477
11. Bostwick DG, Kindrachuk RW, Rouse RV (1985) Prostatic adenocarcinoma with endometrioid features. Clinical, pathologic, and ultrastructural findings. Am J Surg Pathol 9:595–609
12. Christensen WN, Steinberg G, Walsh PC, Epstein JI (1991) Prostatic duct adenocarcinoma. Findings at radical prostatectomy. Cancer 67:2118–2124
13. Epstein JI, Woodruff JM (1986) Adenocarcinoma of the prostate with endometrioid features. A light microscopic and immunohistochemical study of ten cases. Cancer 57:111–119
14. Millar EK, Sharma NK, Lessells AM (1996) Ductal (endometrioid) adenocarcinoma of the prostate: a clinicopathological study of 16 cases. Histopathology 29:11–19
15. Ro JY, Ayala AG, Wishnow KI, Ordóñez NG (1988) Prostatic duct adenocarcinoma with endometrioid features: immunohistochemical and electron microscopic study. Semin Diagn Pathol 5:301–311
16. Kunju LP, Mehra R, Snyder M, Shah RB (2006) Prostate-specific antigen, high-molecular-weight cytokeratin (clone 34betaE12), and/or p63: an optimal immunohistochemical panel to distinguish poorly differentiated prostate adenocarcinoma from urothelial carcinoma. Am J Clin Pathol 125:675–681
17. Lane BR, Magi-Galluzzi C, Reuther AM et al (2006) Mucinous adenocarcinoma of the prostate does not confer poor prognosis. Urology 68:825–830
18. Owens CL, Epstein JI, Netto GJ (2007) Distinguishing prostatic from colorectal adenocarcinoma on biopsy samples: the role of morphology and immunohistochemistry. Arch Pathol Lab Med 131:599–603
19. Ro JY, Grignon DJ, Ayala AG et al (1990) Mucinous adenocarcinoma of the prostate: histochemical and immunohistochemical studies. Hum Pathol 21:593–600
20. Saito S, Iwaki H (1999) Mucin-producing carcinoma of the prostate: review of 88 cases. Urology 54:141–144
21. Herawi M, De Marzo AM, Kristiansen G, Epstein JI (2007) Expression of CDX2 in benign tissue and adenocarcinoma of the prostate. Hum Pathol 38:72–78
22. Aprikian AG, Cordon-Cardo C, Fair WR, Reuter VE (1993) Characterization of neuroendocrine differentiation in human benign prostate and prostatic adenocarcinoma. Cancer 71:3952–3965
23. Evans AJ, Humphrey PA, Belani J et al (2006) Large cell neuroendocrine carcinoma of prostate: a clinicopathologic summary of 7 cases of a rare manifestation of advanced prostate cancer. Am J Surg Pathol 30:684–693
24. Freschi M, Colombo R, Naspro R, Rigatti P (2004) Primary and pure neuroendocrine tumor of the prostate. Eur Urol 45:166–169; discussion 169–170
25. Ro JY, Têtu B, Ayala AG, Ordóñez NG (1987) Small cell carcinoma of the prostate. II. Immunohistochemical and electron microscopic studies of 18 cases. Cancer 59:977–982
26. Shariff AH, Ather MH (2006) Neuroendocrine differentiation in prostate cancer. Urology 68:2–8
27. Têtu B, Ro JY, Ayala AG et al (1987) Small cell carcinoma of the prostate. Part I. A clinicopathologic study of 20 cases. Cancer 59:1803–1809
28. Weinstein MH, Partin AW, Veltri RW, Epstein JI (1996) Neuroendocrine differentiation in prostate cancer: enhanced prediction of progression after radical prostatectomy. Hum Pathol 27:683–687
29. Yao JL, Madeb R, Bourne P et al (2006) Small cell carcinoma of the prostate: an immunohistochemical study. Am J Surg Pathol 30:705–712
30. Shah RB, Mehra R, Chinnaiyan AM et al (2004) Androgen-independent prostate cancer is a heterogeneous group of diseases: lessons from a rapid autopsy program. Cancer Res 64:9209–9216
31. Adlakha H, Bostwick DG (1994) Paneth cell-like change in prostatic adenocarcinoma represents neuroendocrine differentiation: report of 30 cases. Hum Pathol 25:135–139
32. Casella R, Bubendorf L, Sauter G et al (1998) Focal neuroendocrine differentiation lacks prognostic significance in prostate core needle biopsies. J Urol 160:406–410
33. Tamas EF (2006) JI Epstein: Prognostic significance of paneth cell-like neuroendocrine differentiation in adenocarcinoma of the prostate. Am J Surg Pathol 30:980–985
34. Weaver MG, Abdul-Karim FW, Srigley J et al (1992) Paneth cell-like change of the prostate gland. A histological, immunohistochemical, and electron microscopic study. Am J Surg Pathol 16:62–68
35. Weaver MG, Abdul-Karim FW, Srigley JR (1992) Paneth cell-like change and small cell carcinoma of the prostate. Two divergent forms of prostatic neuroendocrine differentiation. Am J Surg Pathol 16:1013–1016
36. Zarkovic A, Masters J, Carpenter L (2005) Primary carcinoid tumour of the prostate. Pathology 37:184–186
37. Dundore PA, Cheville JC, Nascimento AG et al (1995) Carcinosarcoma of the prostate. Report of 21 cases. Cancer 76:1035–1042
38. Hansel DE, Epstein JI (2006) Sarcomatoid carcinoma of the prostate: a study of 42 cases. Am J Surg Pathol 30:1316–1321
39. Huan Y, Idrees M, Gribetz ME, Unger PD (2008) Sarcomatoid carcinoma after radiation treatment of prostatic adenocarcinoma. Ann Diagn Pathol 12:142–145
40. Ray ME, Wojno KJ, Goldstein NS et al (2006) Clonality of sarcomatous and carcinomatous elements in sarcomatoid carcinoma of the prostate. Urology 67:423 e5–423 e8
41. Shannon RL, Ro JY, Grignon DJ et al (1992) Sarcomatoid carcinoma of the prostate. A clinicopathologic study of 12 patients. Cancer 69:2676–2682

42. Esrig D et al (1996) Transitional cell carcinoma involving the prostate with a proposed staging classification for stromal invasion. J Urol 156:1071–1076
43. Greene LF, O'Dea J, Dockerty MB (1976) Primary transitional cell carcinoma of the prostate. J Urol 116:761–763
44. Njinou NB, Lorge F, Moulin P et al (2003) Transitional cell carcinoma involving the prostate: a clinicopathological retrospective study of 76 cases. J Urol 169:149–152
45. Oliai BR, Kahane H, Epstein JI (2001) A clinicopathologic analysis of urothelial carcinomas diagnosed on prostate needle biopsy. Am J Surg Pathol 25:794–801
46. Schellhammer PF, Bean MA, Whitmore WF Jr (1977) Prostatic involvement by transitional cell carcinoma: pathogenesis, patterns and prognosis. J Urol 118:399–403
47. Shen SS, Lerner SP, Muezzinoglu B et al (2006) Prostatic involvement by transitional cell carcinoma in patients with bladder cancer and its prognostic significance. Hum Pathol 37:726–734
48. Wood DP Jr, Montie JE, Pontes JE et al (1989) Transitional cell carcinoma of the prostate in cystoprostatectomy specimens removed for bladder cancer. J Urol 141:346–349
49. Miller VA, Reuter V, Scher HI (1995) Primary squamous cell carcinoma of the prostate after radiation seed implantation for adenocarcinoma. Urology 46:111–113
50. Moyana TN (1987) Adenosquamous carcinoma of the prostate. Am J Surg Pathol 11:403–407
51. Orhan D, Sak SD, Yaman O et al (1996) Adenosquamous carcinoma of the prostate. Br J Urol 78:646–647
52. Parwani AV, Kronz JD, Genega EM et al (2004) Prostate carcinoma with squamous differentiation: an analysis of 33 cases. Am J Surg Pathol 28:651–657
53. Ro JY, el-Naggar A, Ayala AG et al (1988) Signet-ring-cell carcinoma of the prostate. Electron-microscopic and immunohistochemical studies of eight cases. Am J Surg Pathol 12:453–460
54. Ali TZ, Epstein JI (2007) Basal cell carcinoma of the prostate: a clinicopathologic study of 29 cases. Am J Surg Pathol 31:697–705
55. Devaraj LT, Bostwick DG (1993) Atypical basal cell hyperplasia of the prostate. Immunophenotypic profile and proposed classification of basal cell proliferations. Am J Surg Pathol 17:645–659
56. Grignon DJ, Ro JY, Ordoñez NG et al (1988) Basal cell hyperplasia, adenoid basal cell tumor, and adenoid cystic carcinoma of the prostate gland: an immunohistochemical study. Hum Pathol 19:1425–1433
57. Iczkowski KA, Ferguson KL, Grier DD et al (2003) Adenoid cystic/basal cell carcinoma of the prostate: clinicopathologic findings in 19 cases. Am J Surg Pathol 27:1523–1529
58. McKenney JK, Amin MB, Srigley JR et al (2004) Basal cell proliferations of the prostate other than usual basal cell hyperplasia: a clinicopathologic study of 23 cases, including four carcinomas, with a proposed classification. Am J Surg Pathol 28:1289–1298

Benign Mimics of Prostate Carcinoma

The diagnosis of prostate carcinoma, especially when present in a limited amount in biopsy, is often challenging because numerous benign conditions have architectural and cytological features overlapping with and mimicking carcinoma [1]. These mimics include various anatomic structures, inflammatory and reactive conditions, and pathophysiological conditions, including atrophy, hyperplasia, and metaplasia. Many of these lesions are readily recognized and separated from malignancy but some may cause potential diagnostic difficulties. A useful approach to classifying benign mimics is based on major growth patterns of prostate carcinoma outlined in the Gleason grading system. This approach provides a conceptual framework for considering differential diagnoses. Three major growth patterns are encountered: small gland pattern mimicking Gleason score 4–6 carcinomas; large gland/cribriform growth pattern mimicking Gleason score 7–8 carcinomas; and fused glands/solid growth/single cells pattern mimicking Gleason score 8–10 carcinomas. Most benign lesions mimic small gland (acinar) adenocarcinoma. Before establishing a cancer diagnosis, pathologists should always consider and rule out various benign lesions that mimic carcinoma. This chapter outlines an overall approach, classification, description of pathologic features, and diagnostic pitfalls of each benign entity.

7.1 Classification of Benign Mimics of Prostate Carcinoma using Architectural Pattern-Based Approach

Classification of benign mimics of prostate carcinoma using architectural pattern-based approach

Predominant pattern at low power

- **Well-formed small to mid-sized discrete glands** (Mimic of Gleason score 5–6 carcinoma)
  - **Circumscribed (lobulated) proliferation**
    - **Normal anatomical structures:**
      - Seminal vesicle/ejaculatory duct
      - Cowper's glands
      - Verumontanum mucosal gland hyperplasia
      - Glandular crowding
    - **Pathophysiological conditions:**
      - Post-atrophic hyperplasia
      - Partial atrophy
      - Adenosis
      - Basal cell adenoma
  - **Haphazard proliferation**
    - Partial atrophy
    - Complete atrophy
    - Basal cell hyperplasia
    - Nephrogenic adenoma
    - Radiation atypia

- **Large cribriform glands** (Mimic of Gleason score 7–8 carcinoma)
  - Reactive benign glands
  - Central zone glands
  - Clear cell cribriform hyperplasia
  - Adenoid cystic-type basal cell hyperplasia

- **Poorly formed or fused glands/nests/single cells** (Mimic of Gleason score 8–10 carcinoma)
  - Sclerosing adenosis
  - Malakoplakia
  - Paraganglion
  - Granulomatous prostatitis

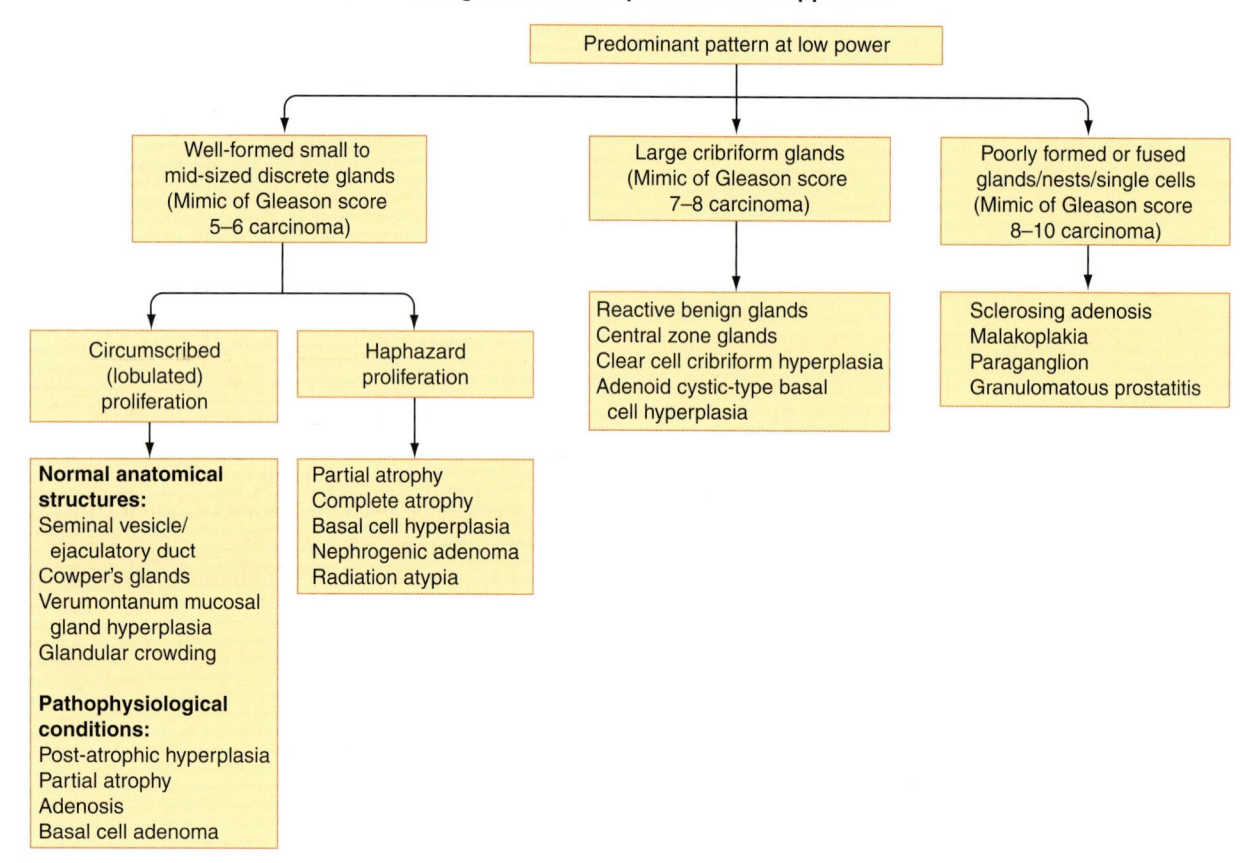

Fig. 7.1 Classification of benign mimics using an architectural pattern-based approach

7.2 Histological Features Commonly Associated with Benign Mimics

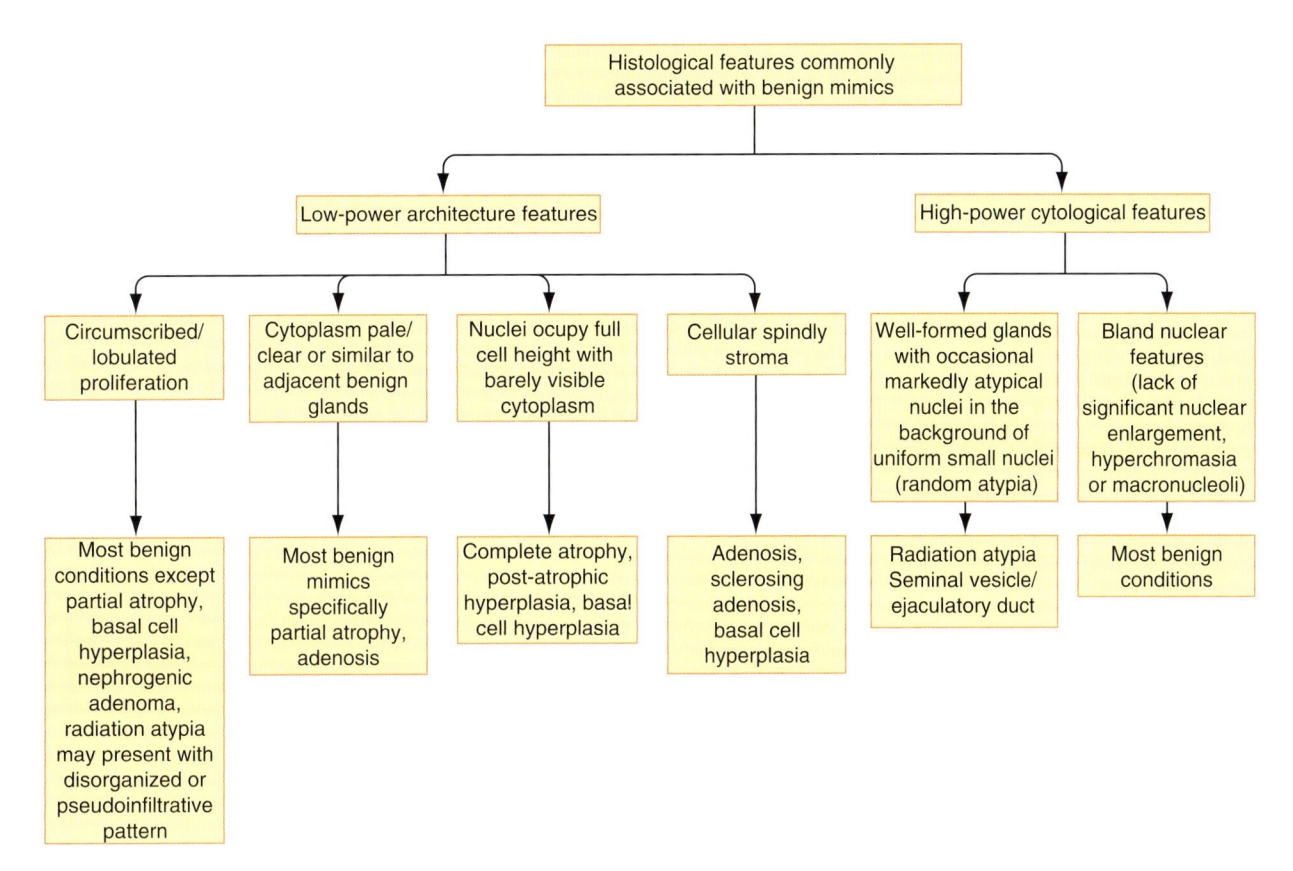

Fig. 7.2 Histological features that are commonly associated with and helpful in recognition of benign mimics

7.3 Atypical Morphological Features Commonly Encountered in Various Benign Mimics of Prostate Cancer

Table 7.1 Summary of atypical morphological features commonly encountered in various benign mimics of prostate cancer

Atypical morphological feature	Type of benign mimic associated with atypical morphological feature
Low-power architecture feature	
Haphazard proliferation of glands	Partial atrophy
	Nephrogenic adenoma
	Basal cell hyperplasia
	Radiation atypia
Intraluminal mucin	Adenosis
	Sclerosing adenosis
	Nephrogenic adenoma
Poorly formed glands	Partial atrophy
	Sclerosing adenosis
	Nephrogenic adenoma
High-power cytological feature	
Visible nucleoli (typically, micronucleoli visible only at high power)	Complete atrophy
	Postatrophic hyperplasia
	Partial atrophy
	Inflammation
	Adenosis
	Sclerosing adenosis
	Basal cell hyperplasia
	Radiation atypia
	Nephrogenic adenoma
Marked random nuclear atypia	Seminal vesicle/ejaculatory duct epithelium
	Radiation atypia

7.4 Seminal Vesicle/Ejaculatory Duct Epithelium

Table 7.2 Seminal vesicle/ejaculatory duct epithelium [2–5]

Microscopical features

Low-power architecture

Well-formed small branching glands budding from central dilated lumina and may be surrounded by smooth muscle (*see* Fig. 7.3)

Golden brown cytoplasmic lipofuscin pigment

High-power cytology

Presence of scattered pleomorphic nuclei ("monster nuclei") and nuclear pseudoinclusions (*see* Fig. 7.3b)

Pleomorphic nuclei are degenerative in atypia and lack mitotic activity

Immunohistochemical features

Lack expression for prostate-specific antigen (PSA) and prostate acid phosphatase (PSAP)

Positive for high molecular weight cytokeratin (HMWCK) (34βE12) and p63

Antibodies to MUC6, PAX-2, PAX-8 are positive in seminal vesicle/ejaculatory duct epithelium but is negative in prostate cancer

Incidence and location

Present in 4–5% of prostate biopsies

Seminal vesicle tissue is usually sampled in needle biopsies incidentally, but sometimes as a result of targeted sampling

Ejaculatory duct epithelium is morphologically similar to the seminal vesicle but lacks well-formed smooth muscle wall and the distinction between the two may not be possible

Differential diagnosis

Low-grade prostate adenocarcinoma and high-grade prostatic intraepithelial neoplasia (HGPIN)

A well-differentiated adenocarcinoma demonstrates uniform cytological atypia and rarely demonstrates random nuclear pleomorphism

Lipofuscin pigment may be present in normal, hyperplastic, PIN glands, and carcinoma glands. However, pigment in cancer glands is rare and usually not prominent.

Common diagnostic pitfalls

Presence of dark granular cytoplasm, marked cytological atypia in small glands are common pitfalls

Unless specified as the biopsy of seminal vesicle, the presence of adenocarcinoma in a needle biopsy containing "seminal vesicle" type epithelium should not be regarded as evidence of seminal vesicle invasion, as ejaculatory duct and seminal vesicle cannot be reliably separated from each other in needle biopsy

7.5 Verumontanum Mucosal Gland Hyperplasia

Table 7.3 Verumontanum mucosal gland hyperplasia (VMGH) [6, 7]

Microscopical features

Low-power architecture

Circumscribed collection of small, closely packed acini, frequently present in proximity to urethral lining (*see* Fig. 7.4)

Intraluminal brown orange amorphous concretions and corpora (*see* Fig. 7.4b)

High-power cytology

Glands lined by bland cells with small nuclei without prominent nucleoli and contain conspicuous layer of basal cells

Immunohistochemical features

Identical to benign prostate glands

Incidence and location

Frequent finding in radical prostatectomy specimens but an infrequent finding in needle biopsy due to its deep location

Exclusively in the region of the verumontanum and adjacent posterior urethra where the ejaculatory ducts and utricle empty into the urethra

Differential diagnosis

Prostate adenocarcinoma (≤ Gleason score 6)

Adenocarcinoma usually has infiltrative features, contains variable cytologic atypia, and lacks characteristic brown-orange concretions and corpora amylacea of VMGH

Occasionally VMGH may assume a papillary appearance and may resemble ductal adenocarcinoma although the cells lining the papillae are cuboidal without atypia compared to variably atypical stratified epithelium in large ductal adenocarcinoma

Common diagnostic pitfalls

Small glandular architecture and crowding mimic cancer at low magnification

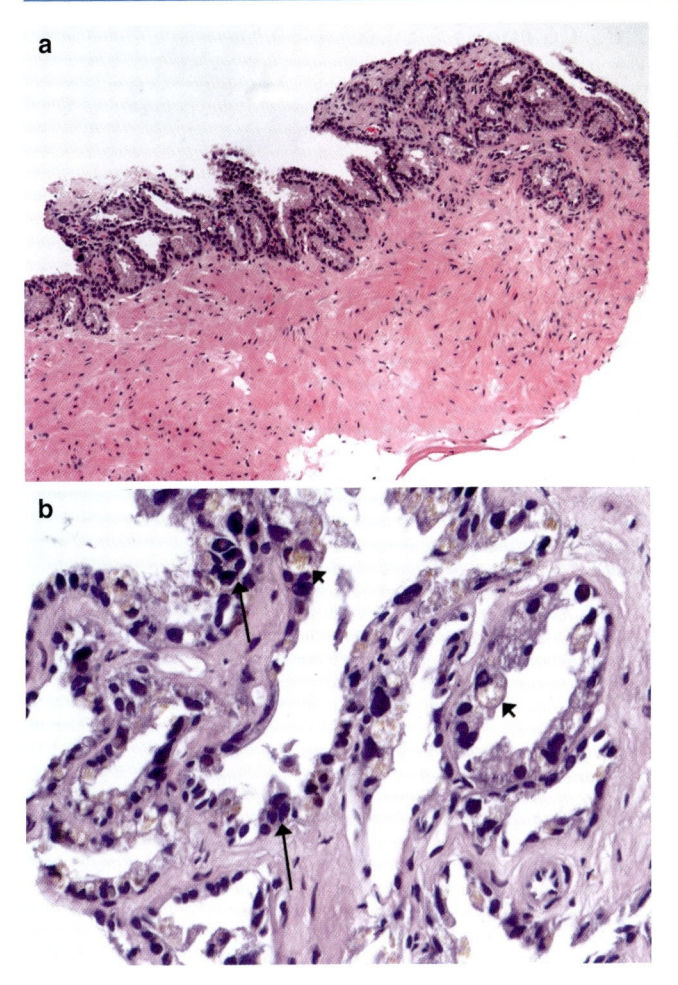

Fig. 7.3 Seminal vesicle/ejaculatory duct epithelium. In small biopsy samples, seminal vesicle and ejaculatory duct structures are usually not distinguishable unless biopsy targeting seminal vesicle is performed. At low power (**a**), peripherally located well-formed small branching glands with cytoplasmic amphophilia, budding from central dilated lumina is a common feature. Well-formed muscular layer surrounding glands favors seminal vesicle tissue but usually is not present in biopsy samples. At higher magnification (**b**), the epithelium lining the lumina and small glands show nuclear hyperchromasia and random pleomorphism (*arrows*), also referred to as "monster nuclei." Nuclear pseudoinclusions are commonly seen. Prominent golden-brown lipofuscin granules (*arrowhead*) are typical. Overall, the random nuclear atypia with prominent lipofuscin pigment in acini is a definitional feature

7.6 Cowper's Glands

Table 7.4 Cowper's glands [8, 9]

Microscopical features
Low-power architecture
A lobulated collection of glands with dimorphic population of a central duct surrounded by tightly packed, round, small acini composed of cells with abundant mucinous cytoplasm (*see* Fig. 7.5)
Skeletal muscle is frequently present in the stroma (*see* Fig. 7.5c)
High-power cytology
Uniform, basally located, bland nuclei
Immunohistochemical features
Intracytoplasmic mucin positive for mucicarmine, periodic acid-Schiff (PAS)-diastase stains
HMWCK 34βE12 stains ducts but the staining is variable in acini
PSA variably positive, prostatic acid phosphatase (PSAP) negative
Incidence and location
Cowper's glands are paired bulbourethral (periurethral) glands located within the urogenital diaphragm below the prostate apex
Rarely sampled in prostate biopsy from the apex
Differential diagnosis
May be confused with small acinar adenocarcinoma, particularly foamy gland cancer (*see* Fig. 6.1a–b). The presence of infiltrative borders, lack of dimorphic ductal–acinar architecture, and variable cellular atypia distinguish it from Cowper's glands.
Adenocarcinoma typically lacks cytoplasmic mucin but contains intraluminal mucin
The majority of lesions mimicking Cowper's gland are mucinous metaplasia of prostatic acini associated with atrophy (*see* Fig. 7.7)
Common diagnostic pitfalls
Small well-formed glands with cytoplasmic mucin and round, rigid, acinar architecture may be mistaken for foamy carcinoma

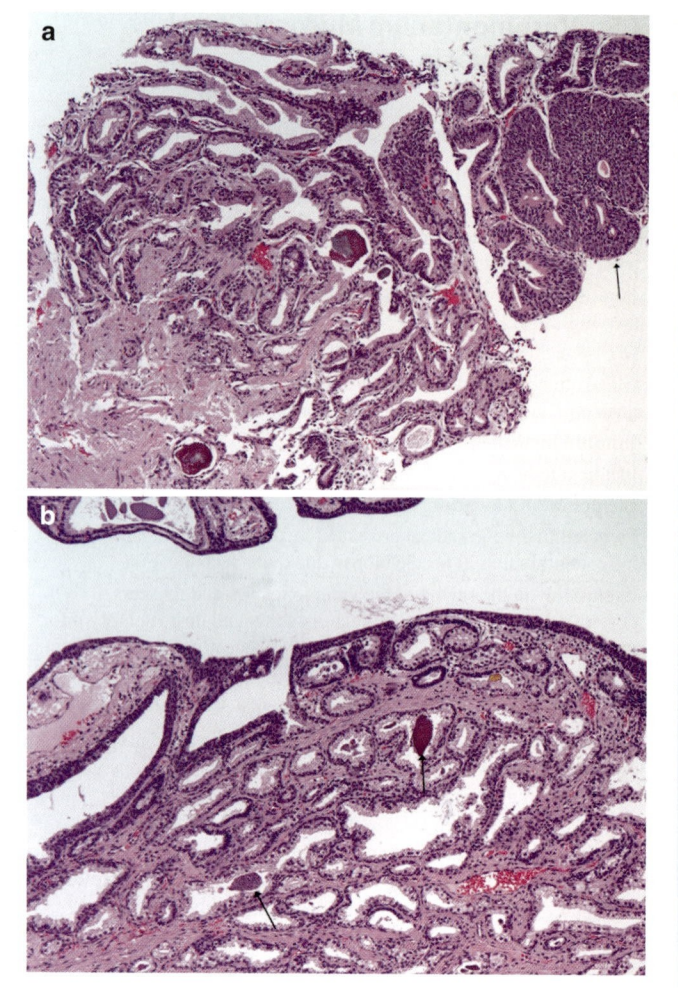

Fig. 7.4 Verumontanum mucosal gland hyperplasia. At low power (**a**), lobulated collection of relatively uniform, closely packed, round, small acini, frequently accompanied by adjacent urothelial epithelium (*arrow*) is a common presentation. Intraluminal brown-orange concretions (*arrow*) are a frequent and distinctive feature. At high magnification (**b**), the luminal cells have small uniform nuclei and inconspicuous nucleoli. An intact basal cell layer is present

7.7 Mesonephric Remnant Hyperplasia

Table 7.5 Mesonephric remnant hyperplasia [10, 11]

Microscopical features

Low-power architecture

Resemble the same lesion encountered in the female genital tract

Majority retains a lobular configuration of glands and tubules but occasionally demonstrating pseudoinfiltrative pattern (*see* Fig. 7.6)

Dense intraluminal eosinophilic secretions are common and occasional papillary tufting is seen (*see* Fig. 7.6)

High-power cytology

Glands/tubules are lined by single cuboidal epithelium with scant atrophic cytoplasm and bland cytology

Immunohistochemical features

Negative for PSA and PSAP and positive for basal cell markers

Incidence and location

More likely present in TURP specimens from the transition zone of the prostate, 0.6% of transurethral resection of the prostate (TURP) specimen. Extremely rare in prostate biopsies

Differential diagnosis

Mimic well to intermediately differentiated Gleason score 6–7 prostate carcinoma

Adenocarcinoma lacks lobular arrangement, demonstrates variable cytoplasm and cytological atypia, and lacks epithelial tufting or micropapillary formations. In addition, the intraluminal eosinophilic material in mesonephric hyperplasia typically has a dense, hyaline appearance in contrast to the more flocculent nature of the intraluminal eosinophilic material in prostate cancer

Mesonephric hyperplasia lacks expression for prostate markers PSA and PSAP. HMWCK (clone 34βE12) stain is expressed in the lining epithelium

Common diagnostic pitfalls

Florid small acinar and tubular architecture; single layer of the lining epithelium; occasional prominent nucleoli; intraluminal eosinophilic material, haphazard appearance in some cases (with some even showing perineural and extraprostatic location) may lead to misdiagnosis of prostate carcinoma

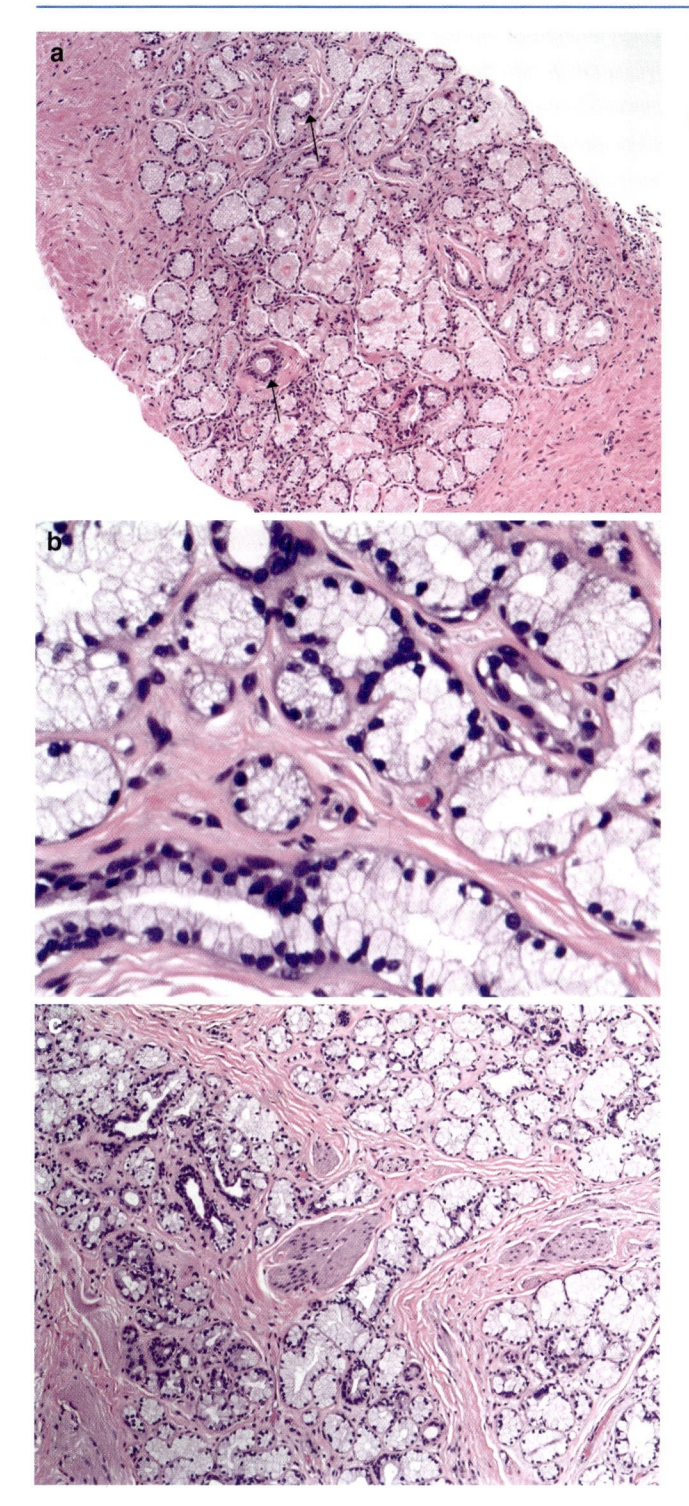

Fig. 7.5 Cowper's glands. At low power (**a**), Cowper's glands are composed of tightly circumscribed or lobulated proliferation of small, uniform acini lined by mucus-containing cells with a central duct. This dimorphic population of ducts (*arrow*) surrounded by acini is a characteristic feature. Cytological features are bland, including small nuclei and inconspicuous nucleoli. Mucin is present in the intracellular compartment in contrast to intraluminal mucin in prostate cancer (**b**). Skeletal muscle is frequently present in stroma (**c**)

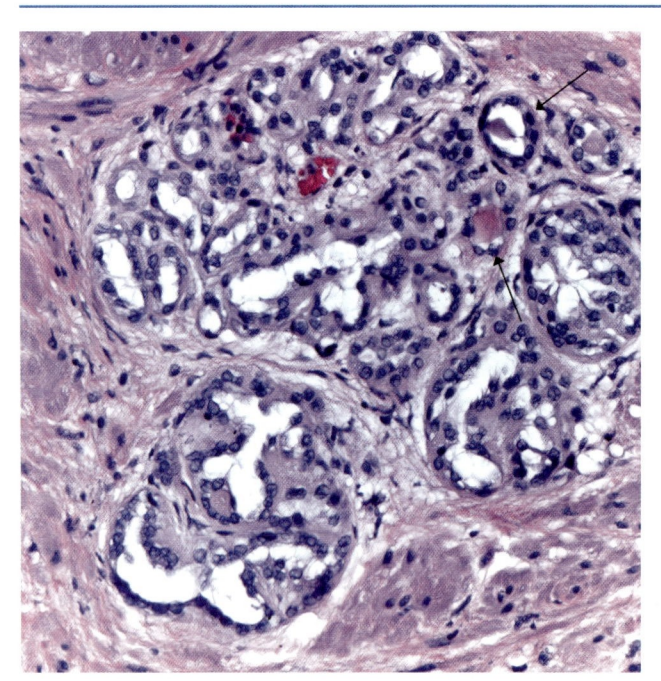

Fig. 7.6 Mesonephric remnant hyperplasia. Glands appear atrophic with attenuated bland epithelium and grow in a lobulated or sometimes infiltrative pattern. Intraluminal dense eosinophilic secretions (*arrows*) and papillary infoldings and tufts are common useful features to distinguish from adenocarcinoma of the prostate (*Image courtesy of* Dr. Anil Parwani, The University of Pittsburgh Medical Center, Pittsburgh, PA)

7.8 Mucinous Metaplasia

Table 7.6 Mucinous metaplasia [12, 13]

Microscopical features

Low-power architecture

Clusters of small glands lined by tall columnar cells with abundant intracytoplasmic blue mucin

Transition to normal glandular epithelium or atrophic glands is frequent, typically does not involve the entire lobule of acini (*see* Fig. 7.7)

High-power cytology

Bland, small, dark, and basally located nuclei, with inconspicuous nucleoli

Immunohistochemical features

Lacks immunoreactivity for PSA and PSAP

An intact basal layer demonstrated by basal cell markers

Cells contain intracytoplasmic acid mucin that stains for mucicarcmine, Alcian blue, and PAS with diastase digestion

Incidence and location

Incidental but relatively common finding

Primarily seen in the peripheral zone of the prostate

Differential diagnosis

Well-differentiated prostate adenocarcinoma with foamy gland feature. The presence of infiltrative features, variable nuclear atypia, and intraluminal rather than cytoplasmic mucin pattern distinguishes foamy gland carcinoma from mucinous metaplasia. Stains are rarely needed to establish definitive diagnosis (*see* Fig. 6.1a–b).

Table 7.6 (continued)

Cowper's glands. Mucinous metaplasia lacks the characteristic dimorphic pattern of duct and acini and is usually focal and does not involve the entire lobule of acini (*see* Fig. 7.5)

Common diagnostic pitfalls

Small, round, acinar architecture and blue mucin

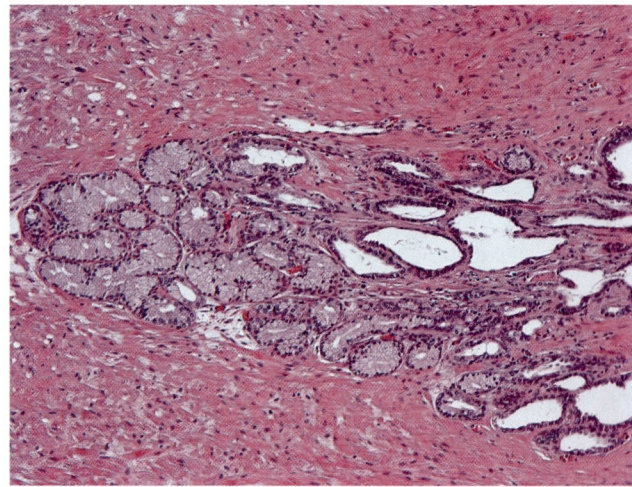

Fig. 7.7 Mucinous metaplasia typically involves part of a lobule. Transition to benign atrophic glands in the background is seen. Note that glands are lined by tall columnar cells with abundant intracytoplasmic mucin. In contrast to Cowper's glands, no dimorphic duct/acini architecture is seen

7.9 Morphologic Classification of Focal Atrophy Lesions

Table 7.7 Classification of focal atrophy lesions of prostate [14–18]

Simple atrophy (lobular atrophy)[a]

Simple atrophy with cyst formation (cystic atrophy)

Postatrophic hyperplasia[a]

Partial atrophy

Combined patterns

[a]Both simple atrophy and postatrophic hyperplasia are commonly associated with inflammation and may demonstrate increased proliferative activity in epithelium. These lesions are also often termed proliferative inflammatory atrophy (PIA) to imply their potential significance in prostate carcinogenesis

7.9 Morphologic Classification of Focal Atrophy Lesions

Table 7.8 Focal atrophy [14–23]

Microscopical features

Low-power architecture

Morphology varies significantly but all forms of atrophy are characterized by well-formed glands that exhibit a reduction in cytoplasmic volume in luminal epithelial cells

Simple atrophy, cystic atrophy, and postatrophic hyperplasia are characterized by dark-blue glands at low power due to marked reduction in cytoplasm, whereas partial atrophy looks pale due to relatively more lateral cytoplasm but reduced apical cytoplasm

Simple atrophy is characterized by isolated, not particularly crowded, atrophic glands of the same size as adjacent nonatrophic glands. The stroma between glands is frequently sclerotic and contains inflammation (*see* Fig. 7.8a)

In cystic atrophy, a varying degree of acinar dilatation is seen. The term *cystic atrophy* is restricted to glands that have a sharp luminal border without infolding (*see* Fig. 7.8b)

Different forms of atrophy commonly coexist in the same specimen

High-power cytology

Cells with bland small hypochromatic nuclei

Mild nuclear enlargement is occasionally seen

Micronucleoli in significant percentage of cases

Immunohistochemical features

Basal cell markers, in general, highlight the basal cell layer but are often fragmented or absent particularly in partial atrophy

Significant percentage of partial atrophy expresses α-Methylacyl-CoA racemase (AMACR)

Incidence, location, and clinical significance

Common, age-related process

Atrophy typically affects the elderly; however; focal atrophy is present in at least 70% of men between the second and third decades of life. Its frequency and extent increase with age

Atrophy is also common in patients receiving anti-androgens and radiation treatment

Most common in the peripheral zone, but also in the transition and central zones of the prostate

Its pathogenesis is still unknown, although inflammation and chronic ischemia are considered important factors. Focal atrophy, particularly when associated with inflammation, contains cells with increased proliferation in the epithelial compartment, demonstrates some of the early genetic changes seen in HGPIN and prostate cancer, and also demonstrates increased expression of the stress-related oxidative enzyme, glutathione S-transferase (GSTP1). *Proliferative inflammatory atrophy* (PIA) has been proposed as a term for these lesions

PIA has recently been proposed as a lesion from which early prostate carcinogenesis develops (*see* Fig. 13.1)

Differential diagnosis

Prostate cancer with Gleason score 6 or 7

Postatrophic hyperplasia and partial atrophy most closely mimic prostate cancer and cause most diagnostic difficulties in routine practice and will be discussed in later sections

Common diagnostic pitfalls

Presence of dark small glands within sclerotic stroma and visible nucleoli are common diagnostic pitfalls of simple atrophy and postatrophic hyperplasia

Pale, poorly formed glands, frequent visible nucleoli, and atypical immunohistochemical presentation are common diagnostic pitfalls of partial atrophy

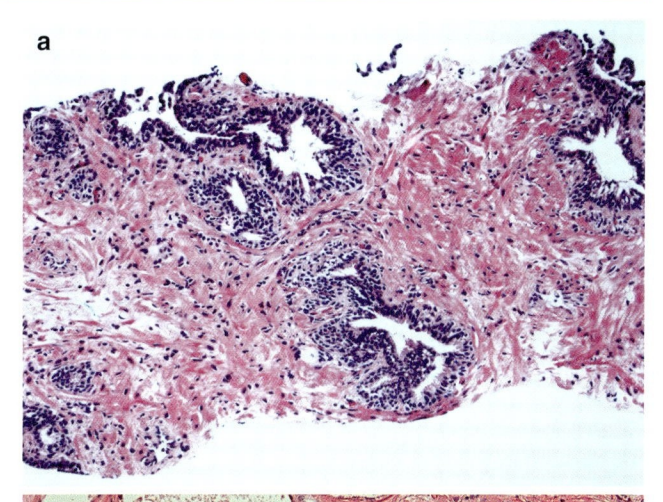

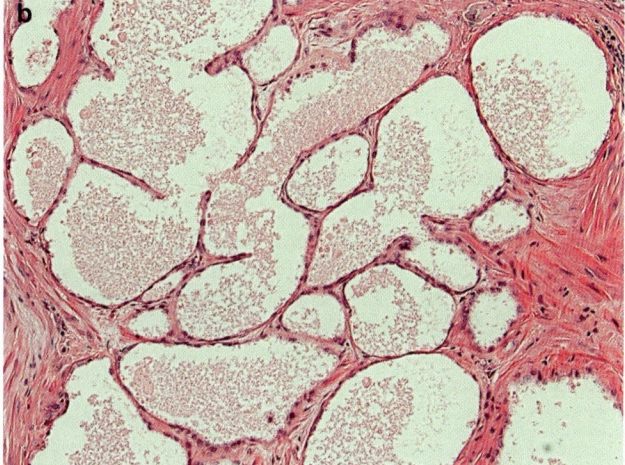

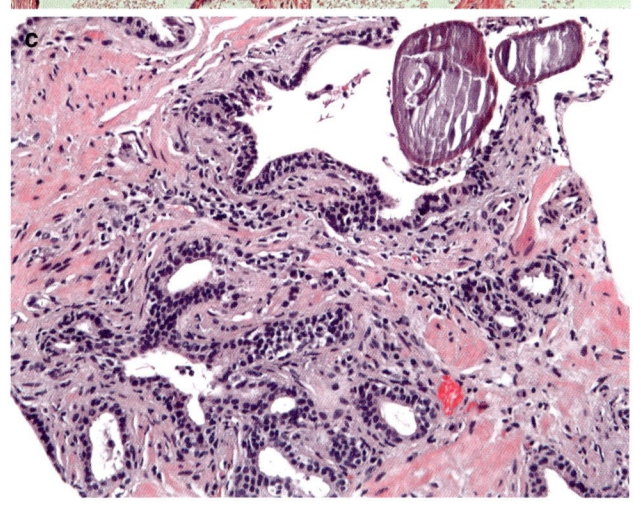

Fig. 7.8 Simple atrophy, cystic atrophy, and PIA lesion. (**a–c**) In simple atrophy, overall architecture of the glands is maintained with marked reduction of cytoplasm, creating a basophilic appearance at low power (**a**). In cystic atrophy, an undulated glandular architecture of the normal gland is lost; glands are round and cystically dilated with attenuated cytoplasm (**b**). Both simple and postatrophic hyperplasia are commonly accompanied by inflammation and sclerotic stroma (**c**). Although glands appear rather atrophic and involuting, they demonstrate higher proliferative activity on immunostain for proliferation marker Ki-67 (*not shown*). Such lesions are also termed PIA and are proposed as an early precursor to prostate carcinoma

7.10 Partial Atrophy

Table 7.9 Partial atrophy [22, 24, 25]

Microscopical features

Low-power architecture

Majority present with circumscribed/lobulated collection of small glands with lumina ranging from undulated stellate-shaped to round (*see* Fig. 7.9a–b)

Occasionally disorganized growth

Lined with cells with reduced cell height but clear pale cytoplasm placed laterally to nuclei rather than an apical distribution pattern, creating a pale appearance at low power (*see* Fig. 7.9d)

Completely atrophic glands within a focus are common (*see* Fig. 7.9c–d.)

High-power cytology

Small bland nuclei, often with micronucleoli; occasionally mild nuclear enlargement is seen (*see* Fig. 7.9f)

Immunohistochemical features

Basal cell markers often patchy and fragmented, occasionally entirely negative

Up to 70% expresses AMACR

Rarely negative for basal cell markers and positive for AMACR

Incidence and location

The most common cancer mimic encountered in contemporary practice

Primarily seen in the peripheral zone of the prostate

Differential diagnosis

Prostate adenocarcinoma (Gleason score 6 or 7)

Most carcinoma demonstrate infiltrative features, round glands with straight luminal borders, relatively abundant, apically distributed amphophilic or foamy cytoplasm, and more pronounced cytological atypia

Partial atrophy was described by some pathologists as postatrophic hyperplasia. Compared with PAH (*see* Fig. 7.11), partial atrophy appears pale due to relatively more cytoplasm; exhibit stellate-shaped glands; and typically lacks stromal sclerosis or inflammation. However, it is common to see different forms of atrophy coexisting within a case

Common diagnostic pitfalls

Disorganized growth pattern (~30%) with predominantly round and poorly formed lumina (~9%)

Frequently (~30%) visible nucleoli at high power, occasional mild nuclear enlargement

Patchy basal cell staining (~70%) and sometimes complete lack of staining

Significant percentage expresses AMACR (10–70%)

7.10 Partial Atrophy

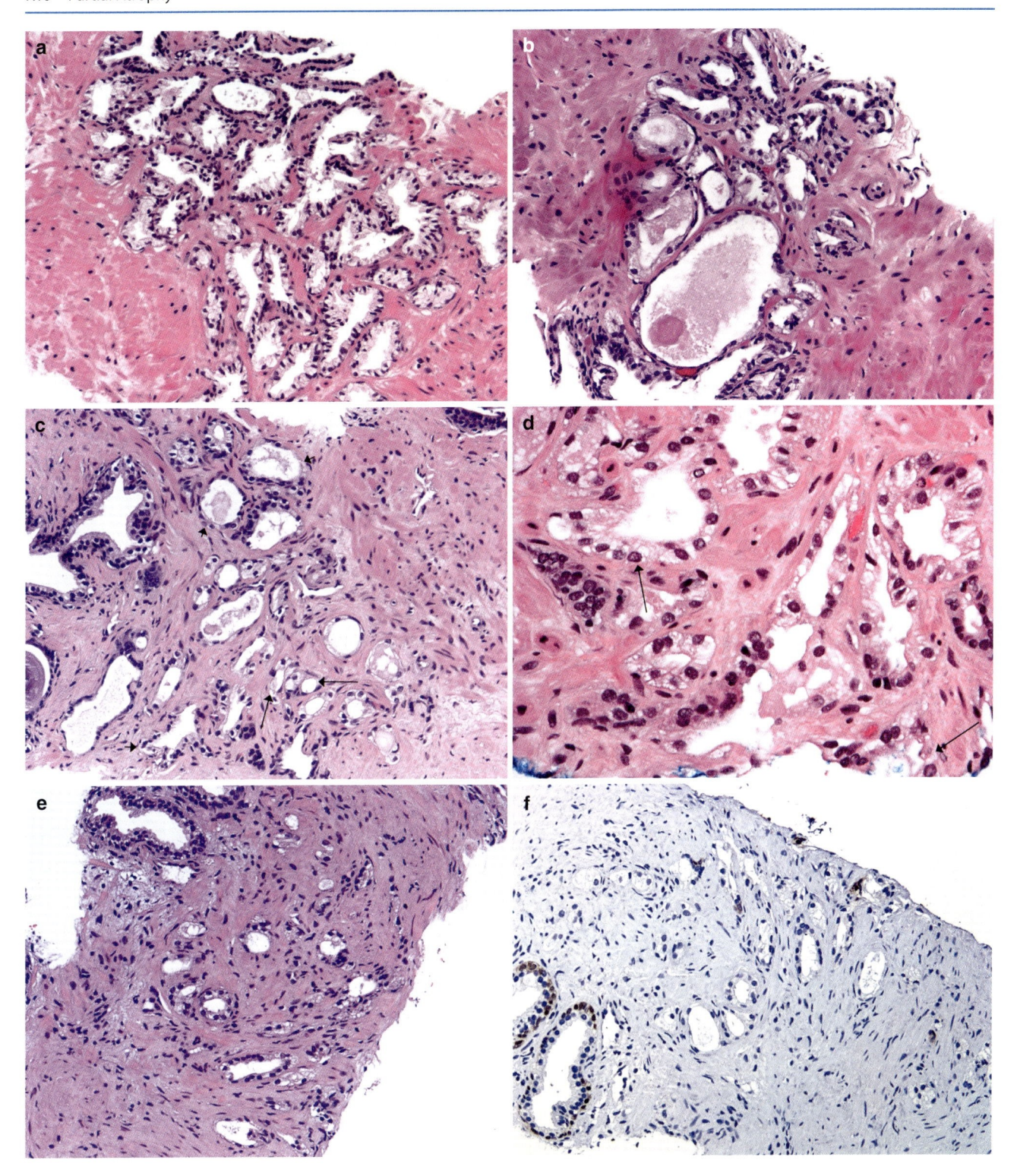

Fig. 7.9 Morphological spectrum of partial atrophy. (**a–f**) The majority of partial atrophy lesions are composed of a lobular arrangement of crowded glands with stellate/undulating gland lumina, and scant pale clear cytoplasm, imparting a distinct pale appearance at low power (**a** and **b**). Partial atrophy composed of a disorganized proliferation of predominantly small, round to occasionally poorly formed glands (*arrows*). In addition to partially atrophic glands, there are several completely atrophic glands (*arrowheads*), a very useful diagnostic clue. Also note that the pale cytoplasm of the lesion is similar to the adjacent benign gland (**c**). At high power, frequent micronucleoli (*arrow*) are visible. Note pale, clear cytoplasm placed laterally to the nuclei, lack of nuclear enlargement and macronucleoli, as well as the presence of few completely atrophic glands within the focus (**d**). (**e**) Another example of partial atrophy showing disorganized growth pattern and predominant poorly formed glands mimicking cancer. Note relatively benign cytology, pale cytoplasm, and few completely atrophic glands within the focus. (**f**) Immunohistochemistry for basal cell markers demonstrates very patchy staining with the lack of staining in the majority of glands

7.11 Postatrophic Hyperplasia

Table 7.10 Postatrophic hyperplasia (PAH) [19]

Microscopical features
Low-power architecture
Lobulated collection of small basophilic and mostly round acini frequently surrounding a central dilated "feeder" duct (*see* Fig. 7.11)
Stroma is sclerotic and contains inflammation
High-power cytology
Acini contain low cuboidal cells with scant cytoplasm
Basal cells may show mild-to-moderate nucleolar enlargement

Immunohistochemical features
Continuous and strong basal cell marker staining but patchy fragmented staining occasionally observed
Lacks AMACR expression

Incidence and location
Common in routine practice
Primarily seen in the peripheral zone of the prostate

Differential diagnosis
Prostate adenocarcinoma, Gleason score ≤6. The presence of infiltrative features, relatively more amphophilic cytoplasm, lack of central dilated duct, and more pronounced cytological atypia suggest adenocarcinoma diagnosis over PAH

In comparison to partial atrophy (*see* Fig. 7.9), PAH lesions appear dark, lack cytoplasm, demonstrate stromal sclerosis, and frequently contain inflammation

Common diagnostic pitfalls
Crowded, dark, and round acini raise concerns for cancer
May occasionally exhibit pseudoinfiltrative growth pattern (*see* Fig. 7.12)
Visible nucleoli are frequent at high-power examination
Stromal sclerosis may mimic desmoplasia

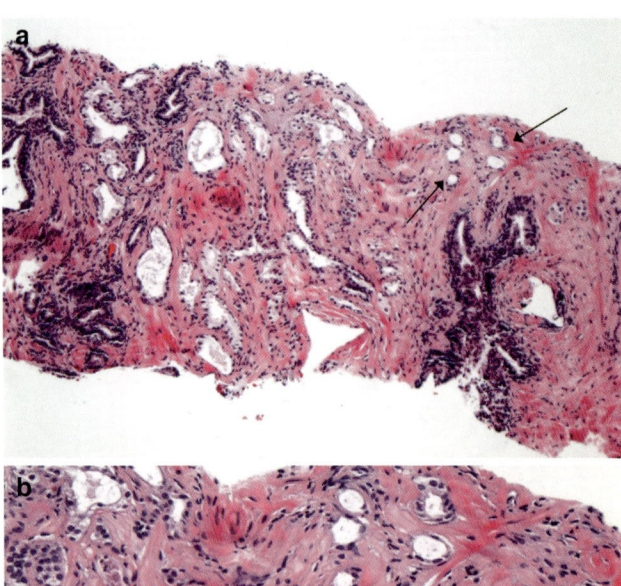

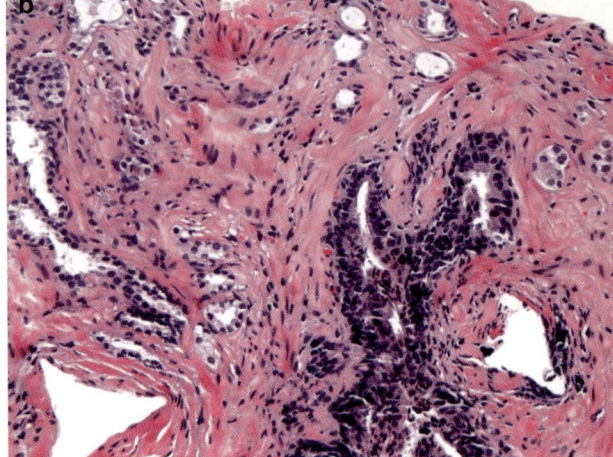

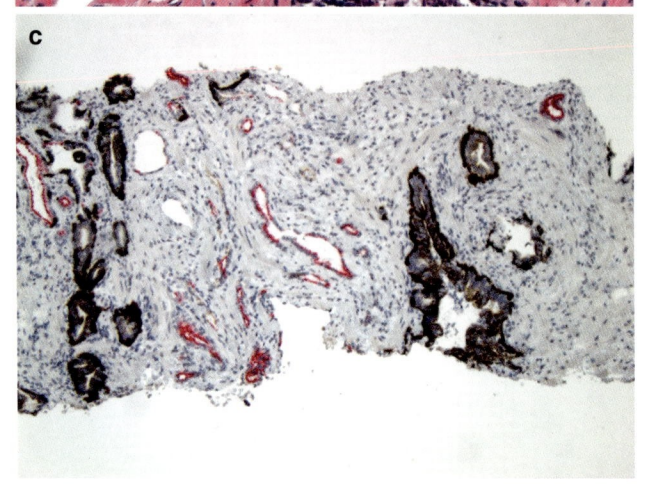

Fig. 7.10 (**a–c**) Partial atrophy with atypical features, suspicious for cancer. At low power, several disorganized glands with partially atrophic cytoplasm are present. A few completely atrophic glands are also present. These features are suggestive of partial atrophy (**a**). At higher magnification, these glands demonstrated bland cytology (**b**). However, the edge of this lesion appears infiltrative (*arrow*, **a**) and it demonstrates immunophenotype identical to cancer (**c**). Despite the presence of several features of partial atrophy, one cannot rule out cancer. Therefore, it is best to diagnose this case as atypical suspicious for cancer

7.11 Postatrophic Hyperplasia

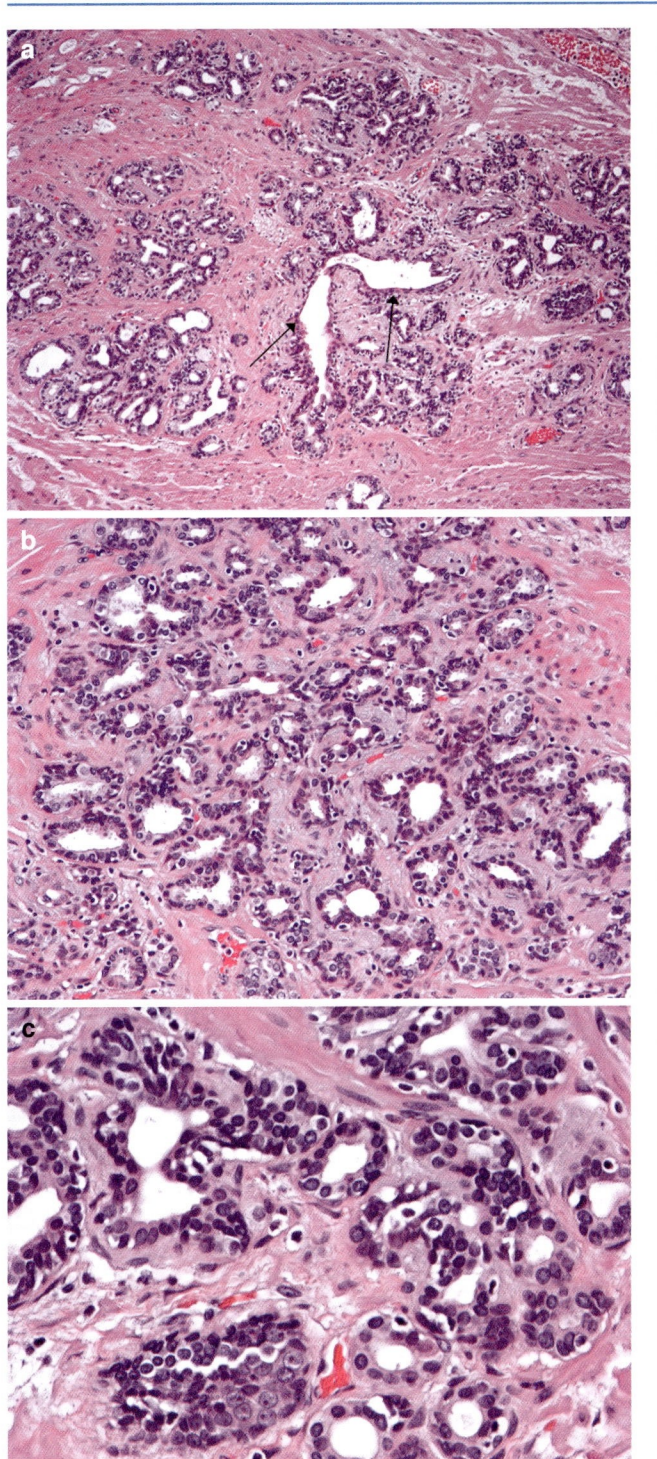

Fig. 7.11 Postatrophic hyperplasia. (**a–c**) At low power, PAH is characterized by a circumscribed/lobulated collection of small dark atrophic acini with round-to-distorted contours arranged around a larger dilated duct (*arrow*; **a** and **b**). The dark appearance of the lesion at low power may arouse a suspicion for cancer but is due to scant cytoplasm rather than abundant amphophilic/granular cytoplasm seen in cancer. At high magnification (**c**), the acini are lined by cuboidal secretory cells with minimal nuclear enlargement, increased nucleus-to-cytoplasmic ratio, and small but visible nucleoli. The stroma is usually sclerotic

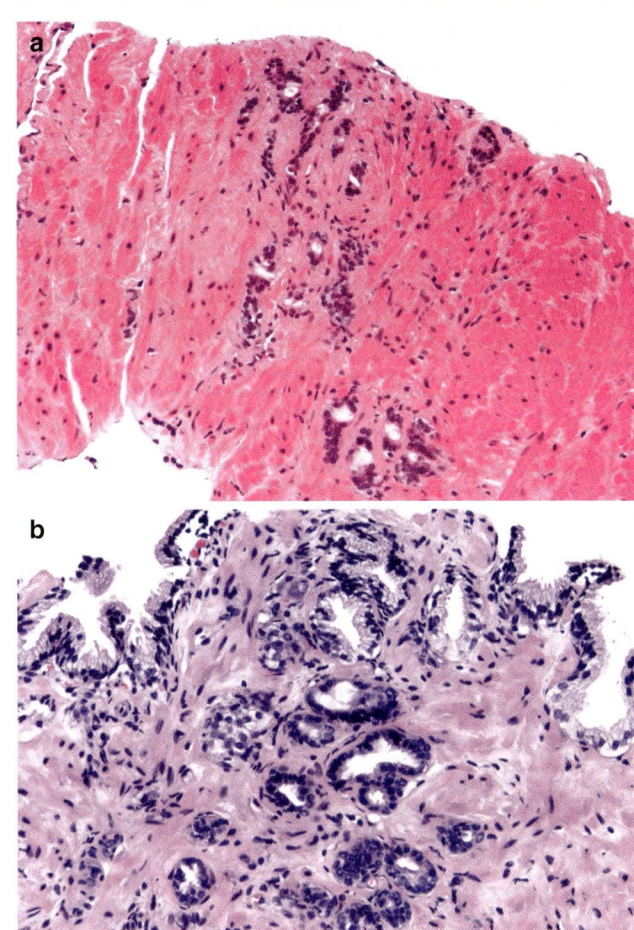

Fig. 7.12 Pseudoinfiltrative growth patterns in focal atrophy. (**a–b**) Benign atrophic glands with haphazard or pseudoinfiltrative growth pattern may raise concern at low-power examination (**a** and **b**). However, note that the pattern of infiltration is like a "patch" different than the true infiltration pattern with cancer glands situated between or on both sides of the benign glands

7.12 Adenosis (Atypical Adenomatous Hyperplasia)

Table 7.11 Adenosis (atypical adenomatous hyperplasia) [26–33]

Microscopical features

Low-power architecture

Well-circumscribed/lobulated lesion comprised of large complex glands typical of hyperplasia admixed and merging with small round glands (*see* Fig. 7.13)

Small and large glands have similar cytoplasmic and cytological features

Stroma is usually cellular and spindly

Crystalloids and basophilic mucin are occasionally present

High-power cytology

The lining cells have small nuclei with fine chromatin

Nucleoli are frequently present but are generally small (<1 μm). Macronucleoli (>3 μm) seen in adenocarcinoma are absent

Immunohistochemical features

Basal cell markers typically demonstrate fragmented or occasionally absent staining (*see* Fig. 7.13e)

AMACR is expressed either focally or diffusely in up to 30% of lesions (*see* Fig. 7.13f)

Incidence, location, and significance

Adenosis represents a part of the morphological spectrum of benign prostate hyperplasia and therefore is primarily encountered in the transition zone of the prostate

Relatively common finding in both radical prostatectomy and transurethral resection specimens. The incidence as a significant lesion, which may be confused as adenocarcinoma in the needle biopsy, is low (~1%)

Referred to as *atypical adenomatous hyperplasia* because of its overlapping features with low-grade adenocarcinoma and therefore has been considered a potential precursor for low-grade cancer. Most experts do not prefer to use the term *atypical* due to its potential misleading clinical implications and insufficient evidence of its preneoplastic potential

Many of the low-grade adenocarcinoma (Gleason grade 2–4) in the past represent examples of adenosis

Diffuse adenosis of the peripheral zone (DAPZ) refers to multiple foci of small, nonlobular proliferation of relatively bland acini diffusely involving the peripheral zone in young patients (average age, 49 y; range, 34–73 y). In needle biopsy, more than 70% of the biopsy cores are involved. Patients with DAPZ are considered at risk for harboring cancer, specifically those also containing foci of atypical glands. Compared to focal adenosis, repeat biopsy is recommended for DAPZ [33]

Differential diagnosis

Prostate cancer with Gleason score ≤6. In adenosis, small glands are admixed with obvious large hyperplastic benign glands; the cytoplasmic and cytological characteristics of small and large glands appear similar and the two essentially merge with each other (*see* Fig. 7.13a–d). Cancer glands, in comparison, invariably demonstrate differences in their cytoplasmic and cytological from the adjacent benign glands. Cellular spindly stroma also favors a reactive/proliferative process such as adenosis

Common diagnostic pitfalls

Visible nucleoli at high power, crystalloids, and occasional luminal mucin

Patchy, sometimes complete lack of staining with basal cell markers

AMACR expression in up to 30% of lesions

7.12 Adenosis (Atypical Adenomatous Hyperplasia) 93

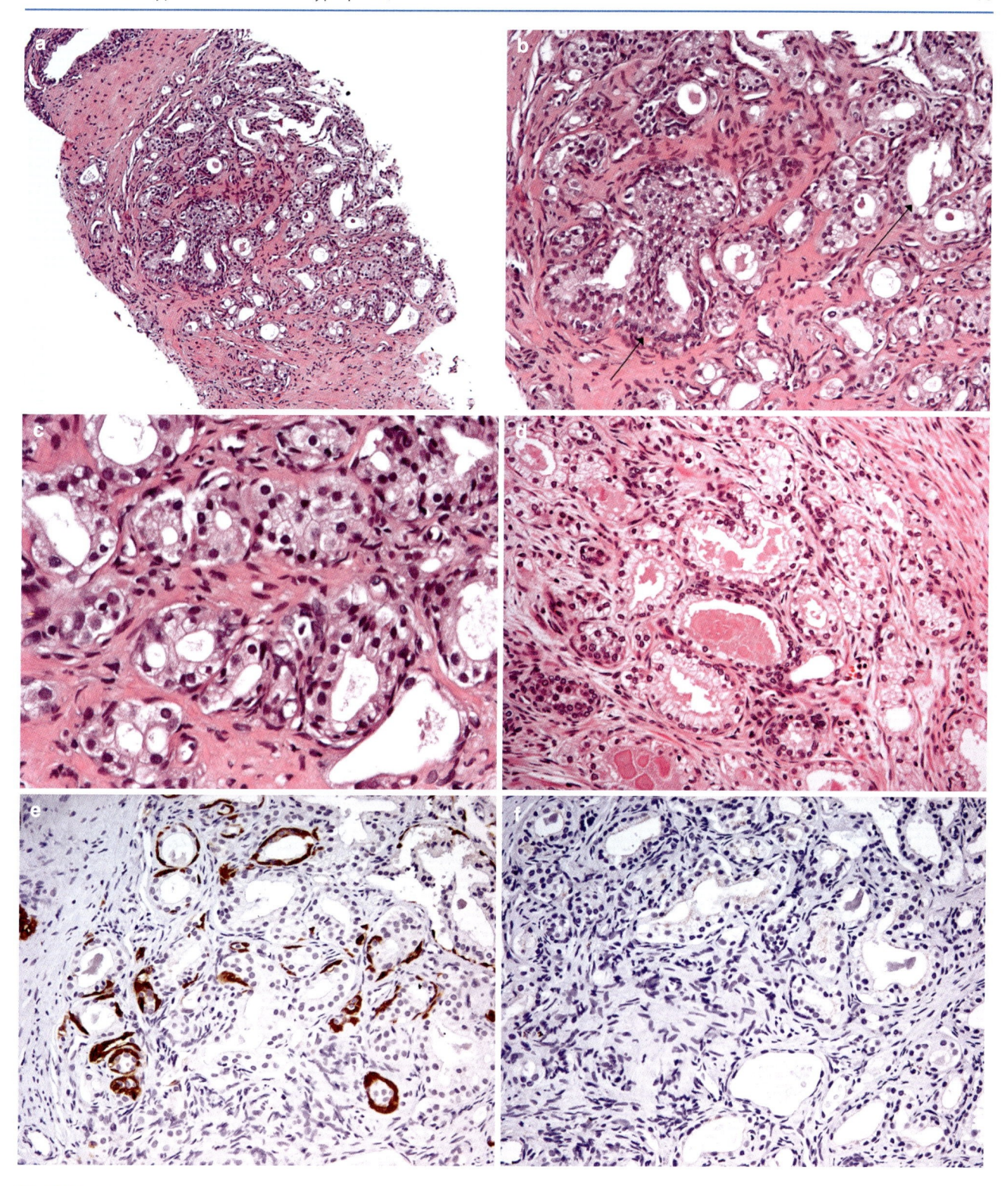

Fig. 7.13 Adenosis (atypical adenomatous hyperplasia). (**a–f**) At low power, adenosis is characterized by a circumscribed collection of variably sized glands (**a**). Within the nodule, small round acini are admixed with larger benign-appearing glands with papillary infolding (*arrows*). There are no obvious cytoplasmic or cytological differences between them. Essentially, small and large glands merge with each other imperceptibly (**b**). At high power, the columnar cells have abundant pale to clear cytoplasm and bland-appearing nuclei with inconspicuous to small nucleoli (**c**). The stroma between the glands is cellular, a feature to suggest a benign reactive nature (**d**). Basal cell markers typically demonstrate a discontinuous/patchy-staining pattern, with some glands lacking the staining (**e**). A small percentage (~30%) of adenosis lesions may demonstrate mild-to-moderate AMACR expression (**f**)

7.13 Basal Cell Hyperplasia

Table 7.12 Basal cell hyperplasia [34–41]

Microscopical features

Low-power architecture

Nodular or sometime haphazard proliferation of uniform round blue glands with stratified nuclei (*see* Fig. 7.14)

In the incomplete form, there are residual small lumina lined by secretory cells with clear cytoplasm that are surrounded by multiple layers of basal cells (*see* Fig. 7.14b). In the complete form, solid nests of dark-blue cells without luminal formation (*see* Fig. 7.14c)

The stroma is very cellular and consists of proliferating fibroblasts and smooth muscle cells similar to those seen in benign prostate hyperplasia

Other growth patterns include cribriform and pseudocribriform architecture (see Fig. 7.14e–f)

Microcalcifications are common

Rarely, intracytoplasmic hyaline globules are present, which is considered to be a specific feature of basal cell hyperplasia

High-power cytology

Oval or somewhat spindly nuclei with homogeneous glassy or vesicular chromatin

Cytoplasm is scant

Nucleoli are usually indistinct but sometimes are prominent and may raise concern for adenocarcinoma

Immunohistochemical features

Strong positivity for basal cell markers

AMACR is typically negative

Weak and focal positivity for PSA and PSAP

Incidence, location, and significance

Basal cell hyperplasia is typically seen as a part of the spectrum of benign prostatic hyperplasia in transition zone specimens; when pronounced, it is referred to as basal cell adenoma

Basal cell hyperplasia may also affect the peripheral zone and may be encountered in needle biopsies

Basal cell hyperplasia also occurs in atrophy, in the setting of anti-androgen therapy

Basal cell hyperplasia, even with atypical morphological presentation, is not associated with an adverse prognosis and therefore the term *atypical basal cell hyperplasia* should not be used

Differential diagnosis

Gleason score 6 prostate cancer demonstrating basaloid features or Gleason score 7–8 cribriform carcinomas. The adenocarcinoma usually demonstrates infiltrative features, round hyperchromatic nuclei with variable cytoplasm, and lacks densely cellular spindly stroma and microcalcifications

p63-positive basal cell prostate adenocarcinoma may be mistaken for basal cell hyperplasia (*see* Fig. 4.5), but negative for HMWCK

Basal cell hyperplasia, usual type or with adenoid cystic morphology, may mimic HGPIN (*see* Fig. 9.2). In basal cell hyperplasia, nucleoli are usually restricted to cells in basal aspect; cells have scant cytoplasm and the nuclei are ovoid, coffee bean–like

Rare adenoid cystic basal cell carcinoma of the prostate (*see* Fig. 6.17). The basal cell carcinoma exhibits infiltrative features such as stromal desmoplasia, necrosis, and mitoses. Immunohistochemical markers are not helpful in this distinction

Common diagnostic pitfalls

Pseudoinfiltrative growth pattern, prominent nucleoli, intraluminal blue mucin, and cellular stroma are common diagnostic pitfalls

7.13 Basal Cell Hyperplasia 95

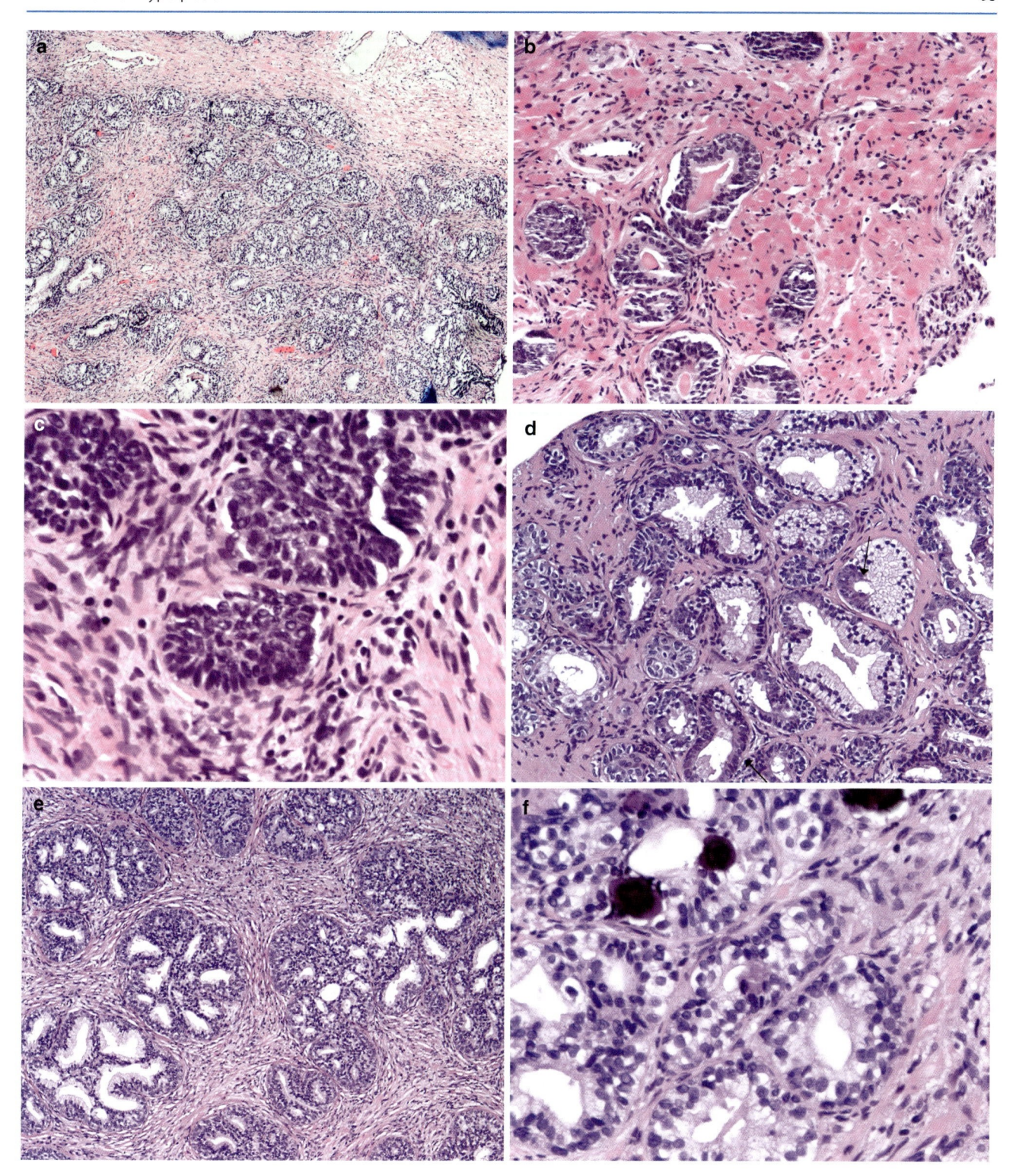

Fig. 7.14 Morphological spectrum of basal cell hyperplasia. (**a–f**) A well-circumscribed nodule of basal cell hyperplasia, also referred to as *basal cell adenoma* in transurethral resection specimen, is a form of epithelial hyperplasia in which glands have markedly stratified lining cells with high N:C ratio, and appears basophilic at low magnification (**a**). In incomplete basal cell hyperplasia, a luminal differentiation is seen (**b**). In complete basal cell hyperplasia, dark-staining nests are seen in a cellular stroma. Note the lack of lumen formation. The presence of cellular spindly stroma is a feature suggestive of the benign proliferative nature (**c**). In basal cell hyperplasia, nuclei are stratified, arranged like a pack of cigar without visible cytoplasm (**c**) and are coffee bean–like with frequent grooves and vesicular glassy chromatin. Prominent nucleoli are frequently seen (*arrows* in **d**). Basal cell hyperplasia can also present with adenoid cystic carcinoma-like cribriform architecture simulating cribriform carcinoma. Also note cellular spindly stroma (**e**). Intraluminal calcifications and cytoplasmic hyaline globules can be seen in basal cell hyperplasia (**f**)

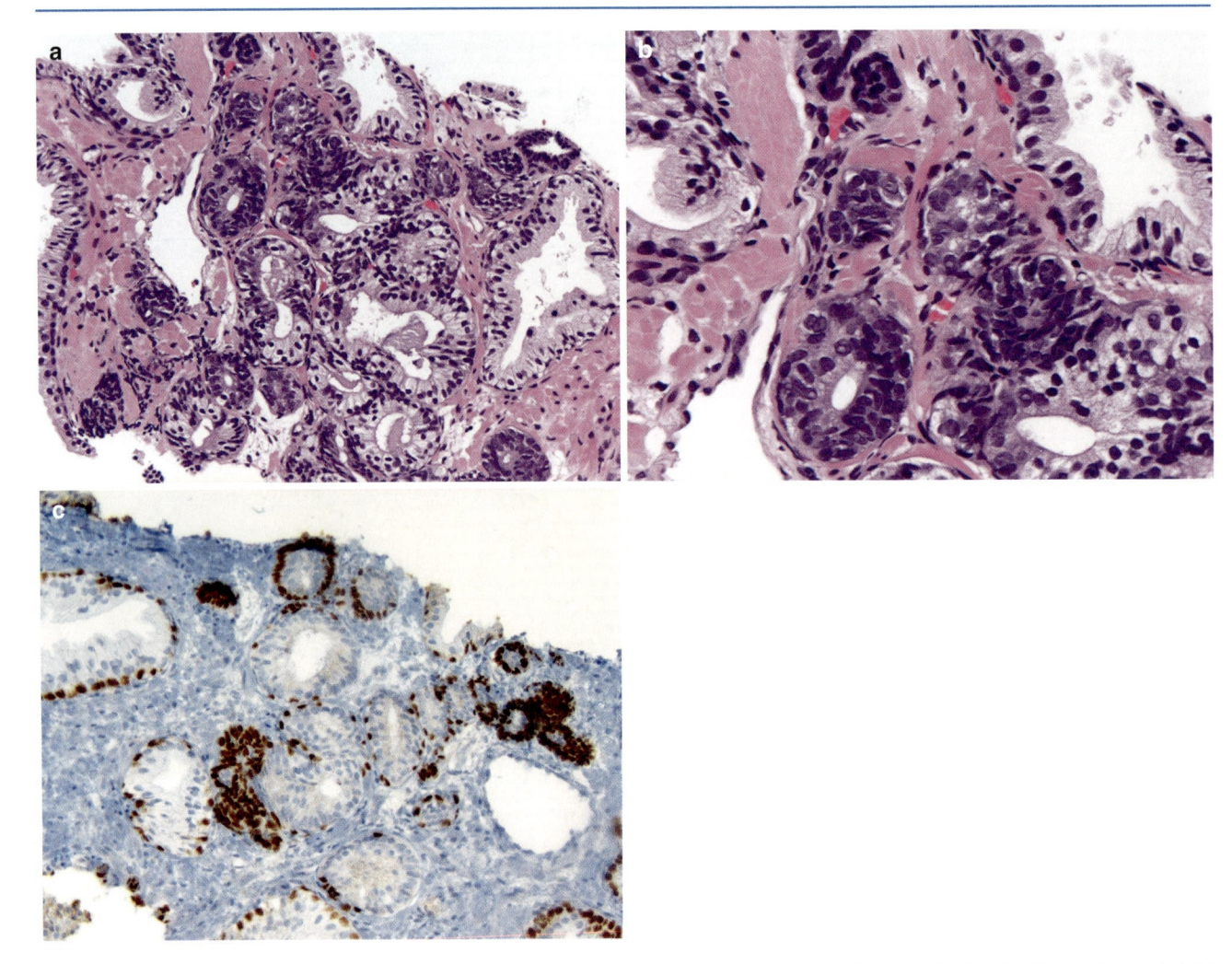

Fig. 7.15 Basal cell hyperplasia in prostate needle biopsy. (**a–c**) Dark-staining nests with stratified epithelium are seen in a haphazard pattern (**a**). Nuclei are stratified with frequent prominent nucleoli (**b**). Immunohistochemical markers for basal cell detection are helpful in difficult cases (**c**, p63)

7.14 Diagnostic Approach to Prostate Basal Cell Lesions

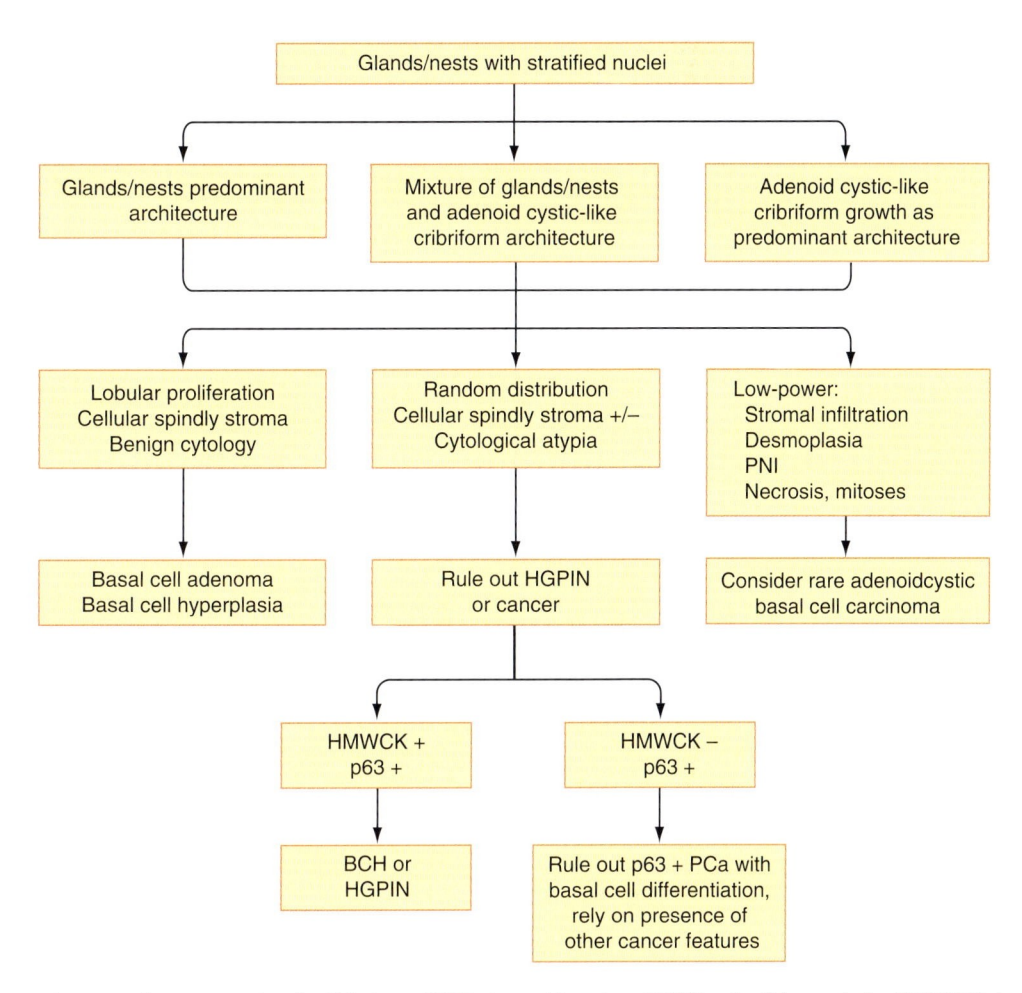

Fig. 7.16 Diagnostic approach to prostate basal cell lesions. *PNI* Perineural invasion, *BCH* Basal cell hyperplasia, *HGPIN* High grade prostatic intraepithelial neoplasia, *HMWCK* High molecular weight cytokeratin

7.15 Postradiation Atypia in Benign Prostate Glands

Table 7.13 Postradiation atypia in benign prostate glands [42–45]

Microscopical features

Low-power architecture

Small-to-medium atrophic glands with minimal cytoplasm are arranged in lobular architecture or random distribution within abundant stroma (*see* Fig. 7.17a–b)

High-power cytology

Presence of scattered marked cytological atypia within well-formed glands (*see* Fig. 7.17c)

Cells appear degenerative with smudgy chromatin, frequent prominent nucleoli, and cytoplasmic vacuolization (*see* Fig. 7.17c)

Immunohistochemical features

Basal cell markers are strongly positive in benign prostate glands with radiation atypia (*see* Fig. 7.17d)

Incidence, location, and significance

Thirty to 36 months following completion of radiation treatment, biopsy may be performed in patients with rising PSA to confirm or rule out the presence of recurrent/persistent tumor

Radiation atypia typically lasts for a prolonged time after radiation treatment. Effects are usually pronounced in the peripheral zone of the prostate

Residual adenocarcinoma in postradiation prostate may become an indication for salvage radical prostatectomy

Differential diagnosis

Benign prostatic tissue with radiation atypia is commonly mistaken for prostate adenocarcinoma with therapy effect or recurrent prostate adenocarcinoma and urothelial carcinoma in situ (CIS)

Residual adenocarcinoma with therapy effect demonstrates relatively small uniform pyknotic nuclei, lacks randomly distributed cytological atypia, and contains abundant vacuolated cytoplasm (*see* Fig. 7.18a). Recurrent adenocarcinoma has features typical of conventional adenocarcinoma

Urothelial CIS fills and expands the prostatic ducts and acini with diffuse cytological atypia (*see* Fig. 6.13)

Common diagnostic pitfalls

Radiation can induce marked nuclear enlargement and prominent nucleoli in benign prostatic tissue that mimics carcinoma

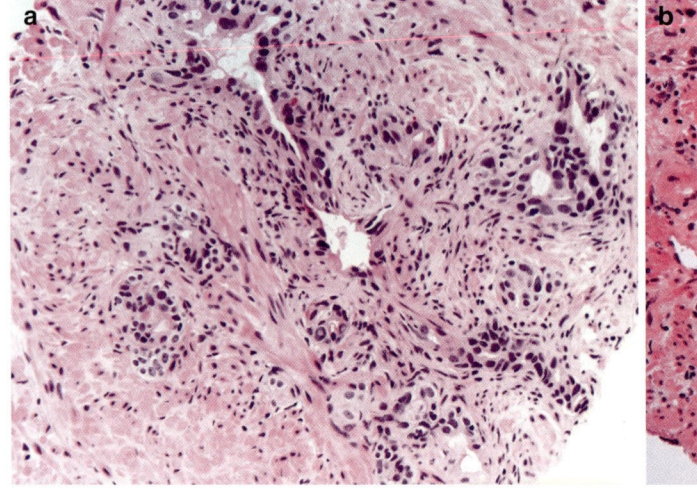

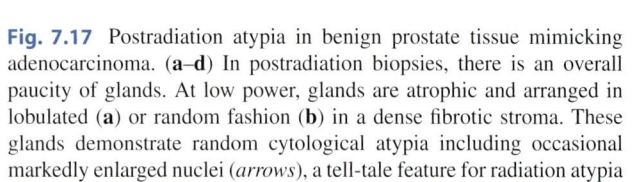

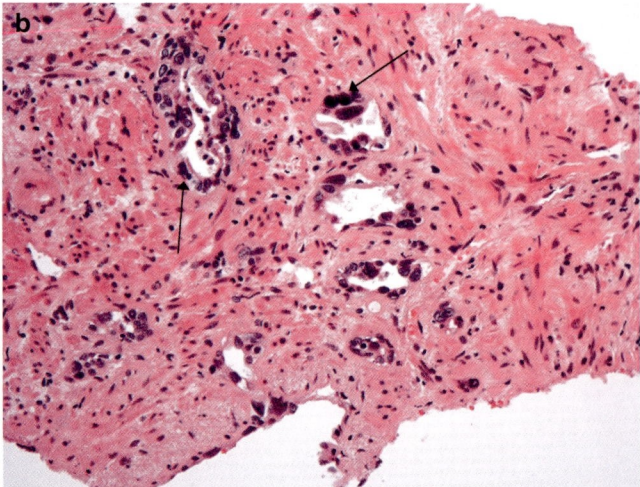

Fig. 7.17 Postradiation atypia in benign prostate tissue mimicking adenocarcinoma. (**a–d**) In postradiation biopsies, there is an overall paucity of glands. At low power, glands are atrophic and arranged in lobulated (**a**) or random fashion (**b**) in a dense fibrotic stroma. These glands demonstrate random cytological atypia including occasional markedly enlarged nuclei (*arrows*), a tell-tale feature for radiation atypia (**b**). At higher magnification, prominent nucleoli are visible, raising concern for cancer. However, the cytological atypia is random and degenerative in nature, and is characterized by hypochromatic nuclei with frequent cytoplasmic vacuolization (*arrow*, **c**). Prostate adenocarcinoma rarely demonstrates this degree of cytological atypia. Basal cell markers are very helpful to confirm the diagnosis in difficult cases (**d**)

7.15 Postradiation Atypia in Benign Prostate Glands

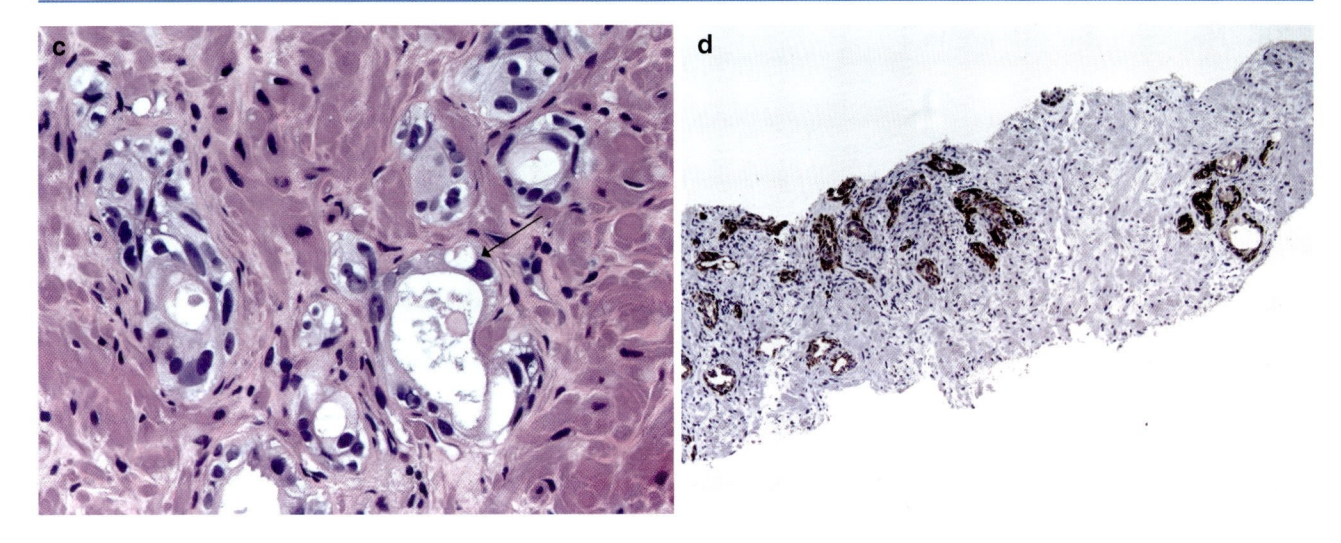

Fig. 7.17 (continued)

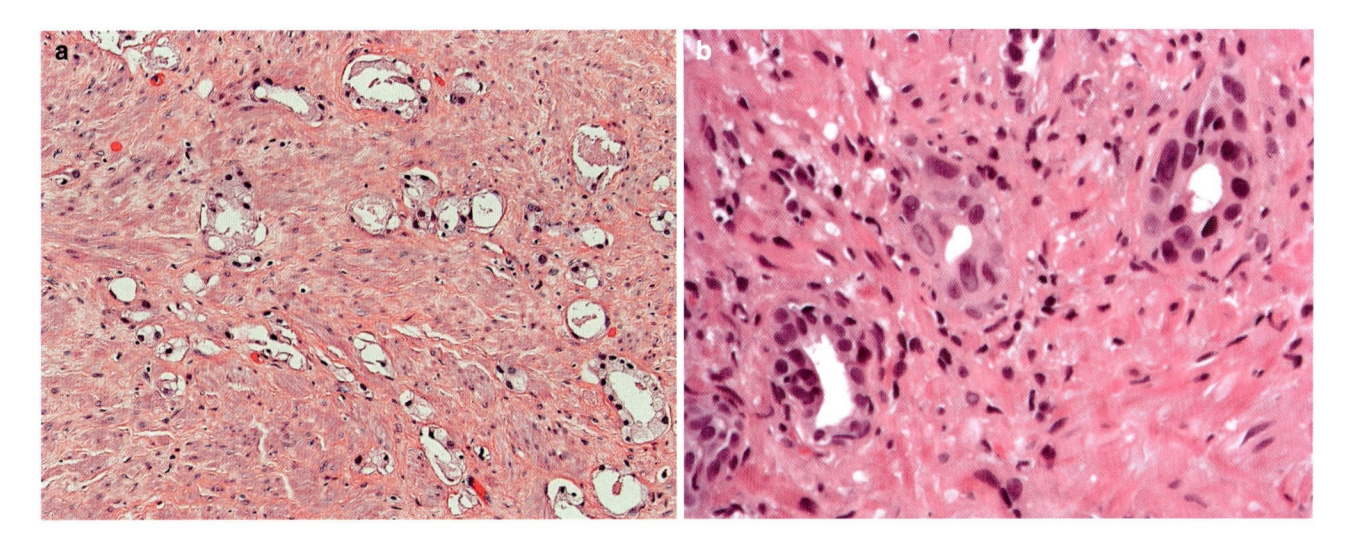

Fig. 7.18 Comparison of morphological features of radiation atypia in benign prostate tissue and adenocarcinoma with radiation therapy effect. (**a–b**) In residual adenocarcinoma demonstrating treatment effect, cancer glands grow in a haphazard manner, show frequent tumor breakdown with poorly formed glands and single cells, relatively abundant cytoplasm, and uniform cytological atypia. Nuclei are small and frequently shrunken (**a**). In contrast, in benign glands with radiation atypia, glands are arranged in lobular configuration and appear atrophic. Nuclear atypia is random and degenerative in nature (**b**)

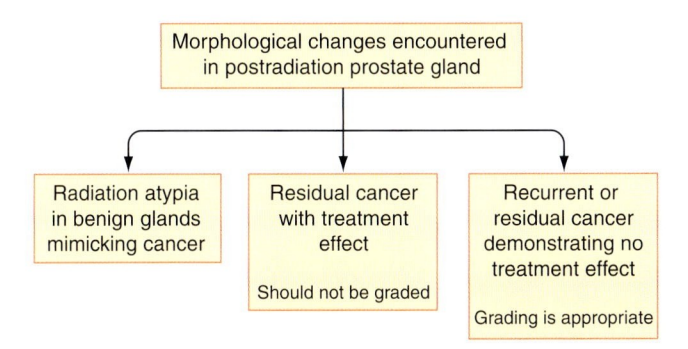

Fig. 7.19 Morphological changes encountered in postradiation prostate gland

7.16 Nephrogenic Adenoma

Table 7.14 Nephrogenic adenoma [46–48]

Microscopical features

Low-power architecture

Presence of both exophytic papillary and infiltrative tubulocystic components is a characteristic feature (*see* Fig. 7.20a)

The tubulocystic architecture ranges from small poorly formed glands, small tubules resembling renal tubules, signet ring–type cells to dilated cystic structures resembling ectatic vessels (*see* Fig. 7.20)

Lining epithelium characteristically is flat cuboidal to hobnail

High-power cytology

Nuclei are uniform with frequent prominent nucleoli; mitosis rare

Nuclear atypia when present is usually degenerative in nature

Intraluminal mucin is frequent

The tubules are frequently surrounded by thick basement membrane (*see* Fig. 7.20a), which can be highlighted with PAS stain

Inflammation is frequent within the lesions

Immunohistochemical features

Majority express PAX-2, PAX-8, and AMACR (*see* Fig. 7.20h–l)

PSA and PAP are usually negative

Cytoplasmic 34βE12 staining in >50% of cases

A panel of PAX-2 or PAX-8, PSA, PAP, and 34βE12 is useful to establish the diagnosis in difficult cases

Incidence and location

It commonly involves the urinary bladder but may occur in any part of the urinary tract including the prostatic urethra (~10%)

Typically encountered in transurethral resections

Rarely seen in prostate needle biopsy

Differential diagnosis

Prostate adenocarcinoma, nested urothelial carcinoma, papillary urothelial carcinoma, and clear cell or adenocarcinoma not otherwise specified (NOS) type

A mixture of papillary and tubulocystic components lined with bland cuboidal cells, periglandular collagen corollate, and inflammatory background are the most useful diagnostic features to distinguish nephrogenic adenoma from its mimics

In urothelial carcinoma, the papillary component demonstrates nuclear stratification

Clear cell adenocarcinoma has infiltrative growth and frank malignant cytology

History of prior treatment, trauma, stones, or other long-standing irritation is present in most cases

Common diagnostic pitfalls

Papillary and tubulocystic components may not be present in the same lesion. In prostatic urethra, the papillary component is often absent, making diagnosis difficult (*see* Fig. 7.20b)

Small percentage of cases present with predominantly nested or poorly formed glands (*see* Fig. 7.20e–f)

Blue mucin and cytological atypia including prominent nucleoli may be present

Extension into stroma or muscle can be rarely seen in a small percentage of cases

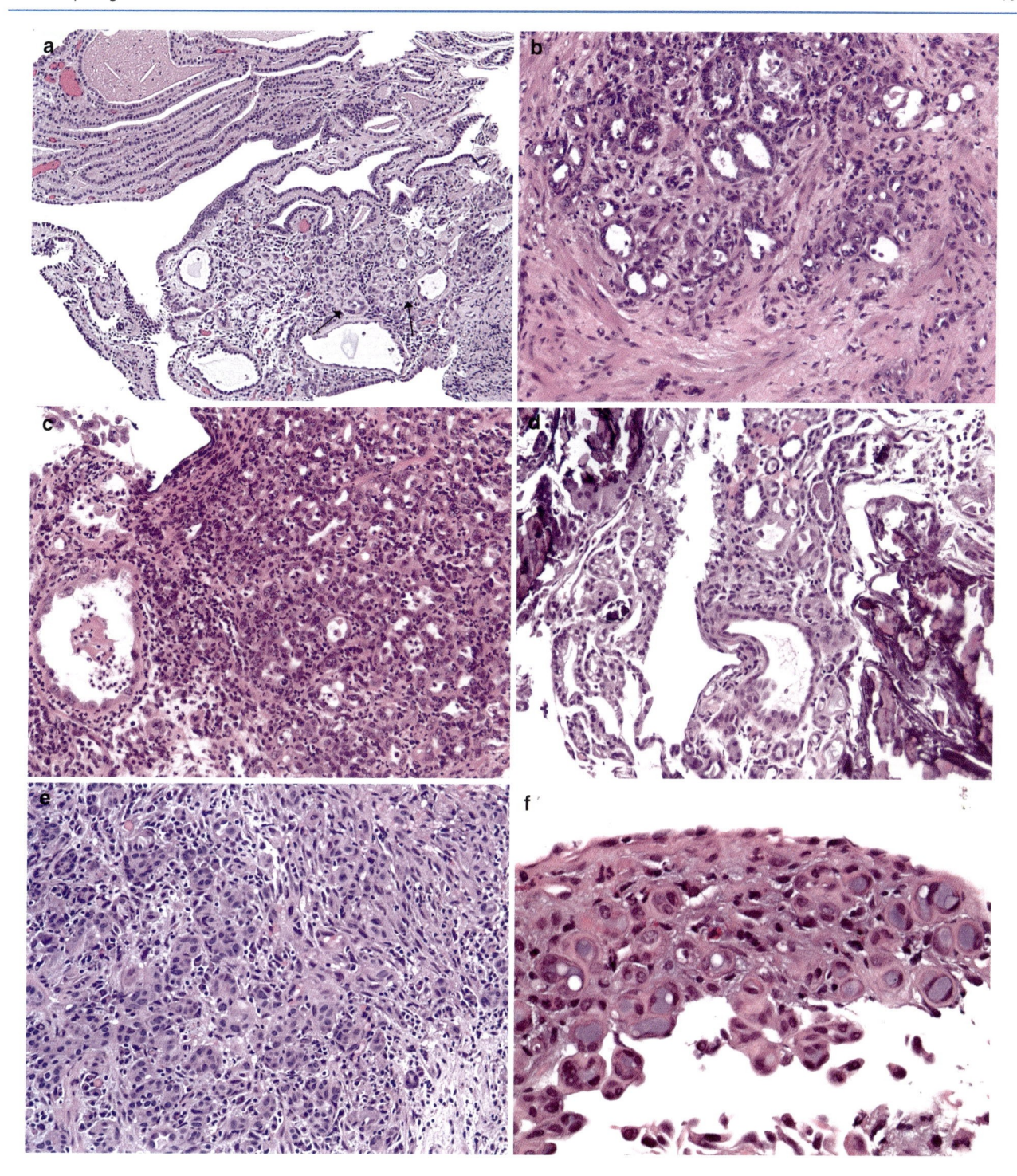

Fig. 7.20 Morphological spectrum of nephrogenic adenoma. (**a**–**i**) A classical nephrogenic adenoma with both papillary and underlying tubular components. Polypoid or papillary component has edematous stroma without well-defined fibrovascular cores and lining epithelium is cuboidal and lacks stratification. Underlying tubules are variably sized and mimic renal tubules. Note thickened eosinophilic basement membrane surrounding tubules (*arrow*), one of the characteristic features of nephrogenic adenoma (**a**). Prostatic urethra biopsy exhibits exclusively a tubular component, mimicking a prostate adenocarcinoma (**b**). In prostatic urethra, this type of presentation is common. The tubules are lined by cuboidal hobnail epithelium. Degenerative cytological atypia and features such as intraluminal blue mucin can be encountered. Background inflammation and calcifications are common (**c** and **d**). Nephrogenic adenoma in transurethral resection specimen, presenting predominantly with nested (**e**) and signet ring cell-like (**f**) pattern. These patterns may be mistaken for nested urothelial carcinoma and poorly differentiated prostate adenocarcinoma. Hyalinized basement membrane surrounding glands (**f**) and superficial nature of the lesion (**e**) are useful features to suggest the diagnosis. Rarely, nephrogenic adenoma may present with prominent fibrous and myxoid component (**g**). Cytoplasmic AMACR expression is present in the vast majority of nephrogenic adenoma, a significant pitfall if this marker is utilized to distinguish nephrogenic adenoma from prostate adenocarcinoma (**h**). Nuclear transcription factors PAX-2 or PAX-8 are expressed in nephrogenic adenoma and are helpful markers to support the diagnosis in difficult cases (**i**)

7.17 Cribriform Proliferations in the Prostate Gland

Table 7.15 Cribriform proliferations encountered in the prostate gland

Benign	Atypical cribriform lesions with basal cells
Central zone glands	Cribriform HGPIN
Reactive glands with pseudocribriform architecture	Intraductal carcinoma of the prostate
Proliferative lesions	*Malignant lesions*
Clear cell cribriform hyperplasia	Cribriform carcinoma spectrum (includes Gleason pattern 3, 4, 5 cancers, large duct, and PIN-like cancers)
Adenoid cystic-like basal cell hyperplasia	Adenoid cystic basal cell carcinoma

7.18 Central Zone Glands

Table 7.16 Central zone glands [49, 50]

Microscopical features

Low-power architecture

Large, complex glands with papillary infoldings that may demonstrate Roman bridges and cribriform pattern (*see* Fig. 7.21)

The glands are lined by tall pseudostratified epithelium with dense eosinophilic cytoplasm and conspicuous basal cell layer

High-power cytology

The cytological atypia is rarely seen and is restricted to the basal cell layer (*see* Fig. 7.21c)

Immunohistochemical features

Immunostains for basal cell markers highlight intact and prominent basal cells

Incidence and location

Commonly encountered in needle biopsies sampled from the base of the prostate

Differential diagnosis

The central zone glands usually mimic HGPIN and, rarely, cribriform carcinoma

Large complex glands with dense eosinophilic cytoplasm; especially when seen in the base of the prostate biopsies raise consideration for central zone glands

HGPIN has significant nuclear enlargement and prominent nucleoli

Cribriform carcinoma has significant nuclear enlargement and prominent nucleoli and lacks basal cell layer

Common diagnostic pitfalls

Complex papillation, Roman bridges, nuclear stratification, cribriform architecture, and cytoplasmic amphophilia raise suspicion for HGPIN or cancer diagnosis

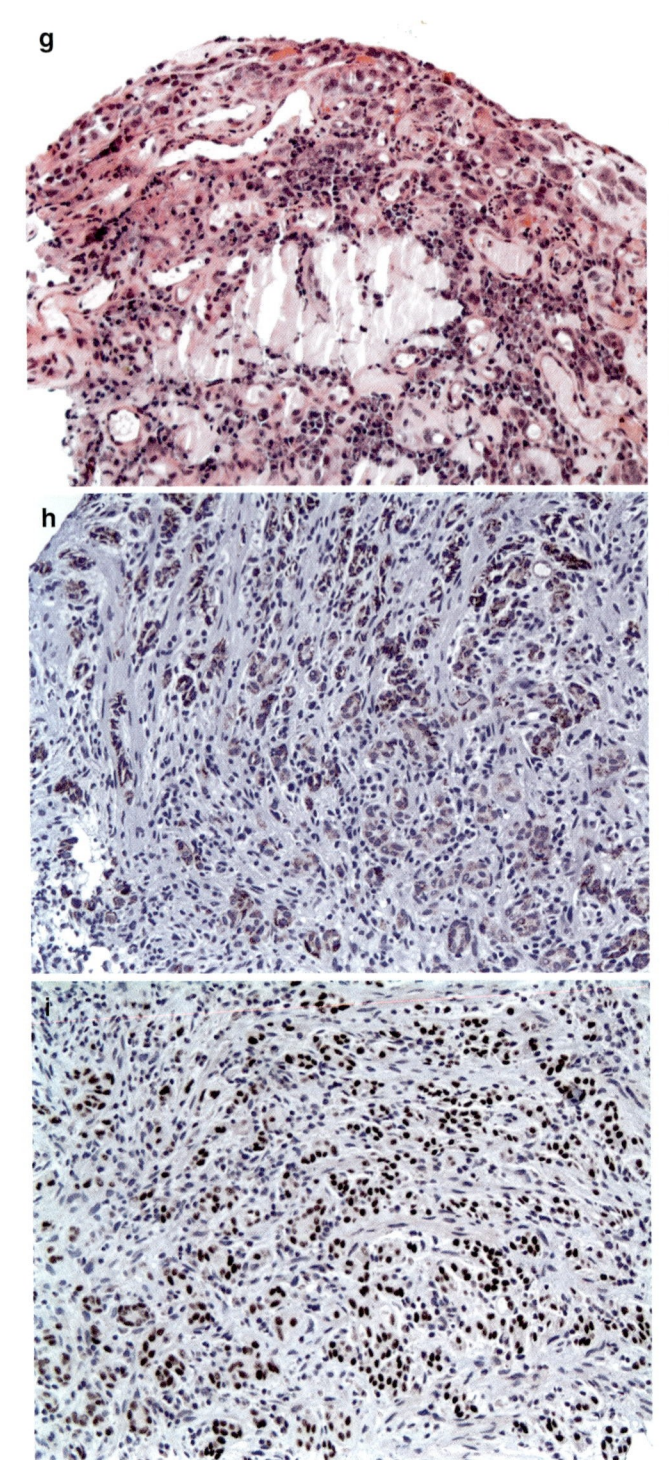

Fig. 7.20 (continued)

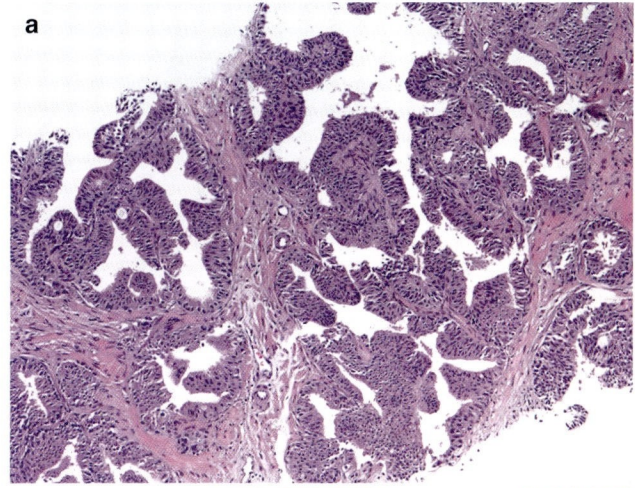

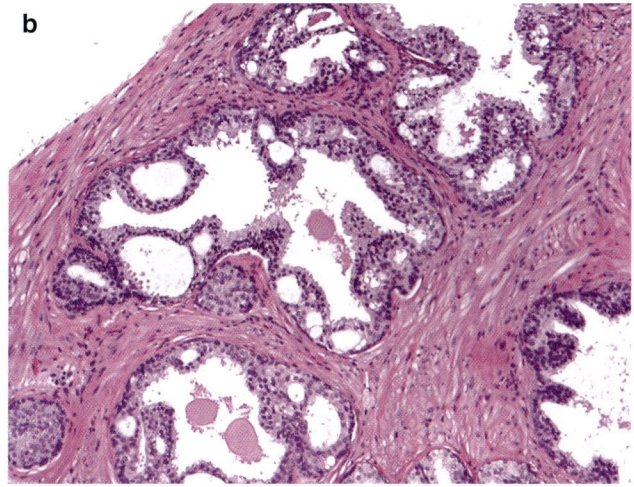

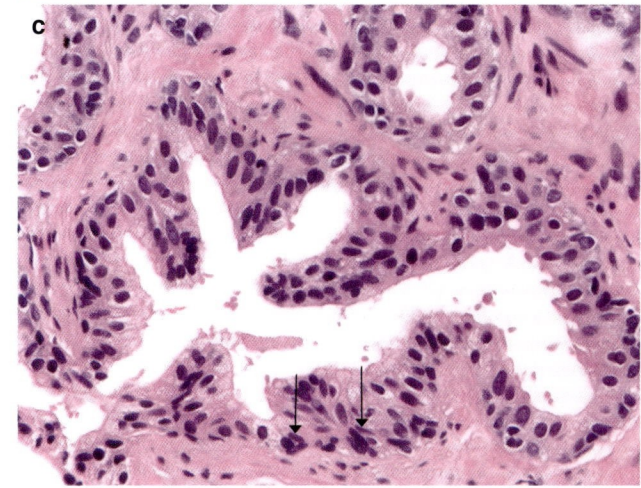

7.19 Clear Cell Cribriform Hyperplasia

Table 7.17 Clear cell cribriform hyperplasia [51]

Microscopical features

Low-power architecture

Nodular proliferation of crowded cribriform glands (*see* Fig. 7.22a)

Cribriform glands have uniform, round lumina and lack complex/confluent architecture (*see* Fig. 7.22)

Strikingly prominent basal cell layer around many cribriform glands (*see* Fig. 7.22b)

High-power cytology

The cells have uniform round nuclei and clear cytoplasm

Immunohistochemical features

Immunostains for basal cell markers highlight prominent continuous layer of basal cells

Incidence and location

Clear cell cribriform hyperplasia represents a spectrum of benign prostate hyperplasia and can occasionally dominate the histological picture

Exclusively seen in TURP specimens from the transition zone of the prostate gland

Differential diagnosis

Differential diagnosis includes central zone glands, HGPIN, and cribriform carcinoma

Central zone glands have prominent eosinophilic cytoplasm

HGPIN exhibits significant nuclear enlargement and prominent nucleoli and often discontinuous basal cell layer

Cribriform carcinoma exhibits significant nuclear atypia and lacks basal cell layer and often is associated with conventional acinar carcinoma

Common diagnostic pitfalls

Cribriform architecture and crowded growth pattern

Fig. 7.21 Central zone histology mimicking HGPIN. (**a**–**c**) Central zone histology is typically a mimicker of HGPIN; however, prominent cribriform architecture in some cases may mimic cancer. This histology is typically seen in biopsies from the base of the prostate. In the central zone, glands are complex with frequent papillation and undulating architecture with pseudostratified lining epithelium (**a**). At low magnification, glands demonstrate distinct cytoplasmic eosinophilia (**a**). Roman bridges and cribriform architecture are common (**b**). In contrast to HGPIN, nuclei stream parallel to bridges in comparison to perpendicular orientation in HGPIN (**b**). The cytological atypia is seen in basal cells (*arrow*), a feature helpful to differentiate from HGPIN or cancer (**c**). Before making a diagnosis of HGPIN or atypia in biopsies from the base area of the prostate, central zone histology should be ruled out

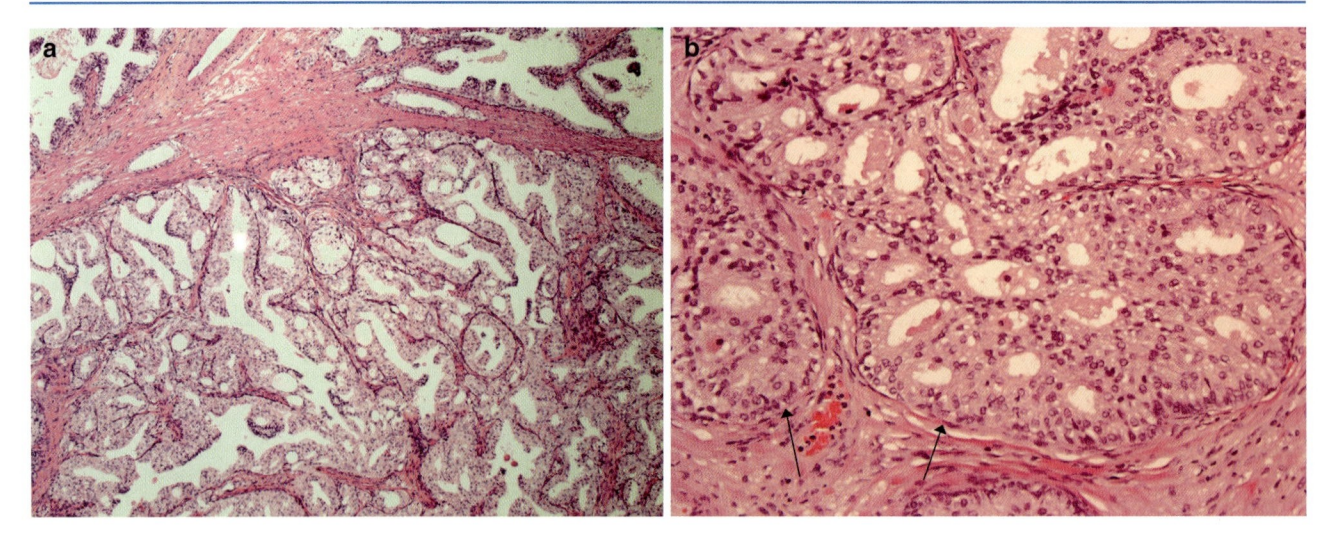

Fig. 7.22 Clear cell cribriform hyperplasia. (**a**–**b**) Clear cell cribriform hyperplasia represents a spectrum of benign prostate hyperplasia and therefore is typically encountered in the transition zone of the prostate. In this transurethral resection specimen, there is a nodular proliferation of nonconfluent cribriform glands with clear to eosinophilic cytoplasm (**a**). The cells forming the central lumina are cuboidal to low columnar secretory-type cells, with uniform round nuclei and clear cytoplasm. The glands (*arrows*) are rimmed with a prominent basal cell layer (**b**)

7.20 Differential Diagnosis of Prostate Cribriform Lesions

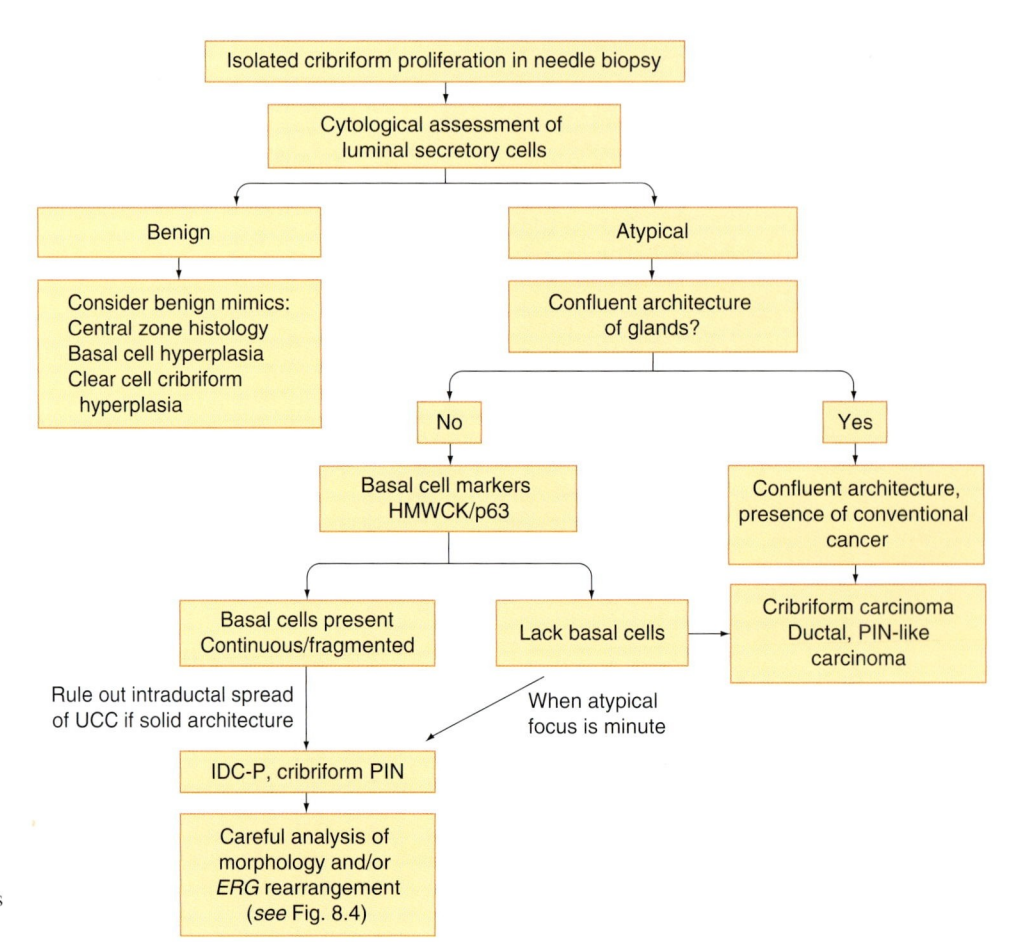

Fig. 7.23 Differential diagnosis of prostate cribriform lesions

7.21 Nonspecific Granulomatous Prostatitis

Table 7.18 Nonspecific granulomatous prostatitis (NSGP) [52–54]

Microscopical features

Low-power architecture

Earlier lesion is characterized by dilated ducts and acini filled with neutrophils, and desquamated epithelial cells and necrotic debris. Focal rupture of these ducts and acini leads to localized chronic granulomatous inflammatory response (*see* Fig. 7.24a)

Advanced lesions are characterized by dense lobular infiltrate of inflammatory cells comprising of lymphocytes, plasma cells, eosinophils, and scattered neutrophils, epithelioid histiocytes, and multinucleated giant cells, obscuring and effacing the ductal and acinar elements (*see* Fig. 7.24b–c)

Older lesions may show a more prominent fibrous component

High-power cytology

Polymorphic inflammatory infiltrate

Many epithelioid histiocytes have a foamy appearance and some are multinucleated; well-formed granulomas are rare

Necrosis is usually rare and noncaseating in nature

Immunohistochemical features

The epithelioid histiocytes are negative for cytokeratin, PSA, PSAP, and positive for histiocytic marker CD-68

Incidence and location

Relatively rare presentation. Incidence < 3% in unselected series of prostate biopsies

Peripheral zones are typically involved but the entire prostate may be affected

Differential diagnosis

High-grade Gleason 8–10 prostate carcinoma. The presence of single cells or nests with infiltrative growth pattern, variable cytological atypia, lack of multinuclear giant cells and mixed inflammatory infiltrates, and positivity for cytokeratins and prostate markers support the diagnosis of carcinoma

Granulomatous inflammation secondary to Bacillus Calmette-Guerin (BCG) therapy in patients with bladder cancer and due to infectious granulomatous prostatitis (*see* Fig. 7.25). Multinucleated giant cells and granulomas easily identified; caseating necrosis may be present; special stains for microorganisms may identify infectious agents

Common diagnostic pitfalls

Granulomatous prostatitis may simulate carcinoma both clinically as well as microscopically. Clinically, the prostate often feels firm to hard. Serum PSA level is often elevated in the range of 30–40 ng/mL with PSA > 4 ng/mL seen in the majority of nonspecific granulomatous prostatitis

When granulomatous and chronic inflammation is florid and diffuse, prostate ducts may not be appreciated and therefore, it may raise the suspicion for a high-grade, Gleason pattern 5 carcinoma. The problem is often amplified if poor preservation or mechanical artifacts are present

106   7   Benign Mimics of Prostate Carcinoma

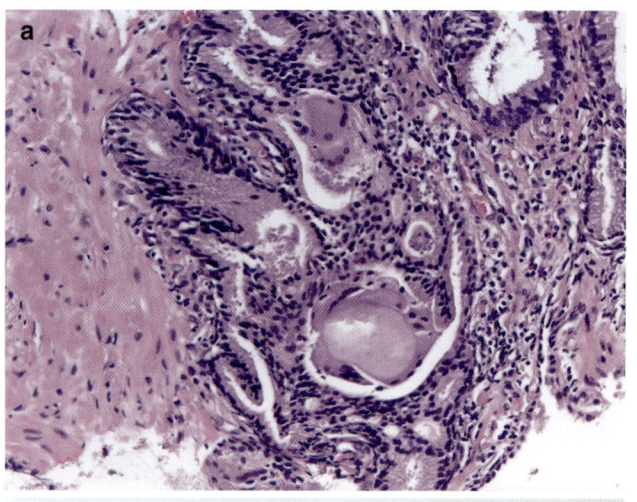

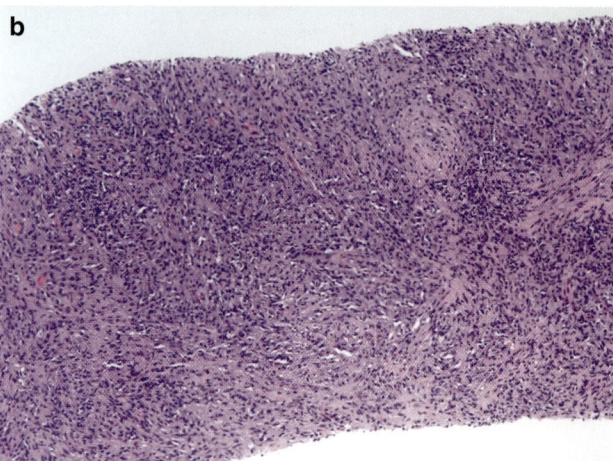

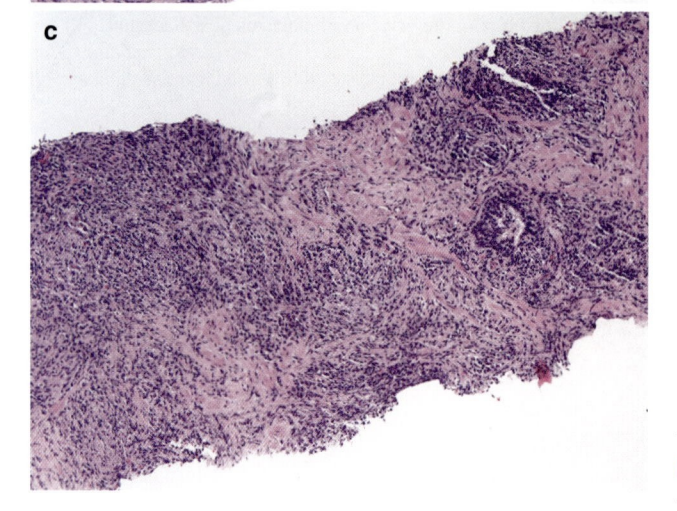

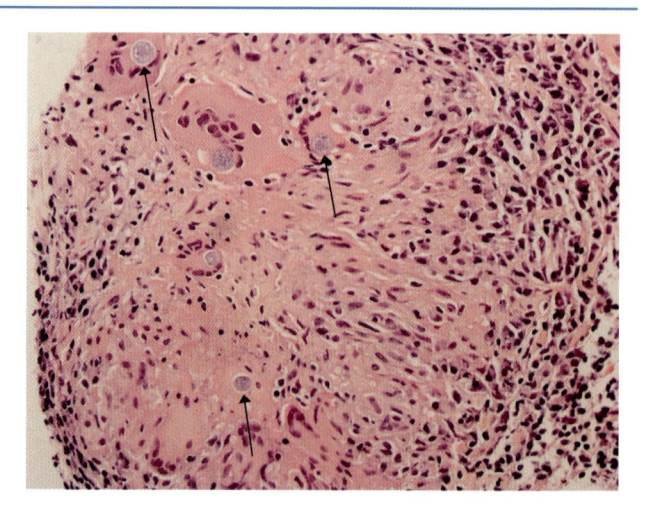

Fig. 7.25 Granulomatous prostatitis secondary to blastomycosis (*arrows*). Nonspecific granulomatous prostatitis should be differentiated from granulomatous inflammation secondary to BCG therapy in patients with bladder cancer or due to infectious granulomatous prostatitis. Clinical history, caseous necrosis, and well-formed granulomas provide clues to infectious etiology. Special stains for microorganisms may identify inciting agents (*arrows*)

Fig. 7.24 Nonspecific granulomatous prostatitis. (**a**) Early lesion is characterized by dilated ducts and acini filled with neutrophils, giant cells, debris, and desquamated epithelial cells. Rupture of these ducts and acini leads to localized chronic granulomatous inflammatory response (**a**). A more advanced lesion is characterized by dense lobular infiltrate of inflammatory cells comprised of lymphocytes, plasma cells, eosinophils and scattered neutrophils, epithelioid histiocytes, and multinucleated giant cells, obscuring and effacing the ductal and acinar structure (**b**). When granulomatous and chronic inflammation is florid and diffuse, prostate ducts may be obliterated, raising suspicion for a high-grade, Gleason pattern 5 carcinoma. This problem is further exaggerated by poor tissue fixation and processing artifact (**c**). Careful examination at high power reveals histiocytic and inflammatory nature of the lesion

7.22 Malakoplakia

Table 7.19 Malakoplakia [55, 56]

Microscopical features

Low-power architecture

Sheet-like proliferation of epithelioid histiocytes with abundant eosinophilic cytoplasm (*see* Fig. 7.27)

In classic and late stages, there is an admixture of inflammatory cells comprising of lymphocytes, plasma cells, neutrophils, and histiocytes, whereas in late stages, there is also a component of fibrosis

High-power cytology

Nuclei are bland, pale, and angulated and cytoplasm is typically eosinophilic and bubbly

Intracytoplasmic targetoid Michaelis-Gutmann bodies are characteristic (*see* Fig. 7.27)

Immunohistochemical features

Positive for CD-68 and negative for cytokeratins and PSA

Michaelis-Gutmann bodies can be highlighted by PAS, iron, and copper stains

Incidence and location

Rare lesion

Differential diagnosis

High-grade Gleason score 8–10 prostate carcinoma. The presence of a diffuse sheet of pink epithelioid histiocytes associated with necrosis may mimic high-grade carcinoma. The problem is amplified if the cellular preservation is poor. The presence of variable acinar differentiation, cytological atypia, and positivity for cytokeratins and prostate markers help establish carcinoma diagnosis in difficult cases

Xanthogranulomatous prostatitis can be ruled out with the recognition of Michaelis-Gutmann bodies, which can be highlighted by a PAS stain

Common diagnostic pitfalls

Diffuse sheet-like arrangement of pink epithelioid histiocytes obscuring the acini and ducts is the common pitfall that may simulate a high-grade malignancy at low power. The problem may be significantly amplified if cellular preservation is poor

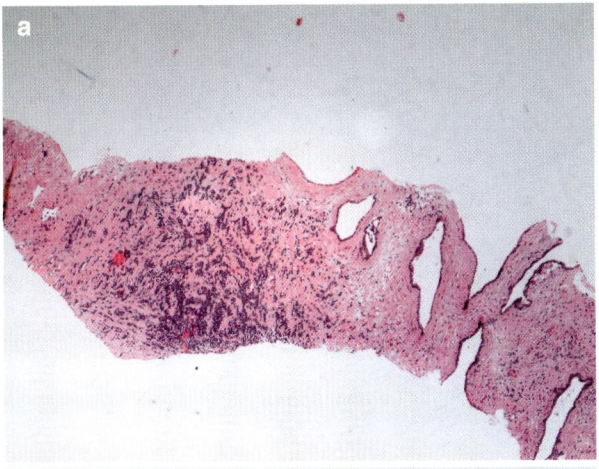

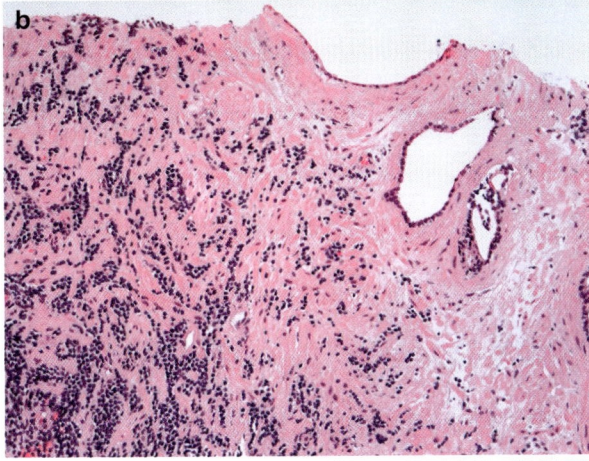

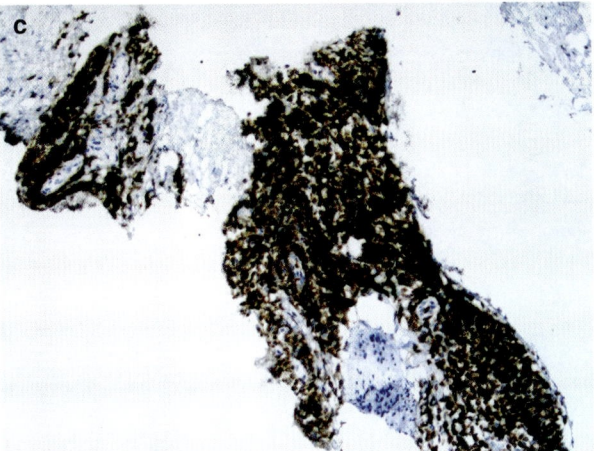

Fig. 7.26 Small lymphocytic lymphoma/chronic lymphocytic leukemia (SLL/CLL) mimicking nonspecific chronic inflammation. SLL/CLL can be infrequently encountered in the prostate biopsies performed for elevated PSA and/or prostate enlargement. Such infiltrate is often overlooked as nonspecific chronic inflammation. If monotonous small lymphocytic infiltrate is multifocal/diffuse in distribution and is not centered around ducts and acini, a lymphoproliferative process should be considered and ruled out (**a** and **b**). Review of clinical history including peripheral blood counts along with a select panel of immunohistochemical markers should be performed to rule out SLL/CLL. In this example, the patient had CLL and small monotonous lymphoid infiltrate in prostate biopsy demonstrated expression for B cell markers CD79a (strong; **c**) and CD20 (weak) with coexpression of CD43 and CD5 and lack of expression for CD3, supporting the diagnosis of CLL involving the prostate gland

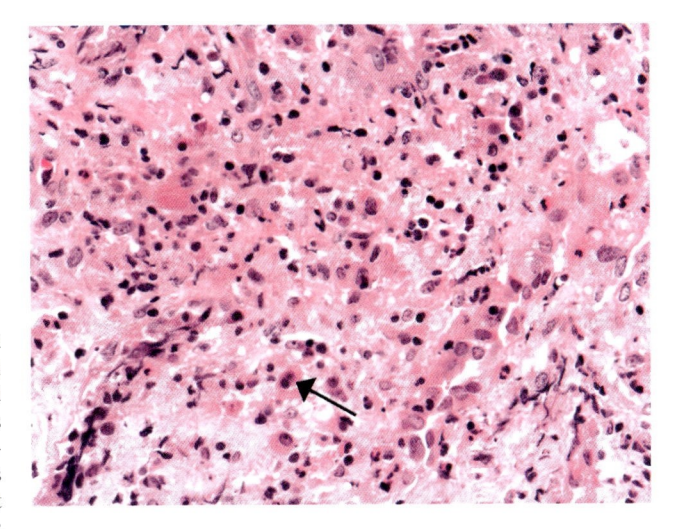

Fig. 7.27 Malakoplakia. In this transurethral resection specimen, there is a diffuse sheet-like proliferation of pink epithelioid histiocytes, accompanied by other inflammatory cells, similar to nonspecific xanthogranulomatous prostatitis. The histiocytic nature of epithelioid cells and the presence of Michaelis-Gutmann bodies (*arrow*) suggest the diagnosis of malakoplakia

7.23 Sclerosing Adenosis

Table 7.20 Sclerosing adenosis [57–60]

Microscopical features
Low-power architecture
Circumscribed proliferation of variably sized and shaped glands and individual cells in a dense spindle cellular stroma (*see* Fig. 7.28)
Glands are frequently compressed with slit-like lumens
High-power cytology
Prominent nucleoli and blue mucin are commonly present
Thick hyaline basement membrane surrounding the glands
Basal cell layer usually present but is difficult to appreciate on hematoxylin and eosin stain examination
Immunohistochemical features
Basal cells undergo myoepithelial metaplasia; coexpress basal cell and myoepithelial markers (muscle-specific actin and S-100)
AMACR is expressed in a small percentage of lesions
Incidence and location
Extremely rare in prostate needle biopsy and largely restricted to the transition zone of the prostate and generally seen as an incidental finding in TURP or radical prostatectomy specimens
Differential diagnosis
High-grade Gleason score 8–10 prostate carcinoma. The lack of circumscription, prominent cytological atypia, and negative basal cell markers suggests a carcinoma diagnosis
Common diagnostic pitfalls
Complex or poorly formed fused glands with slit-like lumina, frequent prominent nucleoli, and blue mucin are often confused with high-grade prostate cancer

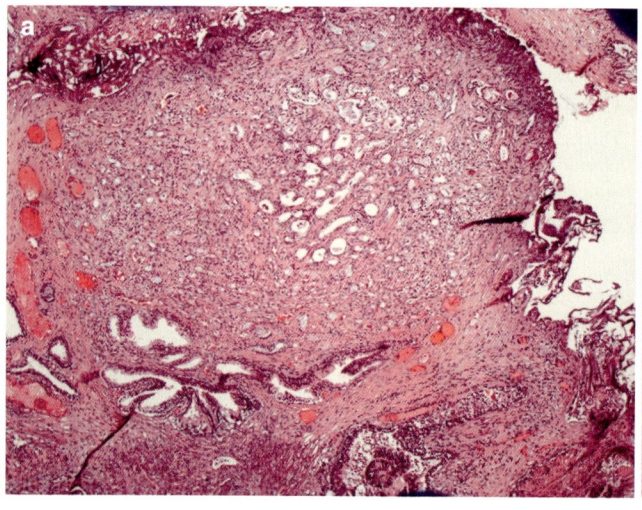

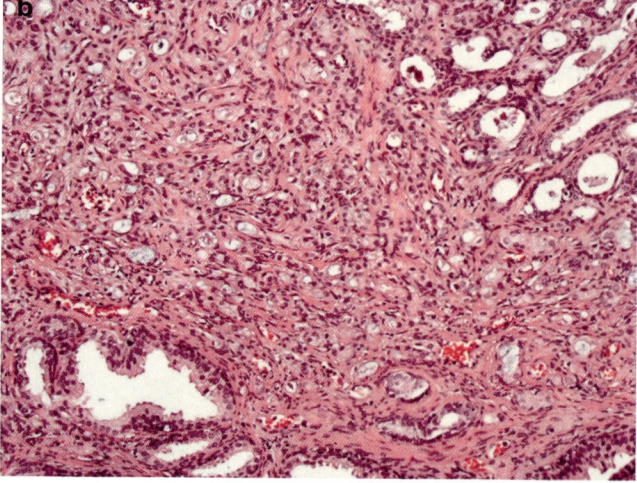

Fig. 7.28 Sclerosing adenosis mimicking high-grade prostate carcinoma. (**a–f**) This TURP specimen demonstrates a proliferation of poorly formed and complex glands mimicking high-grade prostate carcinoma. Low-power recognition is a key. It typically forms a well-circumscribed nodule of tightly packed glands (**a**). At high magnification, glands demonstrate complex proliferation, poorly formed glands with slit-like lumina, fused glands, and even single cells with signet ring cell-like features, mimicking high-grade cancer (**b**). Stroma surrounding the glands is cellular and hyalinized (*arrows*) (**c**). Prominent nucleoli, crystalloids, and blue mucin are common (**d**). Basal cells are highlighted with basal cell marker p63 (**e**). Basal cells undergo myoepithelial metaplasia and show coexpression of basal cell markers and S-100 (**f**) and muscle-specific actin. When one or more well-circumscribed cellular lesions mimicking high-grade prostate cancer are encountered in TURP or biopsies from the transition zone of the prostate, sclerosing adenosis should be ruled out

7.24 Paraganglia

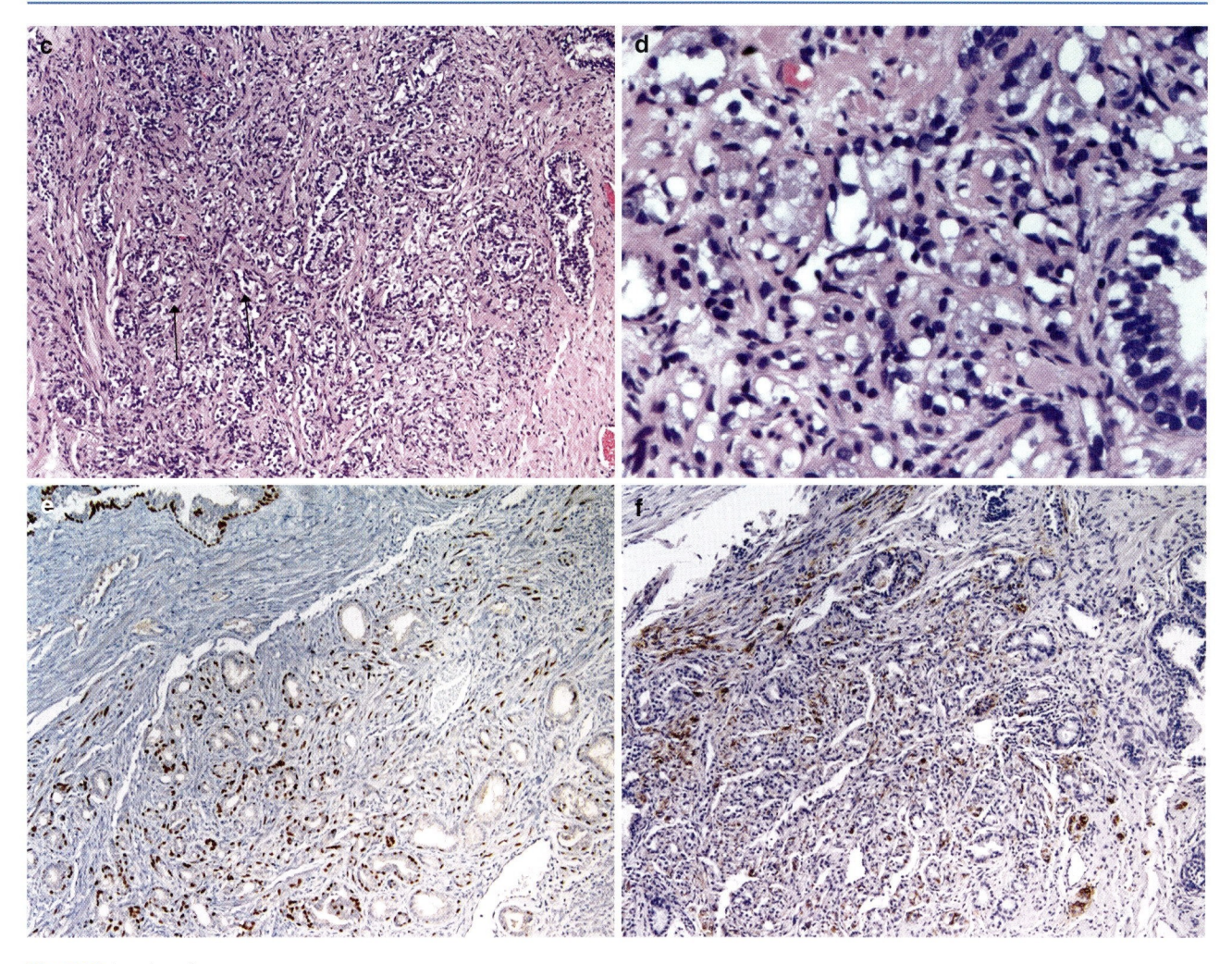

Fig. 7.28 (continued)

7.24 Paraganglia

Table 7.21 Paraganglia [61, 62]

Microscopical features

Low-power architecture

Small clusters or nests of cells with clear to eosinophilic cytoplasm and delicate vasculature pattern commonly referred to as "zellballen" pattern (*see* Fig. 7.29)

Typically seen within the periprostatic space associated with neurovascular bundle but occasionally may be seen in the lateral prostatic stroma

High-power cytology

Random cytological atypia with dense chromatin and degenerative nature is commonly present

Immunohistochemical features

Positive for neuroendocrine markers, chromogranin, and synaptophysin

S-100 stains sustentacular cells

PSA and PSAP and cytokeratins are negative

Incidence and location

Rare in needle biopsy

Mostly paraganglia are encountered in the periprostatic fat of prostatectomy specimens

Differential diagnosis

High-grade Gleason score 8–10 prostate carcinoma invading extraprostatic tissue. The presence of significant nuclear atypia, acini and glands within lesion, and positivity for prostate-specific markers and lack of neuroendocrine markers suggest a carcinoma diagnosis

Common diagnostic pitfalls

Nested cells, with random cytological atypia, and location in the periprostatic soft tissue may lead to misdiagnosis for high-grade prostate cancer and extraprostatic tumor extension

7.25 Xanthomatous Infiltrate

Table 7.22 Xanthomatous infiltrate [63, 64]

Microscopical features	
Low-power architecture	
Localized or diffuse epithelioid histiocytic cells with abundant foamy cytoplasm and small shrunken nuclei (*see* Fig. 7.30)	
Mixed inflammatory infiltrate often seen in the background	
High-power cytology	
Abundant foamy cytoplasm, small uniform nuclei, and inconspicuous nucleoli	
Immunohistochemical features	
Positive for histiocytic marker CD-68	
Prostate markers, PSA and PSAP, and epithelial markers are negative	
Incidence and location	
Uncommon lesion	
May be seen in both peripheral and transition zones of the prostate	
Differential diagnosis	
Poorly differentiated prostate carcinoma with foamy differentiation or hypernephroid morphology	
Foamy carcinoma may contain abundant xanthomatous cytoplasm, but conventional acinar component invariably present; positive for epithelial and prostate markers but negative for CD-68	
Common diagnostic pitfalls	
Xanthoma cells and histiocytes with abundant foamy cytoplasm, especially when infiltrating between benign glands, may be confused for foamy gland carcinoma	

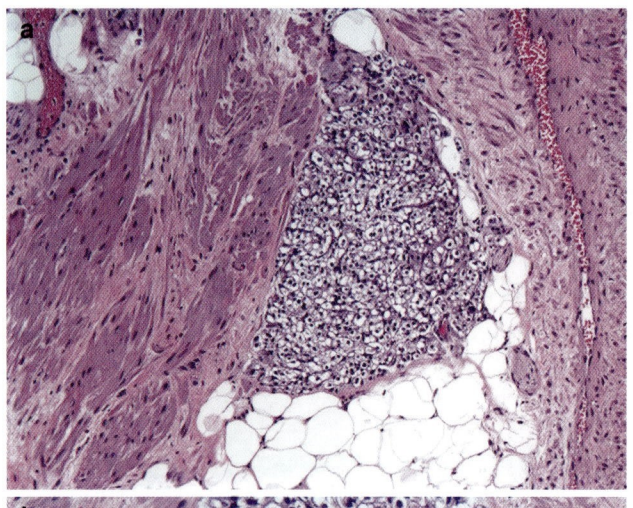

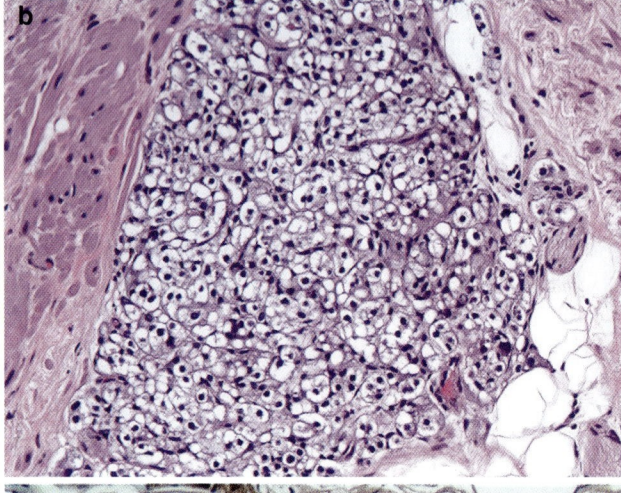

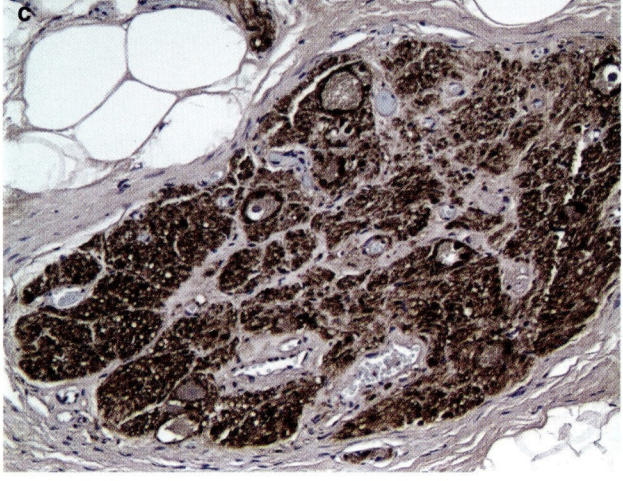

Fig. 7.29 Paraganglia mimicking high-grade prostate carcinoma and extraprostatic extension. (**a**–**c**) At low power, paraganglia consist of small, solid nests of cells with clear cytoplasm separated by a delicate vascular network, mimicking high-grade Gleason pattern 4 or 5 prostate carcinoma. Its presence in adipose tissue may further impart an impression of extraprostatic tumor extension (**a**). At high power, the cells have clear to amphophilic, finely granular cytoplasm. Random cytological atypia may be seen and nuclei are often hyperchromatic, but nucleoli are inconspicuous (**b**). Recognition of the delicate vascular network pattern referred to as the "Zellballen" arrangement is an important clue. In difficult cases, positive neuroendocrine markers support the diagnosis (**c**, synaptophysin)

7.26 Benign Mimics of Prostate Cancer: Take-Home Messages

Table 7.23 Benign mimics of prostate cancer: take-home messages

1. Use a systemic approach to evaluate prostate biopsies: Look for low-power architectural and high-power cytological features; do not rely only on one feature; use benign glands as reference
2. Hesitate to make cancer diagnosis when atypical glands are atrophic
3. Hesitate to make cancer diagnosis when cytoplasm and nuclear features of atypical glands in question are essentially same as surrounding benign glands
4. Presence of very cellular spindle cell stroma within a lesion favors a benign proliferative process
5. Random or scattered cytological atypia in well-formed glands favors a benign process. Well-formed prostate cancer typically has uniform cytological atypia
6. Utilize immunohistochemical markers to support the morphological impression; know the limitations of markers, and make sure stains have appropriate controls
7. Adenosis, atrophy, and HGPIN are typically characterized by fragmented and patchy basal cell staining; many may entirely lack basal cells
8. Majority of HGPIN and nephrogenic adenoma lesions and variable proportion of adenosis and parital atrophy lesions express racemase (AMACR)

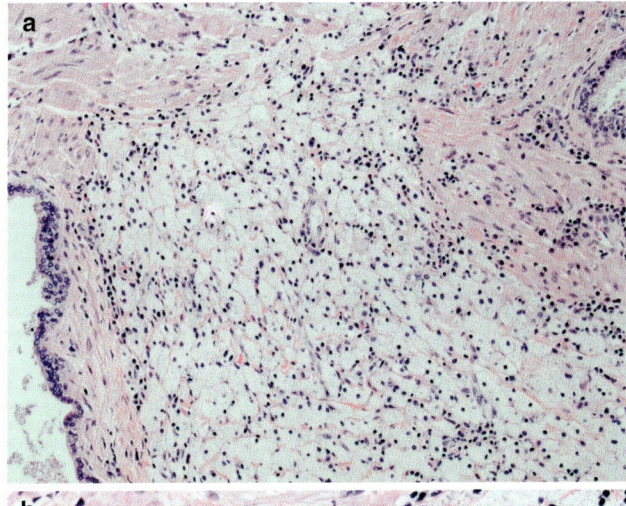

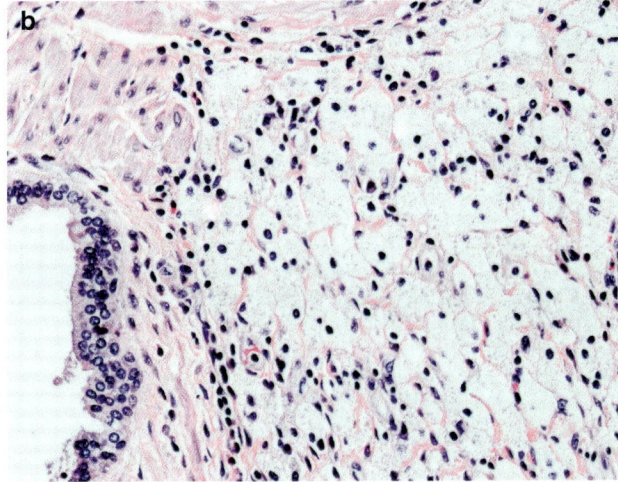

Fig. 7.30 Xanthomatous infiltrate in prostate needle biopsy. (**a–b**) Xanthoma cells grow in a diffuse infiltrative pattern, mimicking poorly differentiated prostate carcinoma with foamy features (**a**). Lack of any glandular differentiation and relatively bland nuclear features suggests the diagnosis of xanthomatous infiltrate (**b**). In small needle biopsy samples, a panel of immunohistochemical markers of histiocytic lineage (CD-68) and pancytokeratin may be necessary to rule out carcinoma. Presence of other inflammatory cells would support the diagnosis of xanthomatous infiltrate

References

1. Srigley JR (2004) Benign mimickers of prostatic adenocarcinoma. Mod Pathol 17:328–348
2. Brennick JB, O'Connell JX, Dickersin GR et al (1994) Lipofuscin pigmentation (so-called "melanosis") of the prostate. Am J Surg Pathol 18:446–454
3. Jensen KM, Sonneland P, Madsen PO (1983) Seminal vesicle tissue in "resectate" of transurethral resection of prostate. Urology 22:20–23
4. Leroy X, Ballereau C, Villers A et al (2003) MUC6 is a marker of seminal vesicle-ejaculatory duct epithelium and is useful for the differential diagnosis with prostate adenocarcinoma. Am J Surg Pathol 27:519–521
5. Arias-Stella J, Takano-Moron J (1958) Atypical epithelial changes in the seminal vesicle. AMA Arch Pathol 66:761–766
6. Gagucas RJ, Brown RW, Wheeler TM (1995) Verumontanum mucosal gland hyperplasia. Am J Surg Pathol 19:30–36
7. Gaudin PB, Wheeler TM, Epstein JI (1995) Verumontanum mucosal gland hyperplasia in prostatic needle biopsy specimens. A mimic of low grade prostatic adenocarcinoma. Am J Clin Pathol 104:620–626
8. Cina SJ, Silberman MA, Kahane H, Epstein JI (1997) Diagnosis of Cowper's glands on prostate needle biopsy. Am J Surg Pathol 21:550–555
9. Saboorian MH, Huffman H, Ashfaq R et al (1997) Distinguishing Cowper's glands from neoplastic and pseudoneoplastic lesions of prostate: immunohistochemical and ultrastructural studies. Am J Surg Pathol 21:1069–1074
10. Gikas PW, Del Buono EA, Epstein JI (1993) Florid hyperplasia of mesonephric remnants involving prostate and periprostatic tissue. Possible confusion with adenocarcinoma. Am J Surg Pathol 17:454–460

11. Bostwick DG, Qian J, Ma J, Muir TE et al (2003) Mesonephric remnants of the prostate: incidence and histologic spectrum. Mod Pathol 16:630–635
12. Grignon DJ, O'Malley FP (1993) Mucinous metaplasia in the prostate gland. Am J Surg Pathol 17:287–290
13. Shiraishi T, Kusano I, Watanabe M et al (1993) Mucous gland metaplasia of the prostate. Am J Surg Pathol 17:618–622
14. De Marzo AM, Marchi VL, Epstein JI et al (1999) Proliferative inflammatory atrophy of the prostate: implications for prostatic carcinogenesis. Am J Pathol 155:1985–1992
15. De Marzo AM, Platz EA, Epstein JI et al (2006) A working group classification of focal prostate atrophy lesions. Am J Surg Pathol 30:1281–1291
16. Palapattu GS, Sutcliffe S, Bastian PJ et al (2005) Prostate carcinogenesis and inflammation: emerging insights. Carcinogenesis 26: 1170–1181
17. Ruska KM, Sauvageot JBS, Epstein JI (1998) Histology and cellular kinetics of prostatic atrophy. Am J Surg Pathol 22:1073–1077
18. Shah R, Mucci NR, Amin A et al (2001) Postatrophic hyperplasia of the prostate gland: neoplastic precursor or innocent bystander? Am J Pathol 158:1767–1773
19. Amin MB, Tamboli P, Varma M, Srigley JR (1999) Postatrophic hyperplasia of the prostate gland: a detailed analysis of its morphology in needle biopsy specimens. Am J Surg Pathol 23:925–931
20. Franks LM (1954) Atrophy and hyperplasia in the prostate proper. J Pathol Bacteriol 68:617–621
21. Gardner WA Jr (1987) Culberson DE: atrophy and proliferation in the young adult prostate. J Urol 137:53–56
22. Oppenheimer JR, Wills ML, Epstein JI (1998) Partial atrophy in prostate needle cores: another diagnostic pitfall for the surgical pathologist. Am J Surg Pathol 22:440–445
23. Postma R, Schroder FH, van der Kwast TH (2005) Atrophy in prostate needle biopsy cores and its relationship to prostate cancer incidence in screened men. Urology 65:745–749
24. Przybycin CG, Kunju LP, Wu AJ, Shah RB (2008) Partial atrophy in prostate needle biopsies: a detailed analysis of its morphology, immunophenotype, and cellular kinetics. Am J Surg Pathol 32: 58–64
25. Herawi M, Parwani AV, Irie J, Epstein JI (2005) Small Glandular proliferations on needle biopsies: most common benign mimickers of prostatic adenocarcinoma sent in for expert second opinion. Am J Surg Pathol 29:874–880
26. Bostwick DG, Srigley J, Grignon D et al (1993) Atypical adenomatous hyperplasia of the prostate: morphologic criteria for its distinction from well-differentiated carcinoma. Hum Pathol 24:819–832
27. Cheng L, Shan A, Cheville JC et al (1998) Atypical adenomatous hyperplasia of the prostate: a premalignant lesion? Cancer Res 58:389–391
28. Gaudin PB, Epstein JI (1995) Adenosis of the prostate. Histologic features in needle biopsy specimens. Am J Surg Pathol 19: 737–747
29. Kunju LP, Rubin MA, Chinnaiyan AM, Shah RB (2003) Diagnostic usefulness of monoclonal antibody p504s in the workup of atypical prostatic glandular proliferations. Am J Clin Pathol 120:737–745
30. Qian J, Jenkins RB, Bostwick DG (1995) Chromosomal anomalies in atypical adenomatous hyperplasia and carcinoma of the prostate using fluorescence in situ hybridization. Urology 46:837–842
31. Shah RB, Kunju LP, Shen R et al (2004) Usefulness of basal cell cocktail (34betaE12+p63) in the diagnosis of atypical prostate glandular proliferations. Am J Clin Pathol 122:517–523
32. Yang XJ, Wu CL, Woda BA et al (2002) Expression of alpha-Methylacyl-CoA racemase (P504S) in atypical adenomatous hyperplasia of the prostate. Am J Surg Pathol 26:921–925
33. Lotan TL, Epstein JI (2008) Diffuse adenosis of the peripheral zone in prostate needle biopsy and prostatectomy specimens. Am J Surg Pathol 32:1360–1366
34. Cleary KR, Choi HY, Ayala AG (1983) Basal cell hyperplasia of the prostate. Am J Clin Pathol 80:850–854
35. Devaraj LT, Bostwick DG (1993) Atypical basal cell hyperplasia of the prostate. Immunophenotypic profile and proposed classification of basal cell proliferations. Am J Surg Pathol 17:645–659
36. Epstein JI, Armas OA (1992) Atypical basal cell hyperplasia of the prostate. Am J Surg Pathol 16:1205–1214
37. Grignon DJ, Ro JY, Ordoñez NG et al (1988) Basal cell hyperplasia, adenoid basal cell tumor, and adenoid cystic carcinoma of the prostate gland: an immunohistochemical study. Hum Pathol 19: 1425–1433
38. Hosler GA, Epstein JI (2005) Basal cell hyperplasia: an unusual diagnostic dilemma on prostate needle biopsies. Hum Pathol 36: 480–485
39. Lin JI, Cohen EL, Villacin AB et al (1978) Basal cell adenoma of prostate. Urology 11:409–410
40. Rioux-Leclercq NC, Epstein JI (2002) Unusual morphologic patterns of basal cell hyperplasia of the prostate. Am J Surg Pathol 26:237–243
41. Yang XJ, Tretiakova MS, Sengupta E et al (2003) Florid basal cell hyperplasia of the prostate: a histological, ultrastructural, and immunohistochemical analysis. Hum Pathol 34:462–470
42. Bostwick DG, Egbert BM, Fajardo LF (1982) Radiation injury of the normal and neoplastic prostate. Am J Surg Pathol 6:541–551
43. Brawer MK, Nagle RB, Pitts W et al (1989) Keratin immunoreactivity as an aid to the diagnosis of persistent adenocarcinoma in irradiated human prostates. Cancer 63:454–460
44. Crook JM, Bahadur YA, Robertson SJ et al (1997) Evaluation of radiation effect, tumor differentiation, and prostate specific antigen staining in sequential prostate biopsies after external beam radiotherapy for patients with prostate carcinoma. Cancer 79:81–89
45. Mahan DE, Bruce AW, Manley PN, Franchi L (1980) Immunohistochemical evaluation of prostatic carcinoma before and after radiotherapy. J Urol 124:488–491
46. Allan CH, Epstein JI (2001) Nephrogenic adenoma of the prostatic urethra: a mimicker of prostate adenocarcinoma. Am J Surg Pathol 25:802–808
47. Malpica A, Ro JY, Troncoso P et al (1994) Nephrogenic adenoma of the prostatic urethra involving the prostate gland: a clinicopathologic and immunohistochemical study of eight cases. Hum Pathol 25:390–395
48. Young RH (1992) Nephrogenic adenomas of the urethra involving the prostate gland: a report of two cases of a lesion that may be confused with prostatic adenocarcinoma. Mod Pathol 5:617–620
49. McNeal JE (1981) Normal and pathologic anatomy of prostate. Urology 17:11–16
50. Srodon M, Epstein JI (2002) Central zone histology of the prostate: a mimicker of high-grade prostatic intraepithelial neoplasia. Hum Pathol 33:518–523
51. Ayala AG, Srigley JR, Ro JY et al (1986) Clear cell cribriform hyperplasia of prostate. Report of 10 cases. Am J Surg Pathol 10:665–671
52. Oppenheimer JR, Kahane H, Epstein JI (1997) Granulomatous prostatitis on needle biopsy. Arch Pathol Lab Med 121:724–729
53. Presti B, Weidner N (1991) Granulomatous prostatitis and poorly differentiated prostate carcinoma. Their distinction with the use of immunohistochemical methods. Am J Clin Pathol 95:330–334
54. Stillwell TJ, Engen DE, Farrow GM (1987) The clinical spectrum of granulomatous prostatitis: a report of 200 cases. J Urol 138: 320–323
55. Long JP Jr, Althausen AF (1989) Malacoplakia: a 25-year experience with a review of the literature. J Urol 141:1328–1331
56. Smith BH (1965) Malacoplakia of the urinary tract: a study of twenty-four cases. Am J Clin Pathol 43:409–417
57. Grignon DJ, Ro JY, Srigley JR et al (1992) Sclerosing adenosis of the prostate gland. A lesion showing myoepithelial differentiation. Am J Surg Pathol 16:383–391

58. Jones EC, Clement PB, Young RH (1991) Sclerosing adenosis of the prostate gland. A clinicopathological and immunohistochemical study of 11 cases. Am J Surg Pathol 15:1171–1180
59. Luque RJ, Lopez-Beltran A, Perez-Seoane C, Suzigan S (2003) Sclerosing adenosis of the prostate. Histologic features in needle biopsy specimens. Arch Pathol Lab Med 127:e14–e16
60. Sakamoto N, Tsuneyoshi M, Enjoji M (1991) Sclerosing adenosis of the prostate. Histopathologic and immunohistochemical analysis. Am J Surg Pathol 15:660–667
61. Kawabata K (1997) Paraganglion of the prostate in a needle biopsy: a potential diagnostic pitfall. Arch Pathol Lab Med 121:515–516
62. Ostrowski ML, Wheeler TM (1994) Paraganglia of the prostate. Location, frequency, and differentiation from prostatic adenocarcinoma. Am J Surg Pathol 18:412–420
63. Chuang AY, Epstein JI (2007) Xanthoma of the prostate: a mimicker of high-grade prostate adenocarcinoma. Am J Surg Pathol 31:1225–1230
64. Sebo TJ, Bostwick DG, Farrow GM, Eble JN (1994) Prostatic xanthoma: a mimic of prostatic adenocarcinoma. Hum Pathol 25:386–389

Atypical Cribriform Lesions of the Prostate Gland: Emerging Concepts of Intraductal Carcinoma of the Prostate (IDC-P)

Atypical cribriform lesions of the prostate gland consist of proliferation of cribriform glands lined by cytologically malignant cells with partial or complete basal cell lining. It may represent cribriform "high-grade prostatic intraepithelial neoplasia" (HGPIN) or "intraductal carcinoma of the prostate" (IDC-P), and are distinguished from cribriform prostate cancer by lack of confluent and/or infiltrative architecture and presence of basal cells [1]. In 1996, IDC-P was first proposed by McNeal and Yemoto [2], and several studies have attempted to further refine histologic definition of IDC-P in the past decade [1, 3–5]. IDC-P is almost always associated with clinically aggressive high-volume prostate carcinoma [1, 6]. However, cribriform HGPIN is a putative neoplastic precursor lesion and recent data have questioned whether HGPIN on needle biopsy is associated with a significantly increased cancer risk in subsequent biopsies, therefore requiring rebiopsy within the first year after its diagnosis [7]. Therefore, distinction between these two lesions has profound clinical significance, especially on needle biopsies. Even though presence of certain morphological features (e.g., pleomorphic nuclei or nuclei 6× of adjacent nuclei, intraluminal necrosis, and dense cribriform architecture) is seen only with IDC-P, HGPIN, and IDC-P overlap at the "low-grade" end of the morphological spectrum [1]. Emerging molecular data on *TMPRSS:ERG* gene fusions further support that these two lesions are biologically distinct [8]. This chapter summarizes the current concepts on morphologic and molecular characteristics of cribriform HGPIN and IDC-P and an approach to workup of atypical cribriform lesions in prostate needle biopsies.

8.1 Intraductal Carcinoma of the Prostate

Table 8.1 Intraductal carcinoma of the prostate

Microscopical features

Low-power architecture

Nonconfluent yet crowded proliferation of large atypical cribriform glands with branching, solid, or dense cribriform, or occasionally micropapillary architecture (*see* Fig. 8.1)

Pleomorphic high-grade nuclei and/or intraluminal necrosis may be present (*see* Fig. 8.1c)

Usually associated with adjacent invasive cancer

High-power cytology

Nuclear enlargement, hyperchromasia, and enlarged nucleoli are present but some of the defining features of IDC-P such as pleomorphic nuclei and/or nuclear enlargement 6× of adjacent nuclei and intraluminal necrosis seen only in a subset of cases [1, 8]

Basal cells may be visible but may require stains for confirmation

Immunohistochemical and molecular features

Positive for prostate-specific antigen (PSA), prostate-specific membrane antigen (PSMA), and prostatic acid phosphatase (PSAP) and negative for thrombomodulin; basal cell markers p63 and high molecular weight cytokeratin highlight residual basal cells

TMPRSS2:ERG gene fusions in up to 70% of cases [8]

Differential diagnosis (*see* Fig. 8.4)

Cribriform PIN

A few small cribriform glands with smooth contour and low-grade nuclei; do not have dense cribriform or solid architecture, pleomorphic nuclei or nuclei 6× of adjacent nuclei and intraluminal necrosis; however, both lesions may overlap at "low-grade" spectrum [1, 5, 8] (*see* Fig. 8.2)

Intraductal spread of urothelial carcinoma

Cribriform and glandular architecture favor IDC-P

A panel of PSA, PSMA, PSAP, thrombomodulin, and basal cell markers are useful to make a definitive diagnosis. IDC-P demonstrates reactivity for PSA, PSMA, and PSAP while negative for other markers, whereas peripheral basal cells are highlighted by basal markers. Urothelial carcinoma has opposite staining pattern (*see* Fig. 8.3)

Ductal adenocarcinoma

Ductal adenocarcinoma and IDC-P share morphological features and frequently coexist, making this distinction particularly problematic in needle biopsies

Confluence, columnar lining epithelium with slit-like lumina favor ductal adenocarcinoma

Lack of basal cell lining supports ductal adenocarcinoma diagnosis

Cribriform acinar cancer

Cribriform carcinoma lacks basal cell lining. Distinction between the two is usually of academic interest

Clinical significance

IDC-P is considered to represent intraductal/acinar spread by invasive cancer

Almost always associated with high-grade and high-volume invasive cancer and has higher likelihood of seminal vesicle invasion and disease progression than prostate cancers without IDC-P. Pure IDC-P without invasive cancer in radical prostatectomy is very rare

Almost always associated with invasive carcinoma in prostate biopsies

Rarely sole finding in prostate biopsies

Recommend definitive therapy even as a sole finding in biopsy (*see* Table 8.4)

8.1 Intraductal Carcinoma of the Prostate

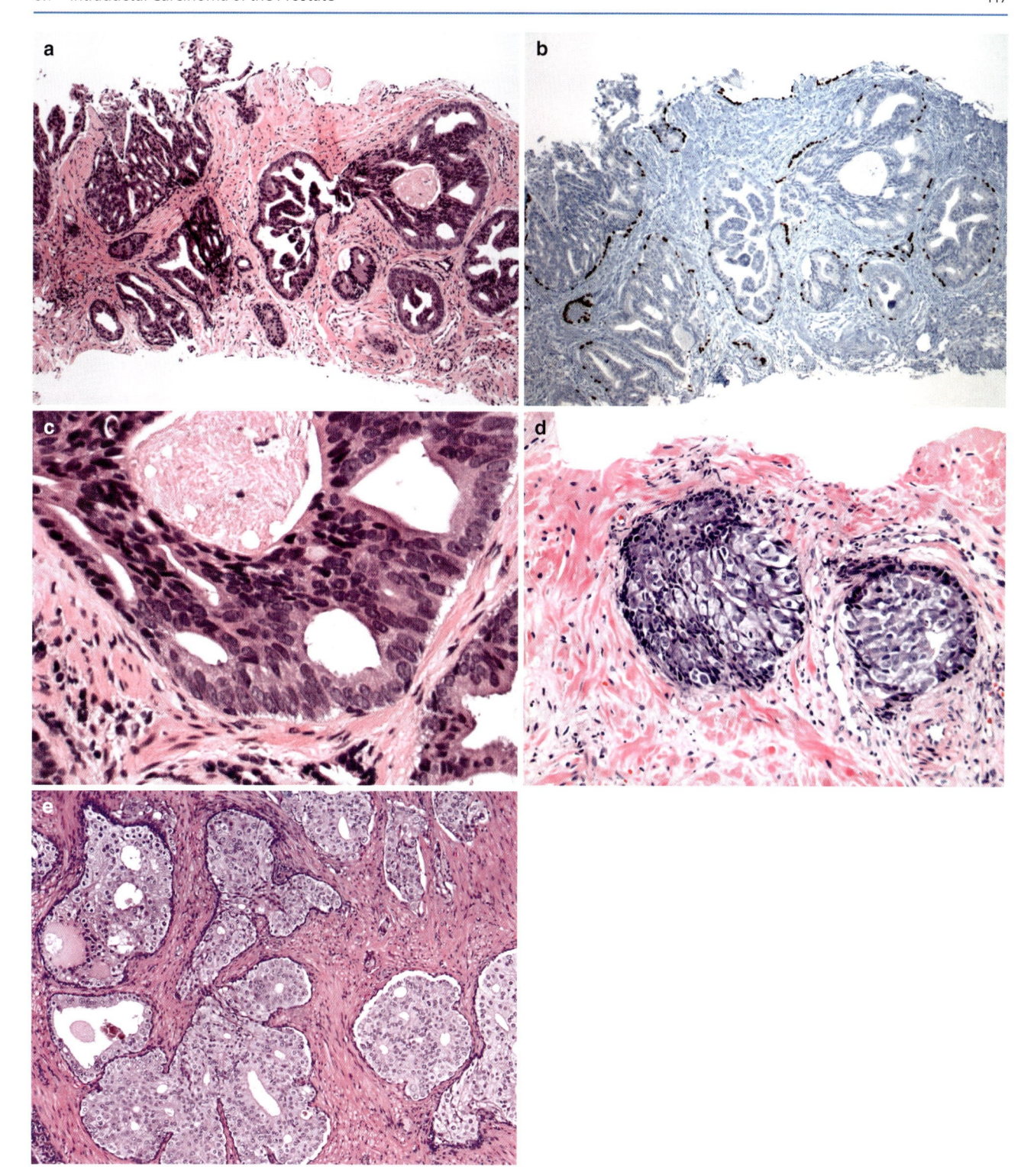

Fig. 8.1 Morphological features of IDC-P. Low-power (**a** and **b**) and high-power (**c**) view of an IDC-P in prostate biopsy showing several large, irregular, branching cribriform glands with dense cribriform architecture and focal intraluminal comedonecrosis; basal cell markers highlight the peripheral layer of basal cells (**b**). (**d**) An IDC-P showing solid architecture and pleomorphic nuclei 6× of adjacent nuclei; basal cells can be appreciated on hematoxylin–eosin stain image but may require immunohistochemistry confirmation. (**e**) An IDC-P with dense cribriform architecture showing punched-out lumina spaces and solid architecture; presence of branching glandular contour, solid or dense cribriform architecture, intraluminal necrosis, and pleomorphic nuclei are characteristic features of IDC-P [1, 3–5, 8]; however, these features are variably present in IDC-P [1]

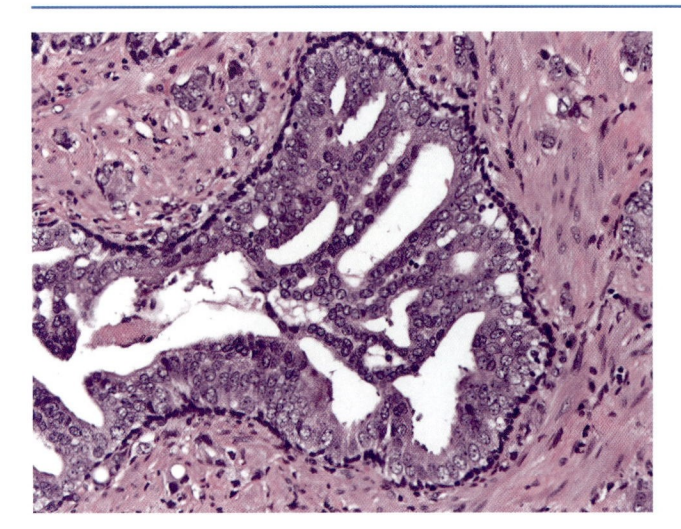

Fig. 8.2 IDC-P overlaps cribriform HGPIN at the "low-grade" end of the morphological spectrum [1, 8]. This cribriform lesion has relatively uniform nuclei and lacks the characteristic cytological features of IDC-P. In our experience, isolated atypical cribriform lesion not associated with cancer (cribriform HGPIN) is uncommon and the majority of atypical cribriform lesions containing basal cells, even when their constituent cells are of low-grade cytology, are associated with cancer and represent a spectrum of IDC-P [1, 8]. In this example, an adjacent invasive acinar cancer is present

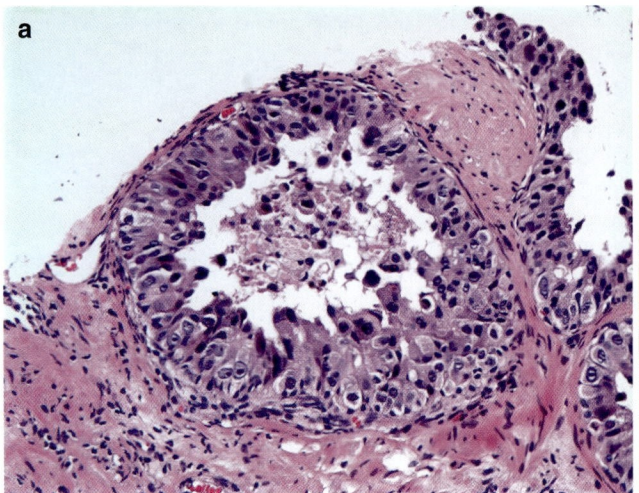

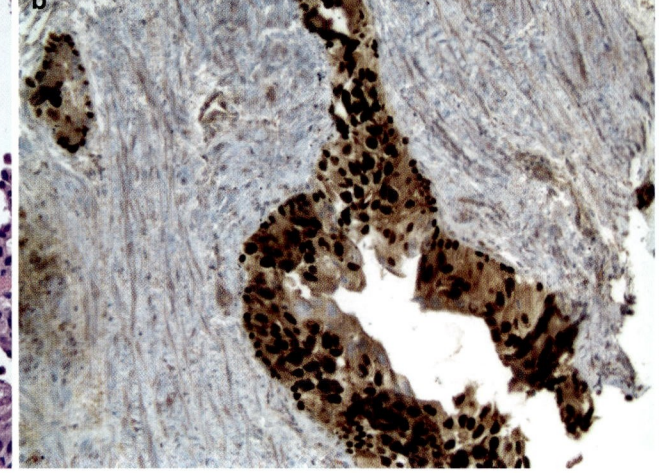

Fig. 8.3 Intraductal spread of high-grade urothelial carcinoma mimicking IDC-P. When atypical cells expand prostate glands and form solid nests with residual basal cells, intraductal spread of high-grade urothelial carcinoma should always be considered and ruled out before diagnosing IDC-P. Associated dense cribriform architecture and/or glandular differentiation favors IDC-P over urothelial carcinoma but immunostains are necessary to confirm the diagnosis. (**a**) Note the relatively uniform high-grade cells and solid architecture. (**b**) Luminal tumor cells demonstrate p63 nuclear reactivity, whereas PSA and PSAP are negative (*not shown*), supporting the diagnosis of intraductal spread of urothelial carcinoma

8.2 General Approach to the Workup of Atypical Cribriform Lesions in Prostate Needle Biopsy

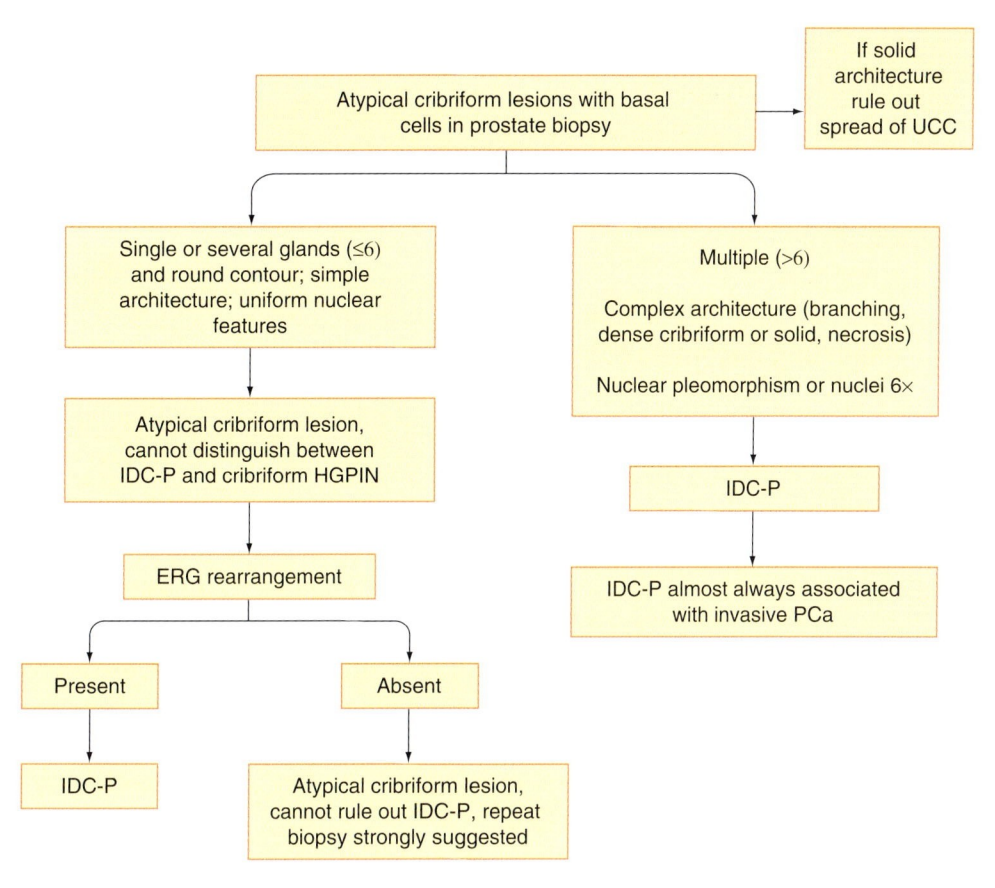

Fig. 8.4 General approach to the workup of atypical cribriform lesions in prostate needle biopsy. *PCa* prostate cancer, *UCC* urothelial cell carcinoma

8.3 Comparisons of Clinical, Morphological and Molecular Characteristics between Cribriform HGPIN and IDC-P

Table 8.2 Comparisons of clinical, morphological, and molecular characteristics between cribriform high-grade PIN and IDC-P [1, 8]

	Cribriform PIN	IDC-P
Frequency in radical prostatectomy specimens	Less common	Relatively common
Characteristics of associated cancer in radical prostatectomy specimens	Low Gleason grade (≤6) and low tumor volume	High Gleason grade ≥ 7 and high tumor volume
Cribriform glands/prostate, *n*	2–3 glands	>6 glands
Size	<1 mm	>1 mm
Glandular contour		
Regular	Typical	Less common
Irregular	Less common	Common
Branching[a]	Rare (<5%)	Typical (~85%)
Architecture		
Dense cribriform[a]	Absent	Infrequent (~15%)
Irregular cribriform	Common	Common
Solid[a]	Absent	Infrequent (~10%)
Comedonecrosis[a]	Absent	Variably present (~33%)
Cytology of atypical cribriform glands		
Uniform or variable nuclei	Typical	Common
Pleomorphic or giant nuclei at least 6× of the adjacent nuclei[a]	Absent	Variably present (~30%)
TMPRSS2:ERG gene fusions[a]	Absent	Enriched (~75%)

[a]Indicates features that are helpful to differentiate between IDC-P and cribriform HGPIN

8.4 Pathologic features of IDC-P

Table 8.3 Pathologic features that distinguish IDC-P and cribriform HGPIN [1, 4, 5]

Number of glands (>6)
Size (>1 mm)
Branching contour
Dense cribriform or solid architecture
Comedo necrosis
Nuclear size 6× of adjacent nuclei or pleomorphic nuclei

8.5 Reporting Recommendations for IDC-P

Table 8.4 Reporting recommendations for prostate biopsies with IDC-P [9]

Diagnostic situations associated with IDC-P in needle biopsy specimens	Reporting recommendations
IDC-P associated with invasive high-grade prostate carcinoma	No need to mention IDC-P
IDC-P associated with Gleason pattern 3 prostate cancer	Document IDC-P and its poor prognostic significance in the report; or grade IDC-P as pattern 4 or 5
IDC-P not associated with any invasive prostate cancer	Diagnose IDC-P and document in the comment that IDC-P is usually associated with high-grade prostate cancer and advise immediate rebiopsy and recommend definitive therapy

References

1. Shah RB, Magi-Galluzzi C, Han B, Zhou M (2010) Atypical cribriform lesions of the prostate: relationship to prostatic carcinoma and implication for diagnosis in prostate biopsies. Am J Surg Pathol 34:470–477
2. McNeal JE, Yemoto CE (1996) Spread of adenocarcinoma within prostatic ducts and acini. Morphologic and clinical correlations. Am J Surg Pathol 20:802–814
3. Cohen RJ, McNeal JE, Baillie T (2000) Patterns of differentiation and proliferation in intraductal carcinoma of the prostate: significance for cancer progression. Prostate 43:11–19
4. Cohen RJ, Wheeler TM, Bonkhoff H, Rubin MA (2007) A proposal on the identification, histologic reporting, and implications of intraductal prostatic carcinoma. Arch Pathol Lab Med 131:1103–1109
5. Guo CC, Epstein JI (2006) Intraductal carcinoma of the prostate on needle biopsy: histologic features and clinical significance. Mod Pathol 19:1528–1535
6. Henry PC, Evans AJ (2009) Intraductal carcinoma of the prostate: a distinct histopathological entity with important prognostic implications. J Clin Pathol 62:579–583
7. Epstein JI, Herawi M (2006) Prostate needle biopsies containing prostatic intraepithelial neoplasia or atypical foci suspicious for carcinoma: implications for patient care. J Urol 175:820–834
8. Han B, Suleman K, Wang L et al (2010) ETS gene aberrations in atypical cribriform lesions of the prostate: implications for the distinction between intraductal carcinoma of the prostate and cribriform high-grade prostatic intraepithelial neoplasia. Am J Surg Pathol 34:478–485
9. Robinson BD, Epstein JI (2010) Intraductal carcinoma of the prostate without invasive carcinoma on needle biopsy: emphasis on radical prostatectomy findings. J Urol 184:1328–1333

High-Grade Prostatic Intraepithelial Neoplasia

Prostatic intraepithelial neoplasia (PIN) is considered to be a precursor lesion to prostate carcinoma [1–3]. It is characterized by secretory epithelial proliferation within the prostate glands and acini that display significant cytological atypia. Based on the degree of atypia, it can be categorized into low- and high-grade PIN (HGPIN). Low-grade PIN (LGPIN) is not associated with increased cancer detection in subsequent follow-up biopsies and its diagnosis is not readily reproducible even among urologic pathologists; therefore, it should not be diagnosed and reported on a prostate biopsy [2]. In contrast, HGPIN diagnosed on needle biopsy carries a 22–25% risk of finding cancer on subsequent rebiopsy as opposed to an 18–20% cancer risk associated with a benign or LGPIN diagnosis. After a biopsy diagnosis of HGPIN, patients are recommended to undergo repeat biopsy within 1–3 years, or within 12 months only if the initial biopsy employs a six-core sextant protocol or contains multifocal HGPIN involving two or more biopsy cores. HGPIN does not result in an abnormal digital rectal examination or elevated serum prostate-specific antigen (PSA) level and can only be diagnosed by histological examination of the prostate tissue. No treatment is required for HGPIN as an isolated finding in prostate needle biopsy.

9.1 Histological Features of Prostatic Intraepithelial Neoplasia (PIN)

Table 9.1 Histological features of PIN

Feature	LGPIN	HGPIN
Architecture	Basophilic appearance	Similar to LGPIN, but more pronounced
	Normal glandular architecture	
	Luminal cell crowding, irregular spacing, multilayering	
Luminal cell cytology		
Nuclei	Enlarged, marked size variation	Enlarged, size and shape variation
Chromatin	Normal	Coarse and clumped
Nucleoli	Inconspicuous	Large and prominent, similar to prostate cancer
Cytoplasm	Amphophilic	Amphophilic
Basal cell layer	Intact	Often discontinuous or absent

Modified from Humphrey [4]

9.2 Diagnostic Criteria for HGPIN

Table 9.2 Diagnostic criteria for HGPIN

Architecture

Darker-appearing glands with benign architecture at low scanning magnification (*see* Figs. 9.1 and 9.2)

Four major architectural patterns: flat, tufting, micropapillary, and cribriform (*see* Fig. 9.5) [5]

Minor histological variants: signet-ring, mucinous, foamy gland, inverted, and small cell neuroendocrine (*see* Fig. 9.6) [6]

Cytology

Nuclear enlargement, crowding, irregular spacing and stratification with chromatin hyperchromasia and clumping (*see* Fig. 9.2)

Prominent nucleoli visible at 20× magnification, or mitosis or pleomorphic nuclei if nucleoli not prominent (*see* Fig. 9.3) [7]

Immunohistochemistry

Secretory cells positive for pan- and low-molecular-weight cytokeratin; often reduced expression of PSA and prostatic acid phosphatase

HGPIN often has discontinuous basal cell layer marked with HMWCK and p63 (*see* Figs. 9.2 and 9.7)

60–80% of HGPIN lesions positive for α-methylacyl-CoA racemase (AMACR) (P504S) (*see* Figs. 9.2 and 9.7) [8, 9]

20% of HGPIN lesions harbor *ERG* gene rearrangement, always adjacent to *ERG*-rearranged cancer (*see* Fig. 9.8) [10–12]

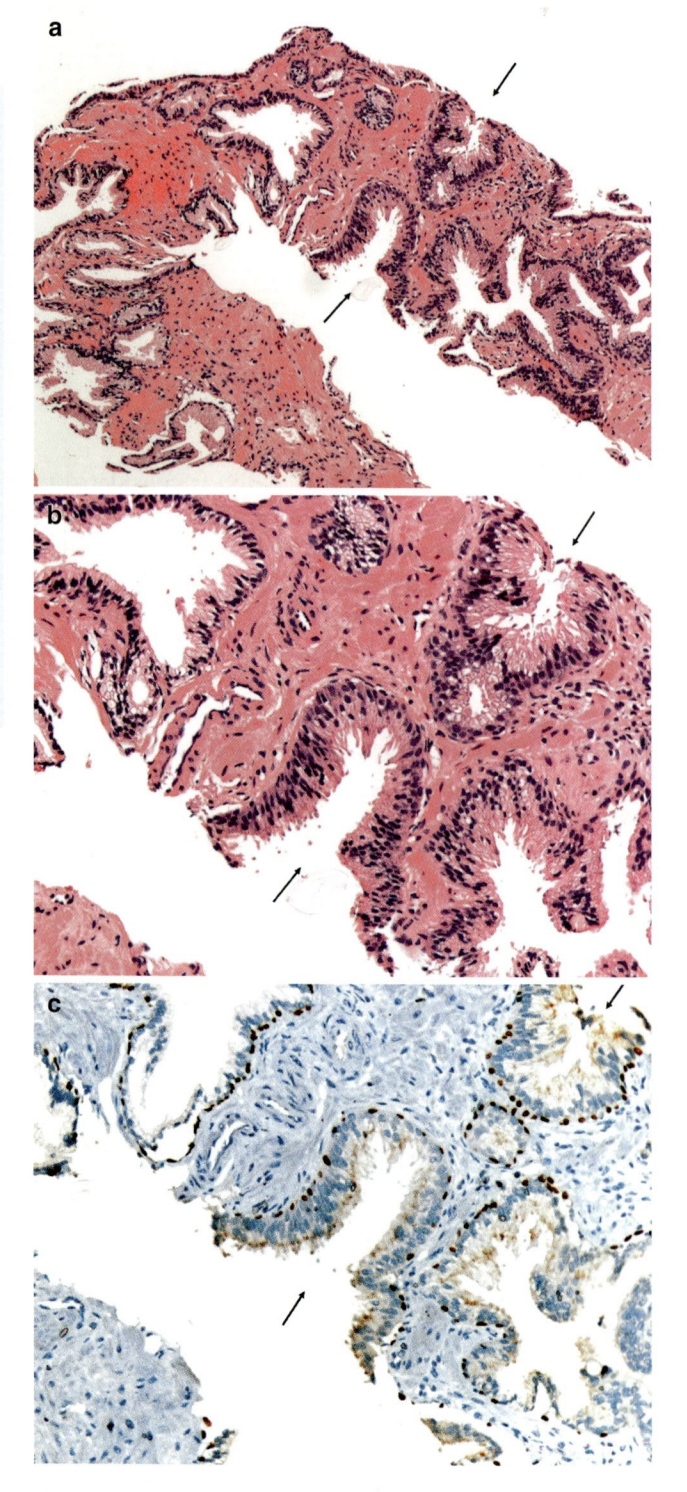

Fig. 9.1 Low-grade PIN. At scanning power, low-grade PIN glands (*arrows*) are architecturally similar to but appear darker than the adjacent benign glands (**a**). At higher magnification, the secretory cells have crowded and stratified nuclei that are enlarged and have variable sizes. No prominent nucleoli are appreciated at this magnification (**b**). p63 immunostain demonstrates continuous basal cell layer (**c**)

9.2 Diagnostic Criteria for HGPIN

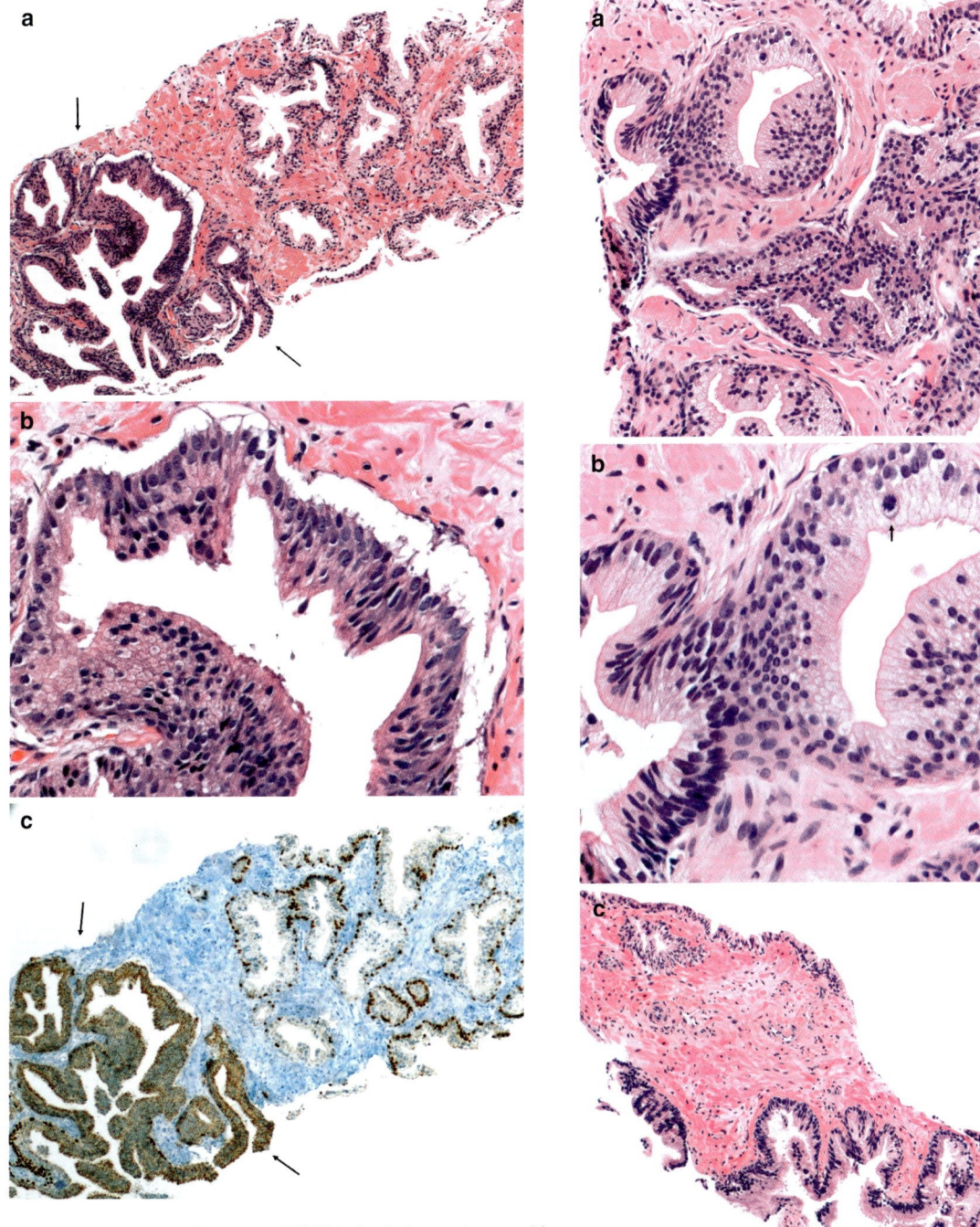

Fig. 9.2 HGPIN. At scanning power, HGPIN glands (*arrows*) are architecturally similar to but appear darker than the adjacent benign glands (**a**). At 20× magnification, the secretory cells have crowded and stratified nuclei that are enlarged and have coarse and clumpy chromatin. Importantly, large and conspicuous nucleoli are present in the secretory cells (**b**). Nuclei toward the center of the gland tend to have less atypia compared with the nuclei at the periphery of the gland. Because the nucleolar prominence is affected by tissue fixation and staining, one should always compare the HGPIN glands to the adjacent benign glands. The nucleoli are considered to be prominent only when they are larger and more conspicuous than those in the benign glands. Cytometric measurement is not reproducible. Glands with more than 10% cells with prominent nucleoli are regarded by some pathologists as diagnostic of HGPIN, a criterion not well accepted. HGPIN glands often have discontinuous basal cell layer, or even absent basal cell layer especially in small glands (**c**). The majority of HGPIN glands are positive for AMACR (**c**)

Fig. 9.3 HGPIN can be diagnosed when there are mitotic figures (**a** and **b**, *arrow*) and/or pleomorphic nuclei (**c** and **d**) in glands with HGPIN-associated morphological features but inconspicuous nucleoli

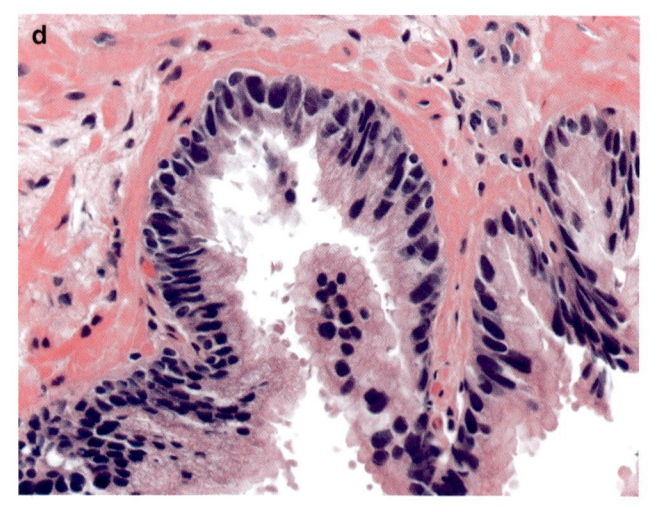

Fig. 9.3 (continued)

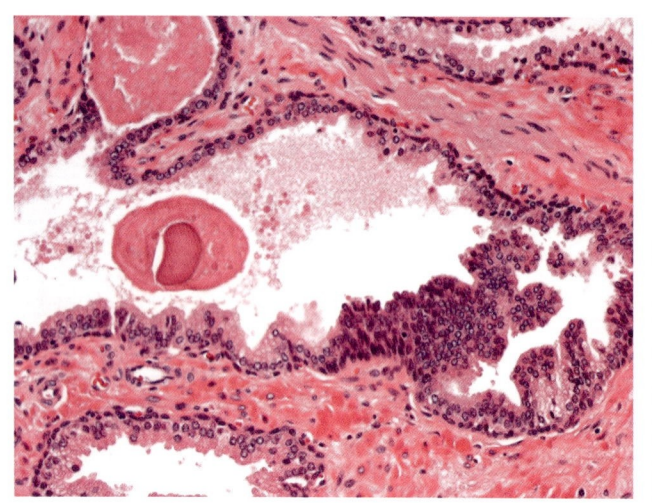

Fig. 9.4 HGPIN partially involves a prostate gland

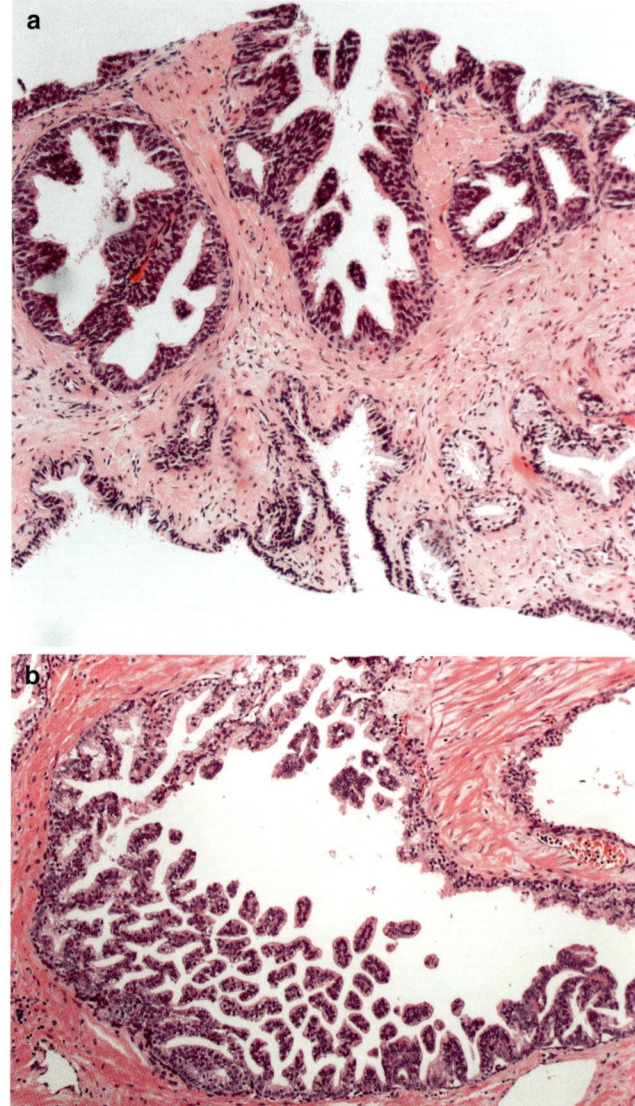

Fig. 9.5 Four major architectural patterns of HGPIN. These patterns often coexist in the same biopsy. Tufting pattern is the most common (**a**). Micropapillary HGPIN has long and slender papillae without fibrovascular core (**b**). Flat HGPIN (**c**). Cribriform HGPIN is least common (**d**). The majority of cribriform glands with atypical cells represent intraductal carcinoma. HGPIN of different architectural patterns has no significant clinical difference and its recognition is for diagnostic consideration only

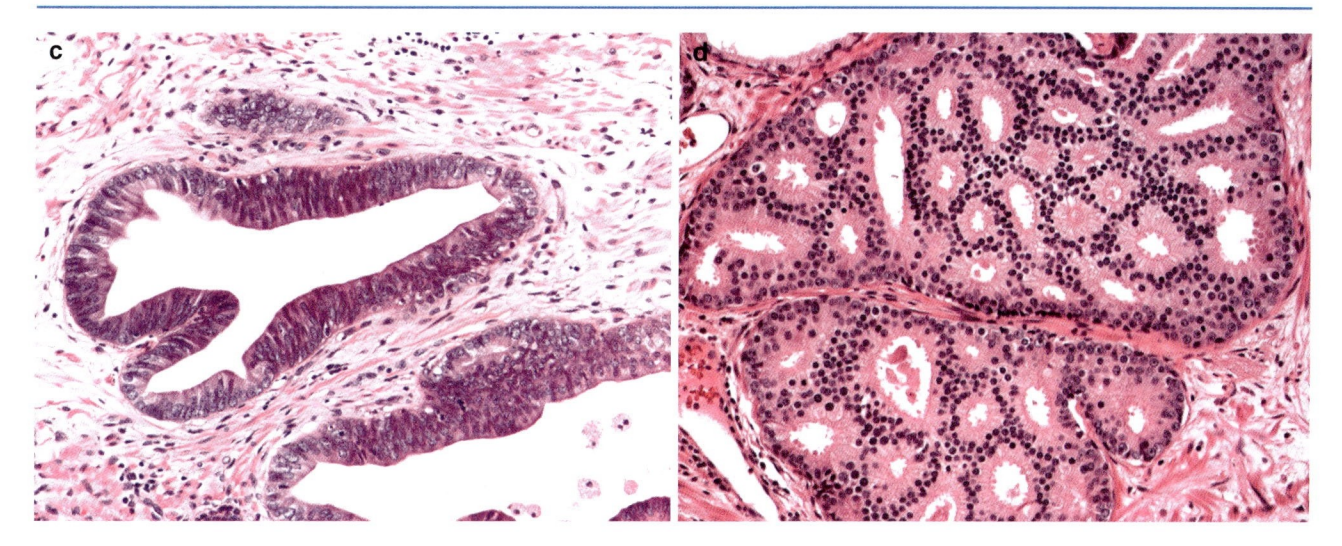

Fig. 9.5 (continued)

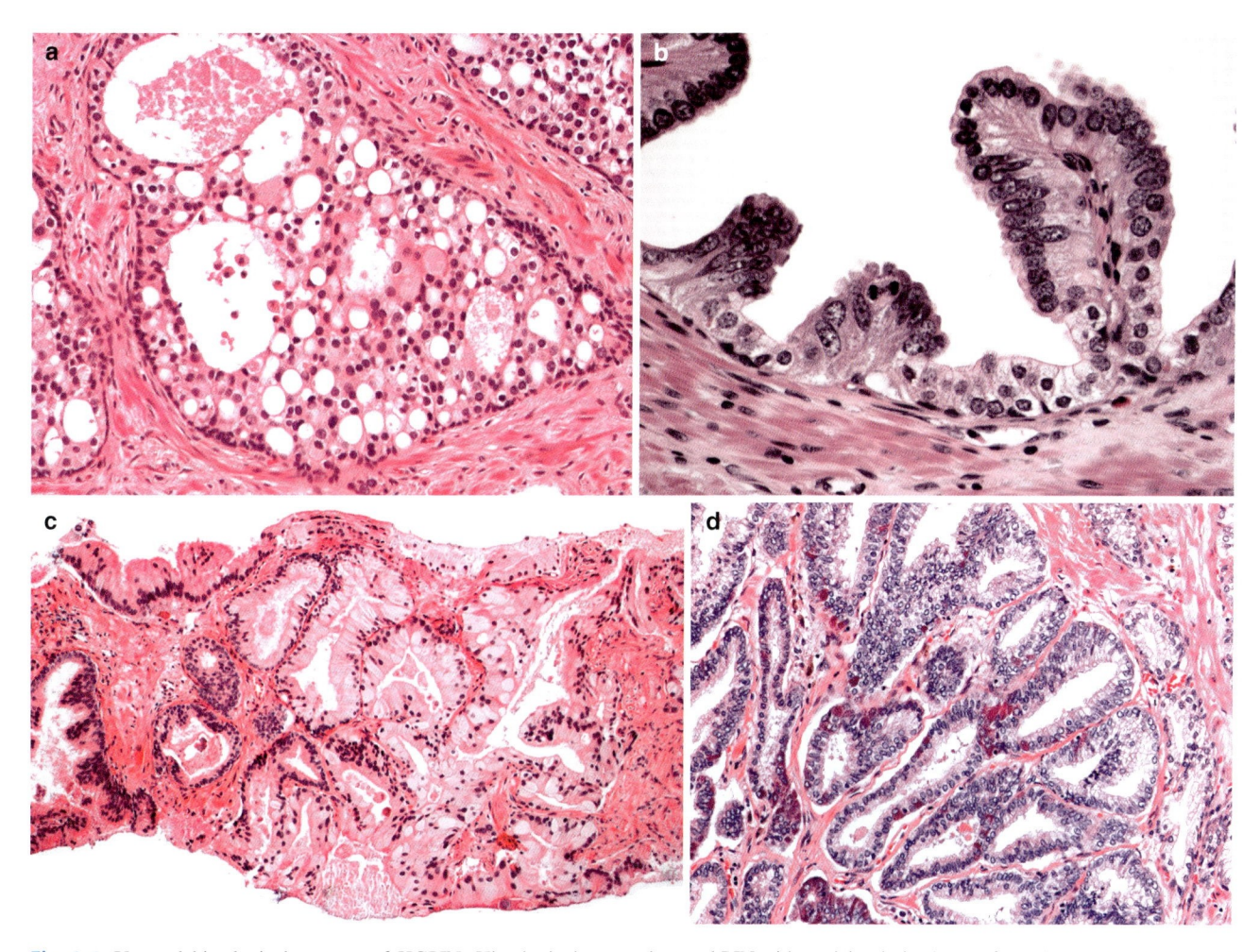

Fig. 9.6 Unusual histological patterns of HGPIN. Histological patterns identified in prostate cancer have also been described in HGPIN, including signet-ring cell PIN with clear vacuoles inside cells (**a**), inverted PIN with nuclei polarized away from the basal to the luminal surface of the gland (**b**), foamy gland PIN with abundant foamy cytoplasm (**c**), and neuroendocrine PIN (**d**)

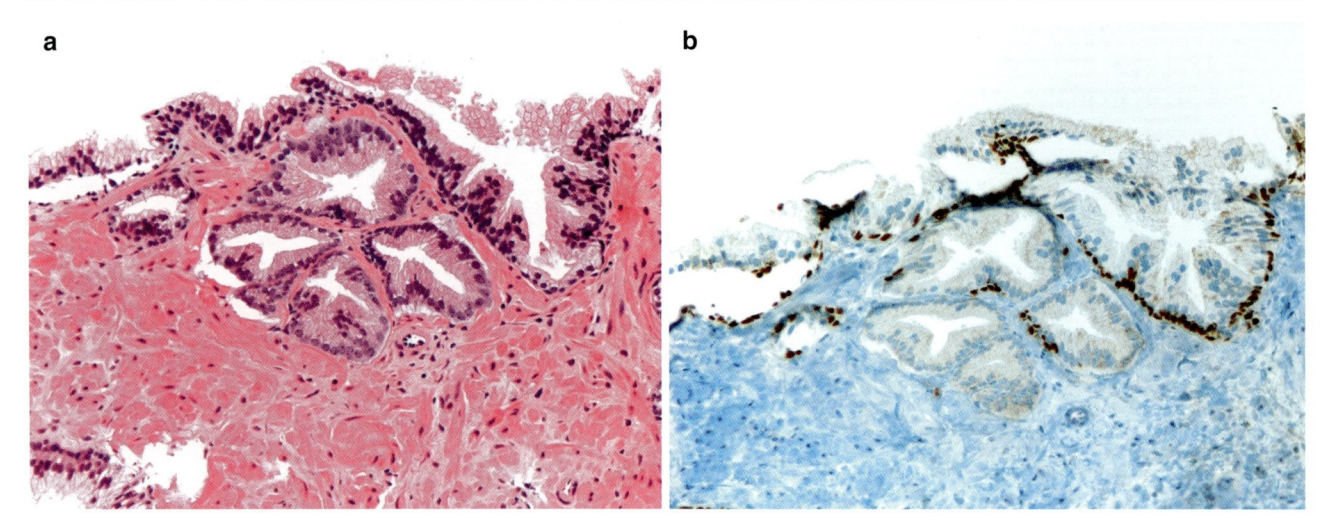

Fig. 9.7 A focus of HGPIN glands (**a**) stained with a cocktail containing p63 and AMACR antibodies. Two glands have focal and discontinuous basal cell lining, whereas the other two glands have no basal cell staining (**b**). The majority of HGPIN is positive, at least weakly, for AMACR (**b**)

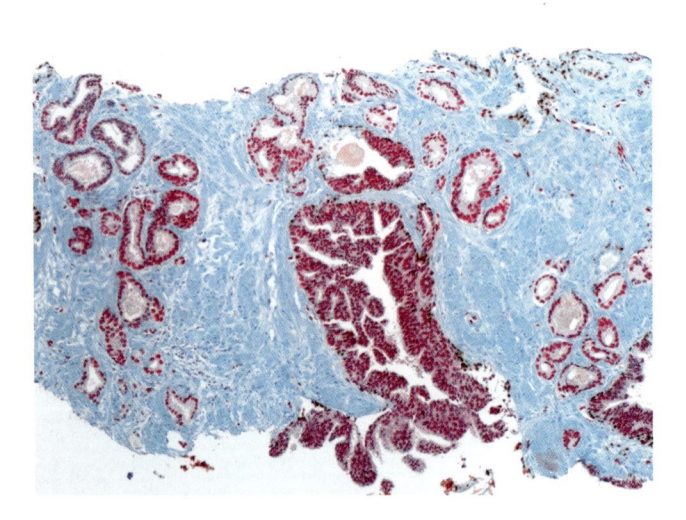

Fig. 9.8 A HGPIN gland adjacent to ERG-positive cancer is also positive for ERG. Positive ERG staining in HGPIN glands distant from cancer is exceedingly rare

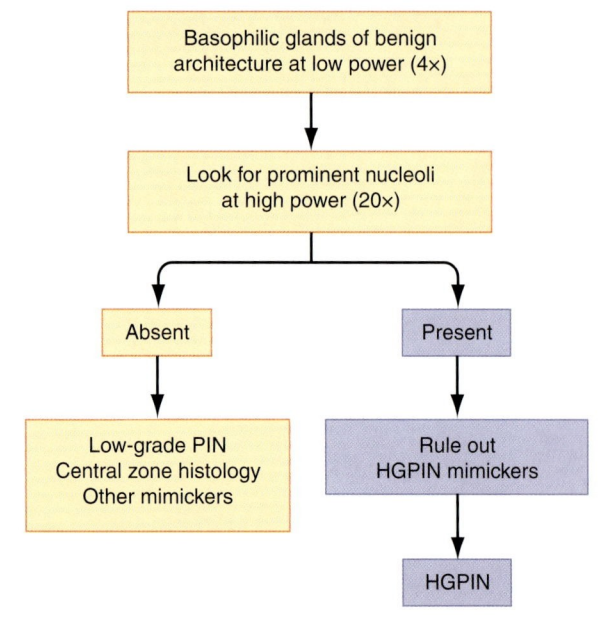

Fig. 9.9 Algorithm for the diagnosis of HGPIN in needle biopsy. When scanning biopsy cores, one should look for dark-appearing glands with architecture similar to the adjacent paler benign glands. If these dark-appearing glands are found, one should switch to 20× magnification and look for nuclear enlargement, stratification, and clumpy, hyperchromatic chromatin. However, the most important diagnostic criterion is prominent nucleoli (compared with adjacent benign glands) visible at 20× magnification in at least some secretory cells. Mimickers of HGPIN should always be considered and ruled out

9.3 Clinical Significance of HGPIN

Table 9.3 Clinical significance of HGPIN

Incidence in biopsy [2]
Mean, 7.7%
Median, 5.2%
Range, 0–24.6%

Short-term (within 1 year) cancer risk in subsequent rebiopsy
Slightly increased cancer risk compared with a benign or low-grade PIN diagnosis in contemporary studies (22% vs 19%) [2, 13, 14]
Focal HGPIN diagnosed on extended biopsy is not associated with increased cancer risk and does not need repeat biopsy within 1 year [2]
Rebiopsy for patients with initial six-core sextant biopsy, or for patients with multifocal HGPIN [2]

Long-term (1–3 years) cancer risk
Scant data
Recommend rebiopsy in 1–3 years [15, 16]

Clinicoradiological parameters predicting cancer risk in repeat biopsy
PSA (total PSA, free PSA, PSA velocity) and digital rectal examination not associated with the cancer risk [2, 14]
Imaging (ultrasound or magnetic resonance imaging) does not predict cancer risk

Pathological parameters predicting cancer risk in repeat biopsy
Morphology (flat vs tufting vs micropapillary vs cribriform) not associated with cancer risk
Number of cores involved by HGPIN [2]
   Unifocal HGPIN not associated with increased cancer risk
   Multifocal (≥2) HGPIN associated with a significantly increased cancer risk

Tumor markers predicting cancer risk in repeat biopsy
May be useful, but not yet in clinical use

Cancer characteristics following an Initial HGPIN diagnosis
Majority have a low Gleason grade and are organ confined [2]

Rebiopsy strategy
Sample the entire gland and more extensively the site and side of the initial HGPIN [17]

9.4 Differential Diagnosis of HGPIN

Table 9.4 Differential diagnosis of HGPIN

Normal prostatic structure
Central zone glands
Seminal vesicle/ejaculatory duct epithelium

Benign lesions
Reactive atypia due to inflammation, infarction, or radiation
Transitional cell metaplasia
Squamous cell metaplasia

Hyperplasia
Clear cell cribriform hyperplasia
Basal cell hyperplasia (see Fig. 9.10)

Prostate carcinoma
Prostate carcinoma with cribriform pattern (see Fig. 9.11)
PIN-like prostate carcinoma (see Fig. 9.12) [18, 19]
Ductal adenocarcinoma (see Fig. 9.13)
Intraductal carcinoma of the prostate (see Fig. 9.14) [20–22]

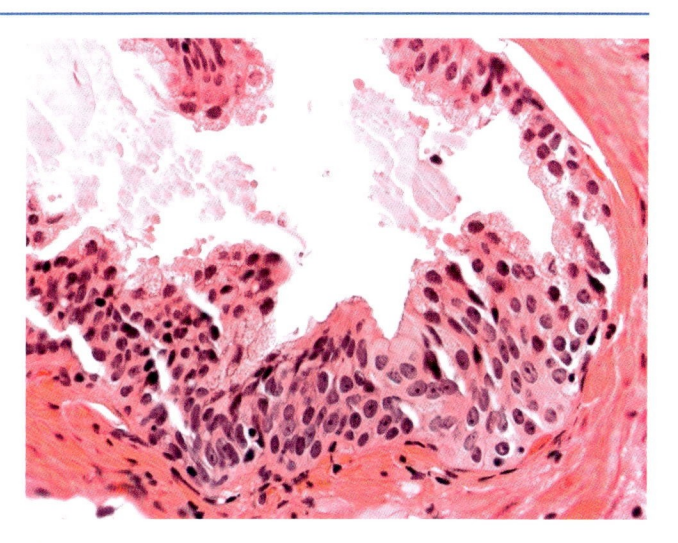

Fig. 9.10 Basal cell hyperplasia mimicking HGPIN. Benign prostate glands rimmed with basal cells with prominent nucleoli. Different from HGPIN, basal cells typically proliferate into the surrounding stroma and do not extend to the luminal surface. Their nuclei appear blue-grayish and smooth as opposed to reddish granular nuclei in secretory cells

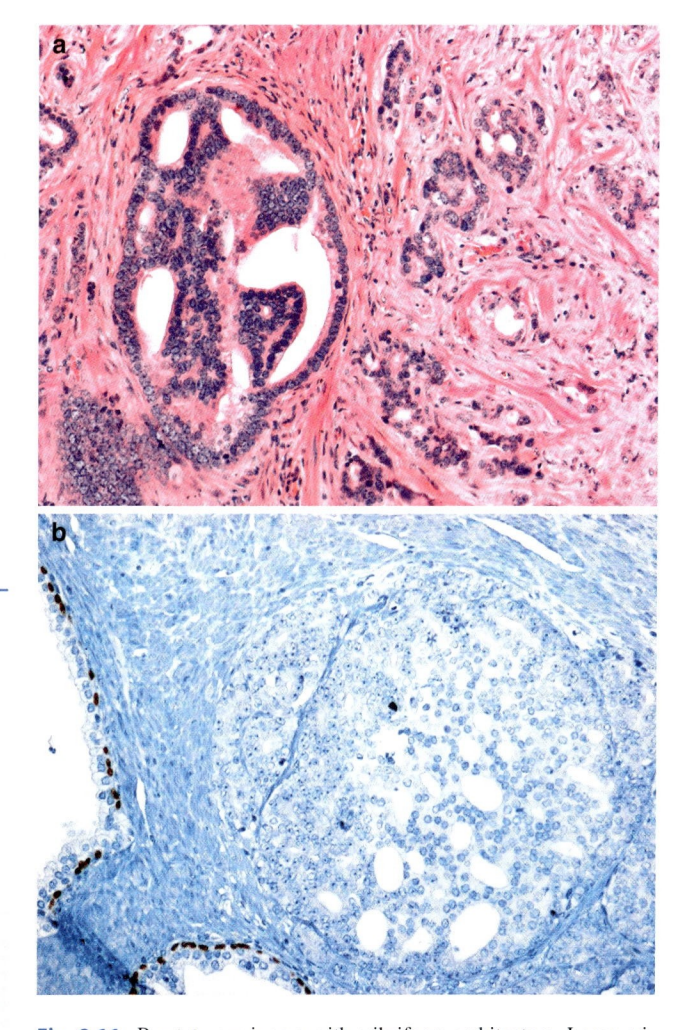

Fig. 9.11 Prostate carcinoma with cribriform architecture. Large cribriform prostate cancer glands may be mistaken for HGPIN (**a**), but they are almost always accompanied by smaller cancer glands. The diagnosis can be confirmed by cancer-specific histological features, such as perineural invasion or extraprostatic extension, or confirmed by the absence of basal cell markers (**b**)

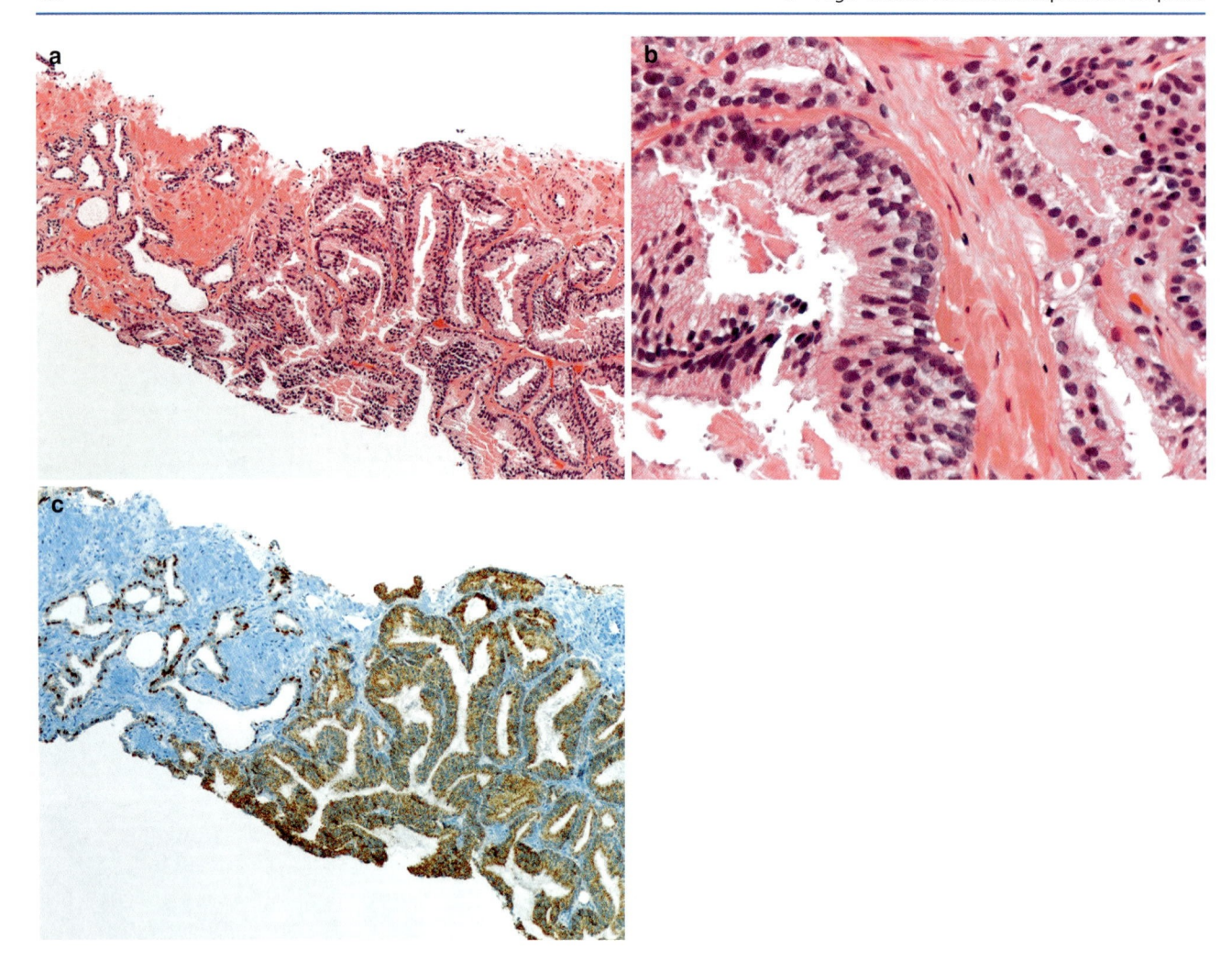

Fig. 9.12 PIN-like prostate cancer mimicking HGPIN. The biopsy contains a focus of closely packed large glands with irregular contour and undulating luminal border (**a**). These glands are lined with stratified nuclei with significant atypia (**b**), raising the suspicion for HGPIN. However, they are negative for basal cell marker p63 and positive for AMACR (**c**). PIN-like cancer has closely packed glands as opposed to PIN glands with a moderate amount of intervening stroma. Absent basal cell staining is required to establish a cancer diagnosis on needle biopsy

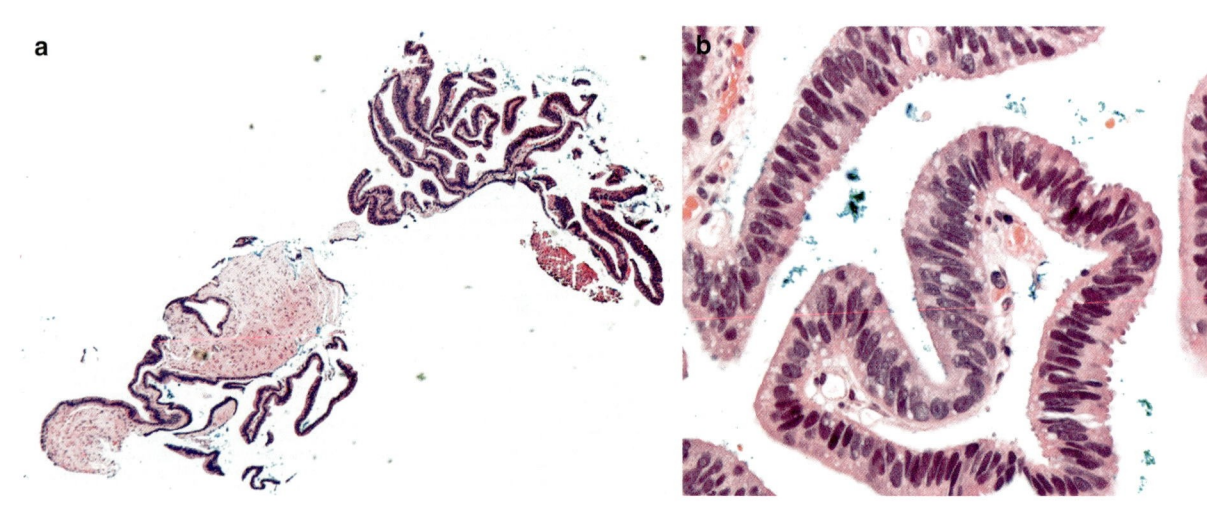

Fig. 9.13 Ductal adenocarcinoma of the prostate. It comprises glands much larger than benign glands (**a**). The cancer glands are lined with stratified columnar cells with or without significant nuclear atypia, superficially resembling endometrial glands (**b**). Necrosis can be present. Stains for basal cell markers can be confusing, as ductal carcinoma may retain basal cells in some cases

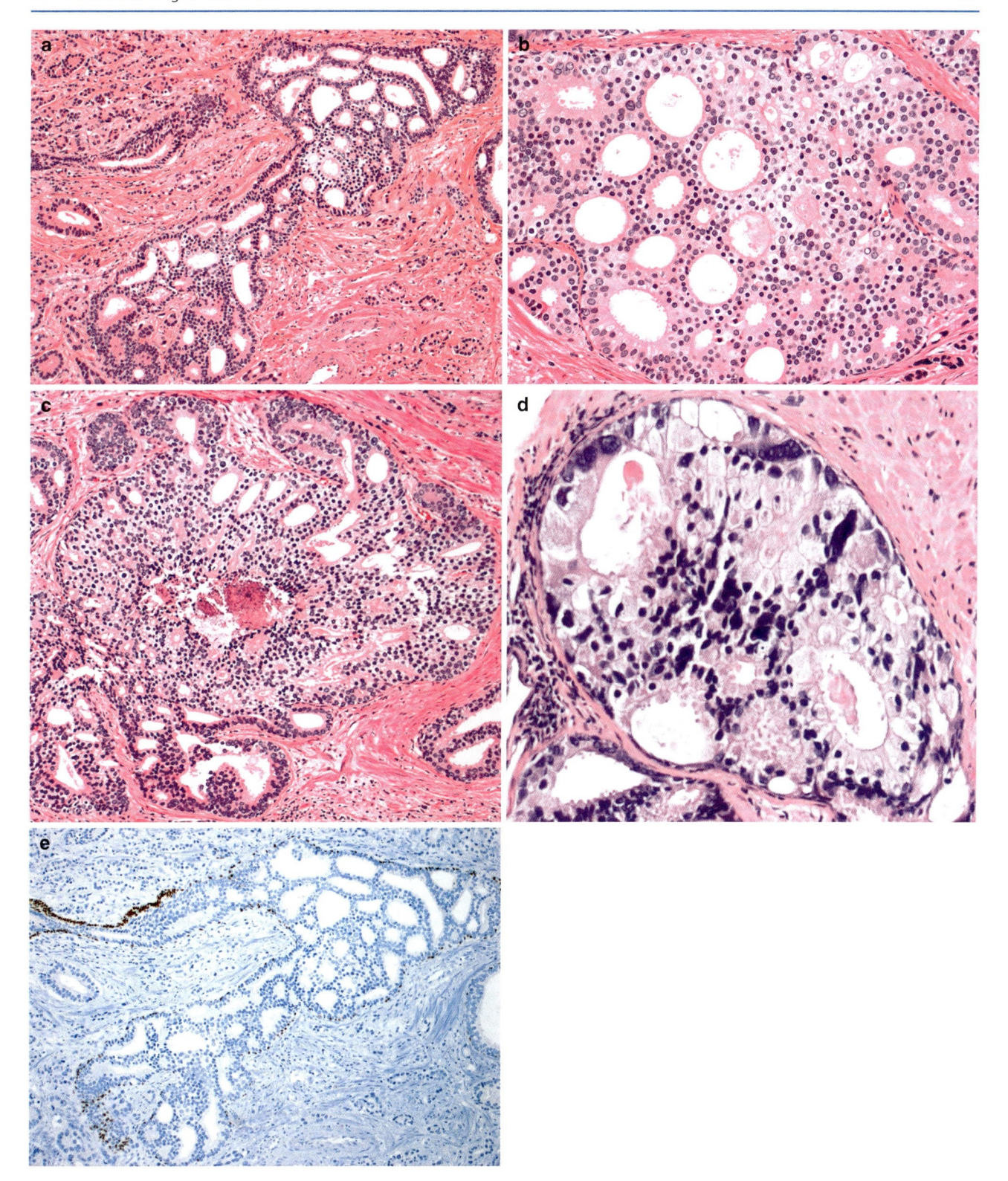

Fig. 9.14 Intraductal carcinoma of the prostate. Large glands with markedly irregular glandular contour intermingle with invasive cancer (**a**). These glands have much larger size and more irregular shape than HGPIN glands and are much more likely to have dense cribriform (**b**) or solid architecture and comedo necrosis (**c**). In addition, the constituent cells in intraductal carcinoma are more likely to exhibit marked nuclear pleomorphism (**d**). Basal cells are always retained in these glands (**e**)

9.5 Reporting of PIN

Table 9.5 Reporting of PIN

Low-grade PIN should not be diagnosed and reported

Quantifying HGPIN optional, but seems to correlate with the cancer risk in subsequent biopsy

   Focal (one core involved) vs multifocal (≥2 cores involved)

References

1. Bostwick DG, Qian J (2004) High-grade prostatic intraepithelial neoplasia. Mod Pathol 17:360–379
2. Epstein JI, Herawi M (2006) Prostate needle biopsies containing prostatic intraepithelial neoplasia or atypical foci suspicious for carcinoma: implications for patient care. J Urol 175(3 Pt 1): 820–834
3. McNeal JE, Bostwick DG (1986) Intraductal dysplasia: a premalignant lesion of the prostate. Hum Pathol 17:64–71
4. Humphrey PA (2003) Prostate pathology. ASCP Press, Chicago, p 186
5. Bostwick DG, Amin MB, Dundore P et al (1993) Architectural patterns of high-grade prostatic intraepithelial neoplasia. Hum Pathol 24:298–310
6. Epstein JI (2009) Precursor lesions to prostatic adenocarcinoma. Virchows Arch 454:1–16
7. Egevad L, Allsbrook WC, Epstein JI (2006) Current practice of diagnosis and reporting of prostatic intraepithelial neoplasia and glandular atypia among genitourinary pathologists. Mod Pathol 19:180–185
8. Rubin MA, Zhou M, Dhanasekaran SM et al (2002) alpha-Methylacyl coenzyme A racemase as a tissue biomarker for prostate cancer. JAMA 287:1662–1670
9. Wu CL, Yang XJ, Tretiakova M et al (2004) Analysis of alpha-methylacyl-CoA racemase (P504S) expression in high-grade prostatic intraepithelial neoplasia. Hum Pathol 35:1008–1013
10. Furusato B, Tan SH, Young D et al (2010) ERG oncoprotein expression in prostate cancer: clonal progression of ERG-positive tumor cells and potential for ERG-based stratification. Prostate Cancer Prostatic Dis 13:228–237
11. Park K, Tomlins SA, Mudaliar KM et al (2010) Antibody-based detection of ERG rearrangement-positive prostate cancer. Neoplasia 12:590–598
12. Perner S, Mosquera JM, Demichelis F et al (2007) TMPRSS2-ERG fusion prostate cancer: an early molecular event associated with invasion. Am J Surg Pathol 31:882–888
13. Godoy G, Taneja SS (2008) Contemporary clinical management of isolated high-grade prostatic intraepithelial neoplasia. Prostate Cancer Prostatic Dis 11:20–31
14. Schlesinger C, Bostwick DG, Iczkowski KA (2005) High-grade prostatic intraepithelial neoplasia and atypical small acinar proliferation: predictive value for cancer in current practice. Am J Surg Pathol 29:1201–1207
15. Lefkowitz GK, Sidhu GS, Torre P et al (2001) Is repeat prostate biopsy for high-grade prostatic intraepithelial neoplasia necessary after routine 12-core sampling? Urology 58:999–1003
16. Lefkowitz GK, Taneja SS, Brown J et al (2002) Followup interval prostate biopsy 3 years after diagnosis of high grade prostatic intraepithelial neoplasia is associated with high likelihood of prostate cancer, independent of change in prostate specific antigen levels. J Urol 168:1415–1418
17. Girasole CR, Cookson MS, Putzi MJ et al (2006) Significance of atypical and suspicious small acinar proliferations, and high grade prostatic intraepithelial neoplasia on prostate biopsy: implications for cancer detection and biopsy strategy. J Urol 175:929–933; discussion 933
18. Hameed O, Humphrey PA (2006) Stratified epithelium in prostatic adenocarcinoma: a mimic of high-grade prostatic intraepithelial neoplasia. Mod Pathol 19:899–906
19. Tavora F, Epstein JI (2008) High-grade prostatic intraepithelial neoplasialike ductal adenocarcinoma of the prostate: a clinicopathologic study of 28 cases. Am J Surg Pathol 32: 1060–1067
20. Guo CC, Epstein JI (2006) Intraductal carcinoma of the prostate on needle biopsy: histologic features and clinical significance. Mod Pathol 19:1528–1535
21. Han B, Suleman K, Wang L et al (2010) ETS gene aberrations in atypical cribriform lesions of the prostate: implications for the distinction between intraductal carcinoma of the prostate and cribriform high-grade prostatic intraepithelial neoplasia. Am J Surg Pathol 34:478–485
22. Shah RB, Magi-Galluzzi C, Han B, Zhou M (2010) Atypical cribriform lesions of the prostate: relationship to prostatic carcinoma and implication for diagnosis in prostate biopsies. Am J Surg Pathol 34:470–477

Atypical Glands Suspicious for Cancer

The diagnostic term "atypical glands suspicious for cancer (ATYP)," or "atypical small acinar proliferation (ASAP)," describes a small focus of prostate glands that exhibits some architectural and cytological atypia and is suspicious for yet falls short of the diagnostic threshold for prostate cancer [1]. It is not a distinct biological entity; rather, it encompasses a broad range of lesions of varying clinical significance, including under-sampled cancer, high-grade prostatic intra-epithelial neoplasia (HGPIN), benign lesions that mimic cancer, and benign prostate glands with reactive atypia [2]. An ATYP diagnosis in prostate needle biopsy is a significant risk factor for detecting prostate cancer in a subsequent biopsy. Such risk ranges from 17% to 70%, with an average of 42%, in published studies [3, 4], compared with the 20–25% risk of cancer associated with an HGPIN diagnosis. Patients with ATYP on initial biopsies are therefore recommended to undergo immediate repeat biopsies [1].

10.1 Histological Features Resulting in ATYP

Table 10.1 Histological features resulting in ATYP

Limited number of atypical glands (lesion minimally sampled in biopsy) (*see* Fig. 10.1)

Biopsy and tissue processing artifact impeding biopsy evaluation
Crush artifact obscuring morphology (*see* Fig. 10.2)
Poorly fixed or stained tissue section (*see* Fig. 10.3)
Atypical glands at the tip or edge of biopsy core (*see* Fig. 10.4)

Atypical morphology that can be seen in both cancer and noncancer lesions
Crowded glands with minimal cytological atypia (cancer vs. adenosis) (*see* Fig. 10.5)
Disorganized and poorly formed glands (cancer vs. partial atrophy)
Atypia in atrophic glands (atrophic cancer vs. benign atrophy) (*see* Fig. 10.6)
HGPIN with adjacent small focus of atypical glands (PINATYP) (microinvasive cancer developing from HGPIN vs. outpouching or tangential sectioning of HGPIN) (*see* Fig. 10.7) [5]
Atypia in the milieu of inflammation (inflamed cancer glands vs. reactive atypia) (*see* Fig. 10.8)

Confusing immunohistochemistry
Negative basal cell markers in a "benign lesion" (*see* Fig. 10.9)
Positive α-methylacyl-CoA racemase (AMACR) in a "benign lesion" (*see* Fig. 10.10)
Focal positive basal cell markers in "cancer glands" (*see* Fig. 10.11)

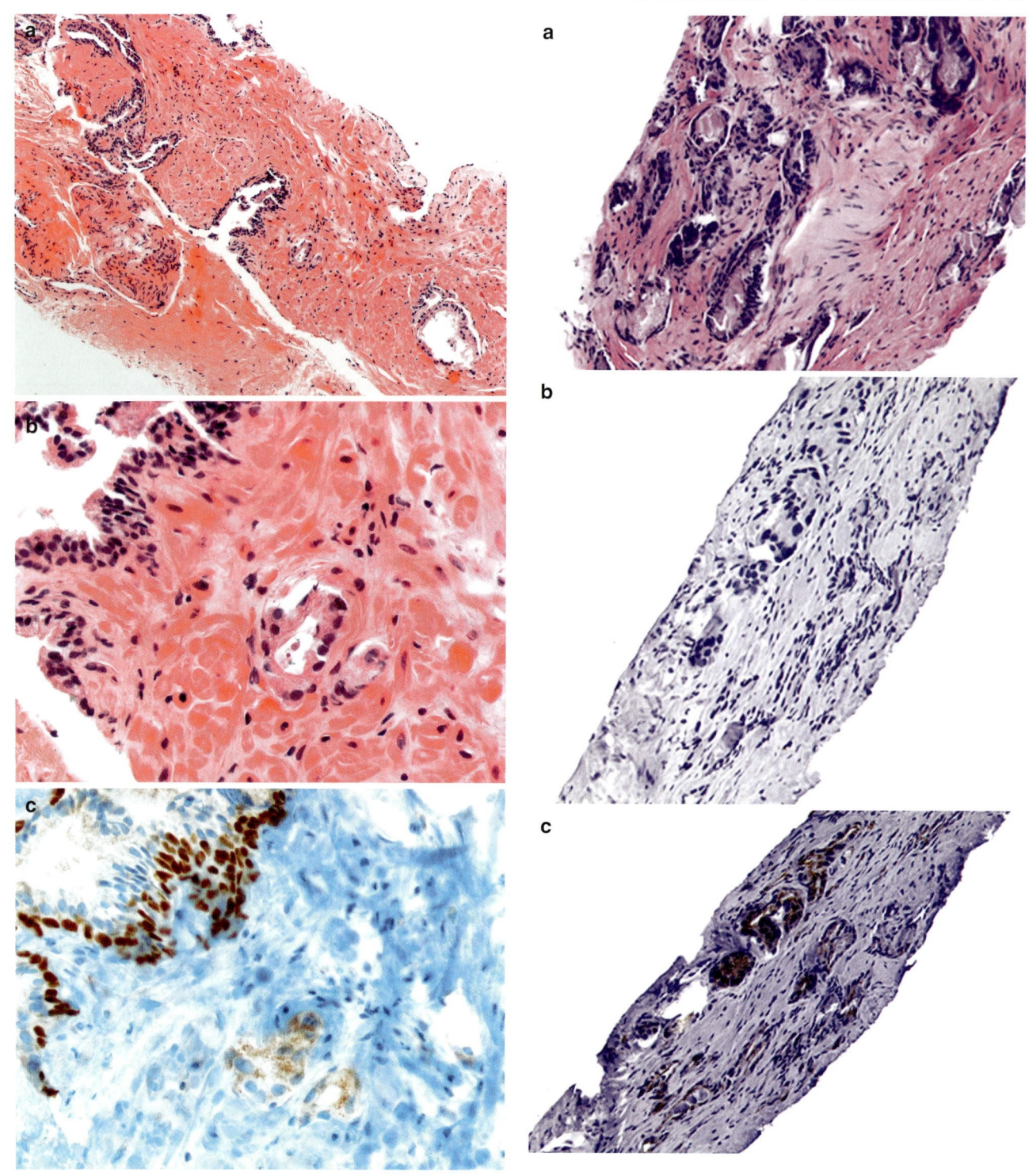

Fig. 10.1 Prostate biopsy with limited number of atypical glands. The biopsy contains two small glands with rigid lumens (**a**) and enlarged nuclei (**b**). They are negative for basal cell marker p63 and positive AMACR (**c**). Although highly suspicious for cancer, a definitive cancer diagnosis cannot be established due to the limited number of atypical glands

Fig. 10.2 Crush artifact obscures the morphology and impedes an adequate evaluation of the biopsy (**a**). Recut and immunohistochemistry may be helpful. In this example, the small crushed glands were negative for basal cell marker, high-molecular-weight cytokeratin (*HMWCK*) (**b**) and positive for AMACR (**c**). A diagnosis of cancer was rendered. Without immunostains, a definitive diagnosis is not possible and likely remains as ATYP

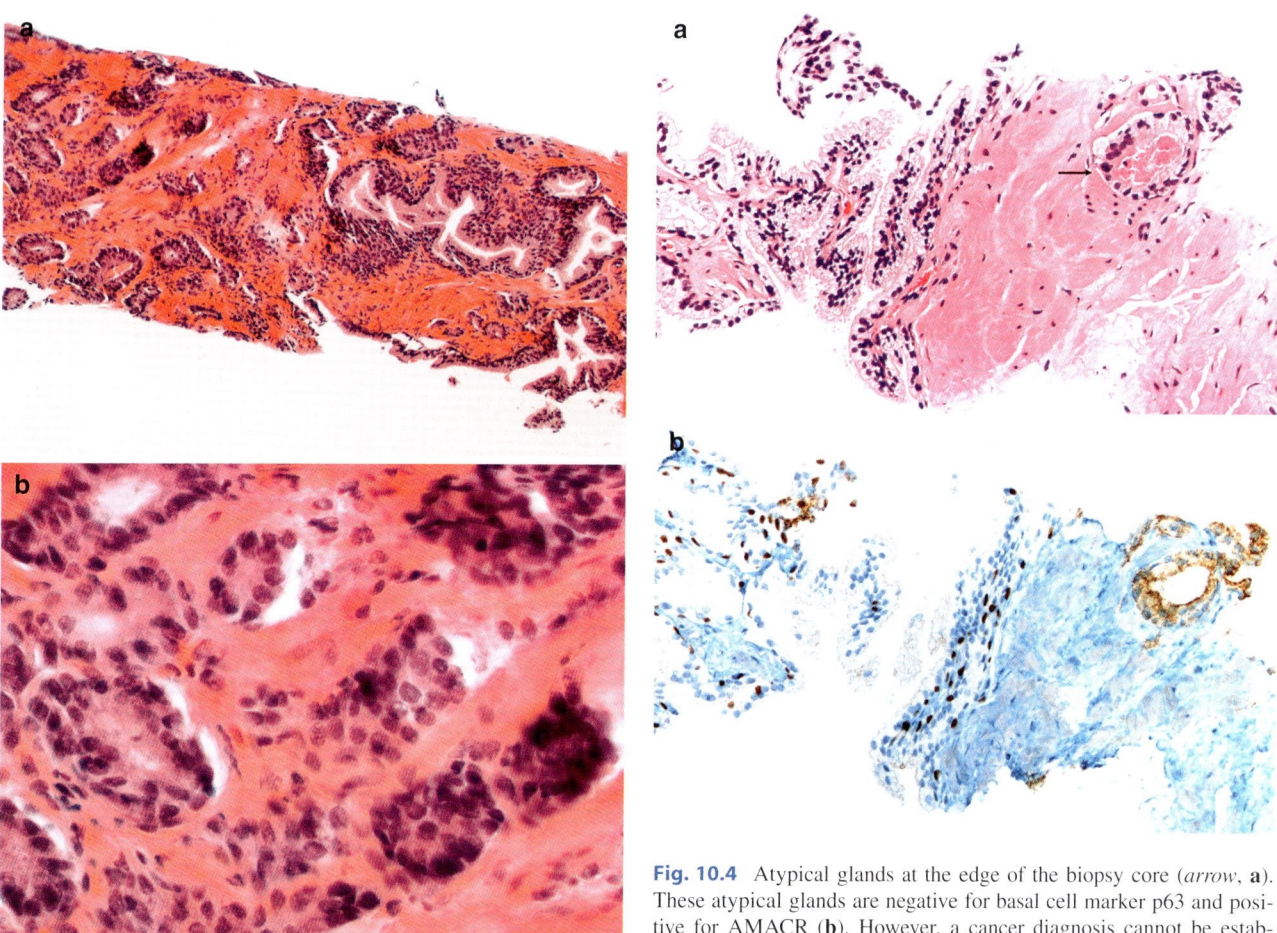

10.1 Histological Features Resulting in ATYP 133

Fig. 10.3 Thick section impedes evaluation of the biopsy. This biopsy contains many small crowded glands that exhibit infiltrative growth (**a**). Evaluation of the cytological features of these glands is hampered by the thick tissue sections (**b**). Recut and immunohistochemistry may be helpful. Without further workup, the diagnosis is ATYP

Fig. 10.4 Atypical glands at the edge of the biopsy core (*arrow*, **a**). These atypical glands are negative for basal cell marker p63 and positive for AMACR (**b**). However, a cancer diagnosis cannot be established because only a limited number of glands are present at the edge of the tissue core

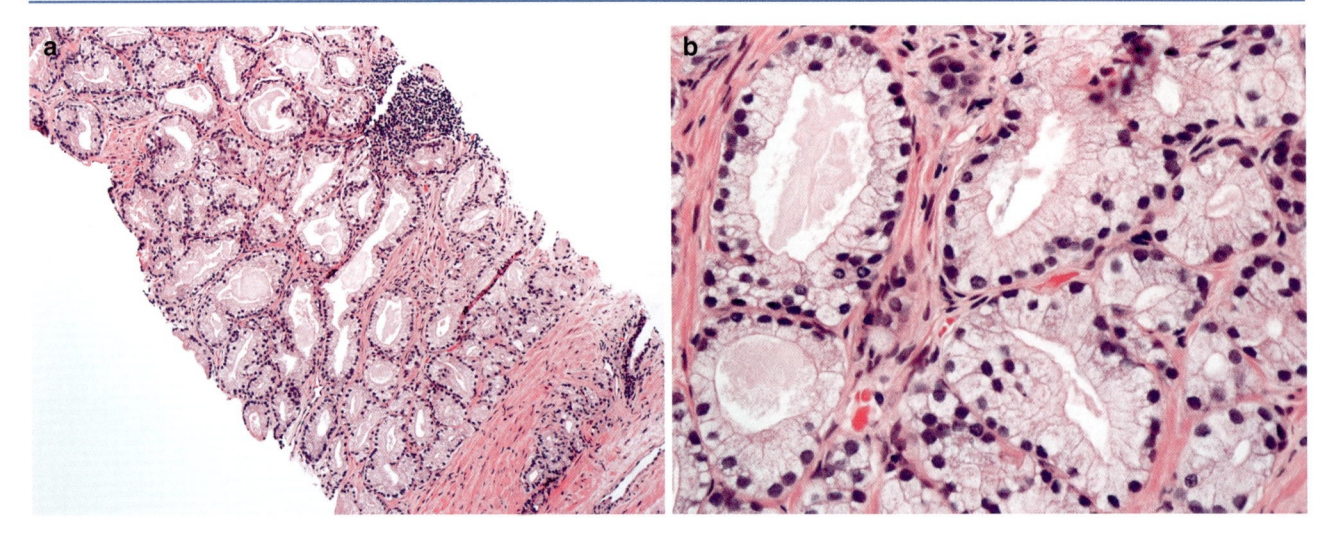

Fig. 10.5 A focus of circumscribed crowded glands (**a**) with slight nuclear enlargement and small nucleoli (**b**). The differential diagnosis includes adenosis and cancer that is typically found in anterior or transition zone of the prostate. Immunostains for basal cell markers and AMACR should be performed in an attempt to reach a definitive diagnosis

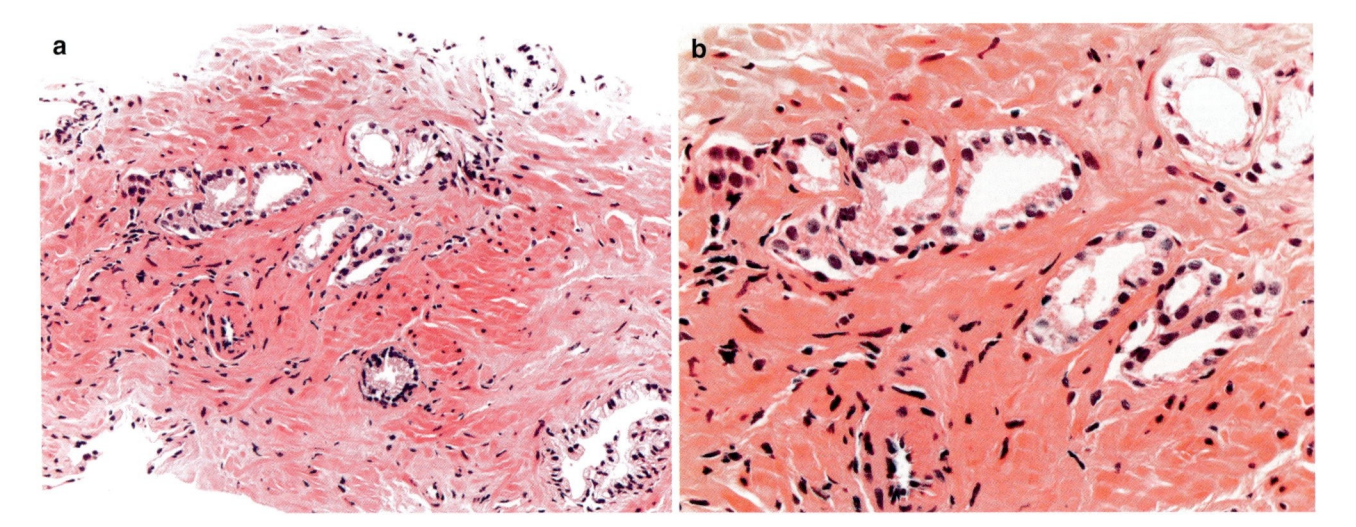

Fig. 10.6 Atrophic glands with crowded growth pattern (**a**) and nuclear enlargement and small nucleoli (**b**). The differential diagnosis includes an atrophic cancer and benign atrophy. Cancer glands may have atrophic cytoplasm. Benign atrophic glands may also exhibit some degree of architectural and/or cytological atypia, including nuclear enlargement and small nucleoli. However, frank nuclear atypia typical of cancer is not seen in benign atrophy. Immunostains for basal cell markers and AMACR should be performed in such borderline cases

10.1 Histological Features Resulting in ATYP

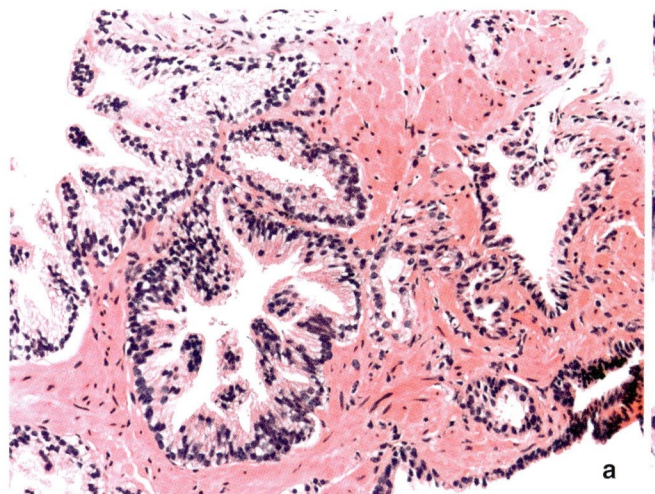

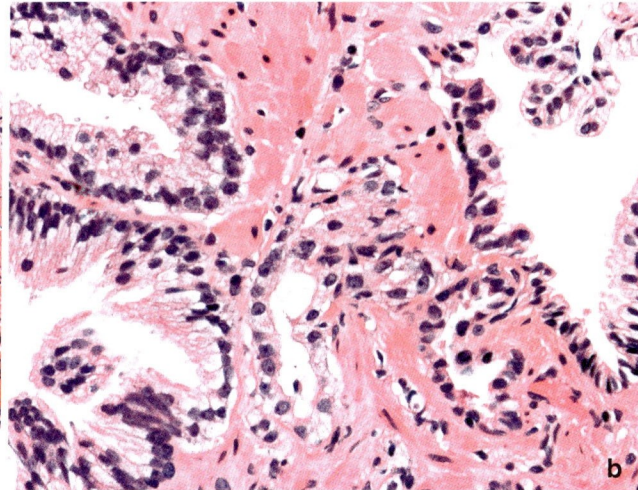

Fig. 10.7 HGPIN with adjacent small focus of atypical glands (PINATYP). Several small atypical glands lie immediately adjacent to a larger HGPIN gland (**a**). The nuclear atypia in these small atypical glands is similar to that in the HGPIN glands (**b**). It is uncertain whether these small atypical glands represent a focus of microinvasive cancer that has developed from HGPIN glands or tangential sectioning and/or outpouching of HGPIN glands. Such distinction may be possible based on the number of the atypical glands and their distance to the HGPIN glands. If the atypical glands are more than a few and not immediately adjacent to the HGPIN glands, they are unlikely the result of tangential sectioning and/or outpouching of the HGPIN glands

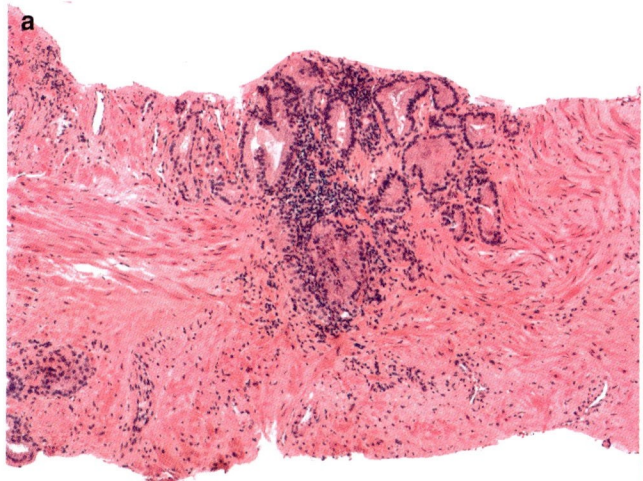

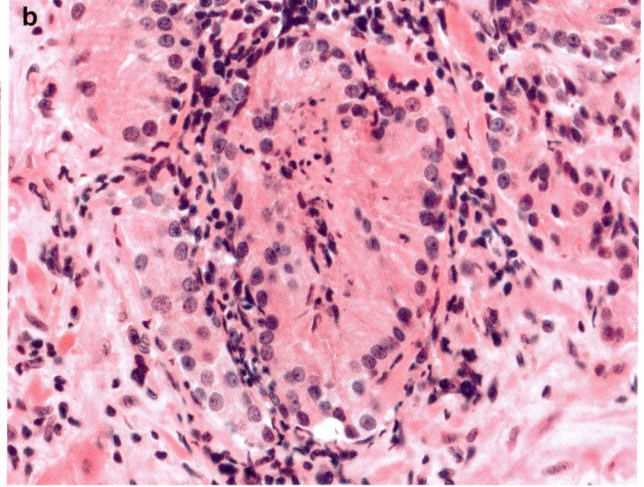

Fig. 10.8 Atypia associated with marked inflammation. This biopsy harbors a group of small glands (**a**) that exhibit nuclear enlargement and prominent nucleoli (**b**). There is marked acute inflammation (**b**). Inflamed benign glands may exhibit architectural and cytological atypia, including cribriform architecture, nuclear enlargement, and prominent nucleoli. On the other hand, cancer glands may be inflamed. Therefore, both conditions should be considered for a focus of atypical glands with inflammation. Immunostains for basal cell markers and AMACR should be performed to reach a definitive diagnosis

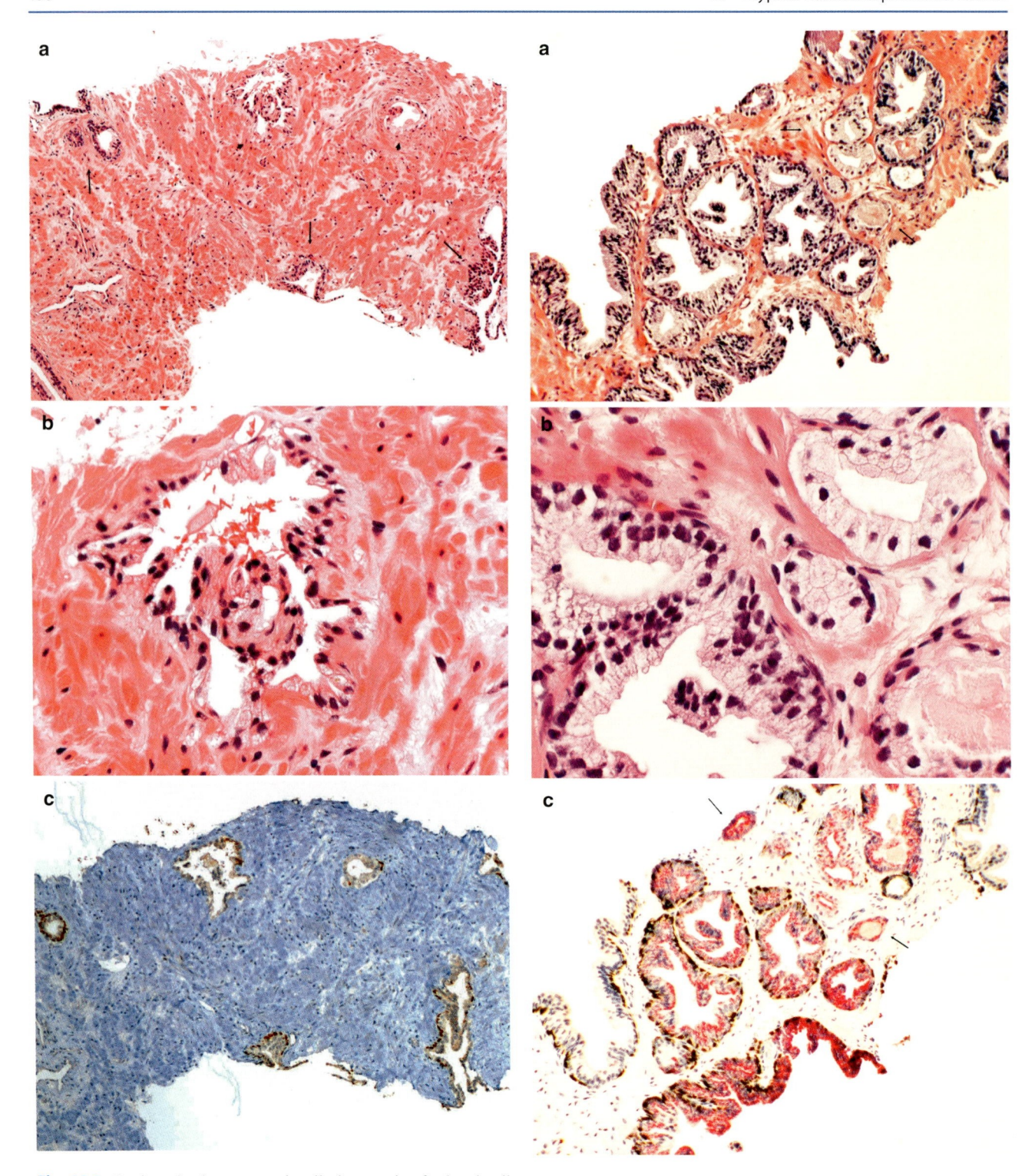

Fig. 10.9 Benign glands can occasionally be negative for basal cell markers. Several small glands (*arrowheads*) are cytologically identical to adjacent, larger, benign glands (*arrows*, **a**). No significant nuclear atypia is observed (**b**). One gland is negative and the other one focally positive for basal cell marker p63 (**c**). Basal cells may be absent in some noncancerous conditions including partial atrophy and adenosis. The lack of basal cells does not equate to cancer. When evaluating atypical glands, one should always use the adjacent benign glands as reference. A cancer diagnosis cannot be rendered in the absence of significant nuclear atypia

Fig. 10.10 Positive AMACR staining in benign prostate glands. Several small glands are adjacent (*arrows*, **a**) and cytologically identical to large benign glands (**b**). These small glands are negative for basal cell markers and positive for AMACR (**c**). Although preferentially expressed in prostate cancer glands, AMACR expression is also found in noncancerous glands, including HGPIN, adenosis, partial atrophy, and morphologically benign glands. When evaluating atypical glands, one should always use the adjacent benign glands as reference. A cancer diagnosis cannot be rendered in the absence of significant nuclear atypia

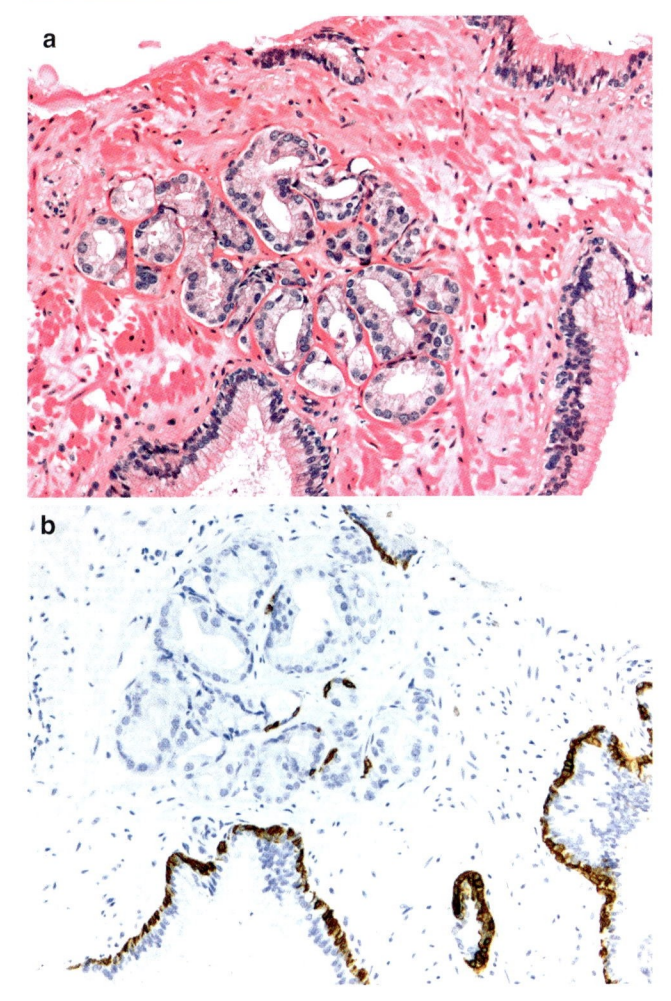

Fig. 10.11 A focus of small atypical glands highly suspicious for cancer with crowded growth pattern and enlarged nuclei and prominent nucleoli (**a**). However, several glands have basal cell marker HMWCK, some in basal cell distribution (**b**). Although basal cells are rarely present in prostate cancer [6], such a diagnosis should be reserved for radical prostatectomy or transurethral resection specimens where a large amount of tissue can be examined

Table 10.3 Diagnosis of ATYP: role of expert consultation

Study	Setting	Cases, n	Initial diagnosis by general pathologists	Final diagnosis by urologic pathologist
Renshaw et al. [7]	Academic	64	ATYP	Cancer, 20.3%
				Benign, 7.8%
Iczkowski et al. [8]	Academic	227	ATYP	Cancer, 2.2%
				Benign, 16.7%
Iczkowski et al. [9]	Urologic Pathology lab	376	ATYP	Cancer, 18%
				Benign 4%
Chan et al. [1]	Referral by pathologists	204	ATYP	Cancer, 45.1%
				Benign, 16.2%

10.3 Clinical Significance of ATYP

Table 10.4 Clinical significance of ATYP [1, 10]

Incidence

Mean, 5.0%

Median, 4.4% (range, 0.7–23.4%)

Trending toward lower incidence in recent studies

Cancer risk in subsequent rebiopsy

Remains relatively constant, 40–50%

Clinical parameters predicting cancer in subsequent biopsy

None, including prostate-specific antigen (PSA) measurements (PSA, free PSA, PSA velocity), digital rectal examination, and transrectal ultrasound imaging findings

Pathological parameters predicting cancer in subsequent biopsy

Categorizing ATYP into "favor cancer," "indeterminate," and "favor benign," based on the degree of suspicion for cancer, may correlate with different cancer risk in rebiopsy in some studies, but is subjective and not routinely done by pathologists

Follow-up scheme

Rebiopsy within 3 months using extended biopsy protocol

Rebiopsy strategy

Sampling the entire gland, with increased sampling of ATYP site and adjacent areas

10.2 Working up Cases with Atypical Diagnosis

Table 10.2 Working up prostate biopsies with atypical glands

Recut or deeper section may improve the histology and increase the number of atypical glands

Ancillary immunohistochemistry reduces the incidence of atypical prostate biopsy and converts ATYP to definitive diagnosis

Expert consultation may lead to definitive diagnosis in some cases (*see* Table 10.3)

References

1. Epstein JI, Herawi M (2006) Prostate needle biopsies containing prostatic intraepithelial neoplasia or atypical foci suspicious for carcinoma: implications for patient care. J Urol 175(3 Pt 1):820–834
2. Cheville JC, Reznicek MJ, Bostwick DG (1997) The focus of "atypical glands, suspicious for malignancy" in prostatic needle biopsy specimens: incidence, histologic features, and clinical follow-up of cases diagnosed in a community practice. Am J Clin Pathol 108:633–640
3. Abouassaly R, Tan N, Moussa A, Jones JS (2008) Risk of prostate cancer after diagnosis of atypical glands suspicious for carcinoma on saturation and traditional biopsies. J Urol 180:911–914; discussion 914
4. Zhou M, Magi-Galluzzi C (2010) Clinicopathological features of prostate cancers detected after an initial diagnosis of 'atypical glands suspicious for cancer'. Pathology 42:334–338
5. Kronz JD, Shaikh AA, Epstein JI (2001) High-grade prostatic intraepithelial neoplasia with adjacent small atypical glands on prostate biopsy. Hum Pathol 32:389–395
6. Oliai BR, Kahane H, Epstein JI (2002) Can basal cells be seen in adenocarcinoma of the prostate?: an immunohistochemical study using high molecular weight cytokeratin (clone 34betaE12) antibody. Am J Surg Pathol 26:1151–1160
7. Renshaw AA, Santis WF, Richie JP (1998) Clinicopathological characteristics of prostatic adenocarcinoma in men with atypical prostate needle biopsies. J Urol 159:2018–2021; discussion 2022
8. Iczkowski KA, Chen HM, Yang XJ, Beach RA (2002) Prostate cancer diagnosed after initial biopsy with atypical small acinar proliferation suspicious for malignancy is similar to cancer found on initial biopsy. Urology 60:851–854
9. Iczkowski KA, Bassler TJ, Schwob VS et al (1998) Diagnosis of "suspicious for malignancy" in prostate biopsies: predictive value for cancer. Urology 51:757; discussion 757–748
10. Schlesinger C, Bostwick DG, Iczkowski KA (2005) High-grade prostatic intraepithelial neoplasia and atypical small acinar proliferation: predictive value for cancer in current practice. Am J Surg Pathol 29:1201–1207

Spindle Cell Lesions of the Prostate Gland

11

Spindle cell lesions of the prostate are encountered infrequently in clinical practice but represent a broad spectrum of diagnostically challenging lesions with varying clinical significance. The spindle cell lesions encompass both primary and secondary processes. A subset of these lesions is thought to be derived from the hormone-responsive stroma of the prostate gland, including stromal hyperplasia, stromal tumors of uncertain malignant potential (STUMP), and prostate stromal sarcoma (PSS). The utility of ancillary studies, including immunohistochemistry, is often limited and the diagnosis relies on careful morphological evaluation.

11.1 Classification of Spindle Cell Lesions of the Prostate

Table 11.1 Classification of spindle cell lesions of the prostate [1–6]

Primary spindle cell lesions unique to prostate gland	Primary spindle cell lesions, not unique to prostate gland	Secondary spindle cell lesions
Stromal hyperplasia (benign prostatic hyperplasia [BPH])	Smooth muscle cell tumors (leiomyoma and leiomyosarcoma)	Gastrointestinal stromal tumors (GIST)
Sclerosing adenosis	Inflammatory myofibroblastic tumor	Other mesenchymal tumors
STUMP	Solitary fibrous tumor	
PSS	Rhabdomyosarcoma	
Sarcomatoid carcinoma of the prostate gland	Other mesenchymal tumors	

R.B. Shah, M. Zhou, *Prostate Biopsy Interpretation: An Illustrated Guide*,
DOI 10.1007/978-3-642-21369-4_11, © Springer-Verlag Berlin Heidelberg 2012

11.2 Specialized Stromal Tumors of the Prostate Gland

Table 11.2 Specialized stromal tumors of the prostate gland [1, 4, 6–19]

Specialized stromal tumors of the prostate gland

Definition

A diverse spectrum of tumors with varying clinical significance arising from hormonally responsive specialized stroma of the prostate

Reported under a variety of terms including prostatic stromal hyperplasia with atypia (PSHA), phyllodes type of atypical stromal hyperplasia, phyllodes tumor, and cystic epithelial-stromal tumors

Stromal tumors of uncertain malignant potential (STUMP) and PSS are preferred terms

Microscopical features

Low-power architecture

STUMP

Four patterns of STUMP are described. Different patterns often coexist.

Degenerative atypia pattern: Most common pattern seen in majority (>50%) of cases. Hypercellular stroma with scattered atypical degenerative cells (symplastic pattern) admixed with benign prostate glands (*see* Fig. 11.2a)

Myxoid pattern: Bland stromal cells embedded in a myxoid stroma; often lacks admixed glands (*see* Fig. 11.2b)

Phyllodes-type growth pattern: Leaf-like hypocellular fibrous stroma covered by benign-appearing prostatic epithelium, similar to benign phyllodes tumor of the breast (*see* Fig. 11.2c)

Hypercellular stroma pattern: Hypercellular fusiform stromal cells with eosinophilic cytoplasm without glands (*see* Fig. 11.2d)

PSS

Monophasic or phyllodes-like biphasic stromal overgrowth with overt infiltration, greater cellularity, pleomorphism, and frequent extraprostatic extension (*see* Fig. 11.3)

High-grade spindle cells may demonstrate solid, stroriform, epithelioid, fibrosarcomatous, or nonspecific pattern that infiltrate between benign prostate glands or may demonstrate stromal predominance

High-power cytology

STUMP

Atypical stromal cells in STUMPs are pleomorphic and hyperchromatic, with a marked degenerative appearance

Mitotic figures are typically absent and atypical mitotic activity should not be present

PSS

Stromal overgrowth with hypercellularity, frank cytologic atypia, mitotic figures, and necrosis

Epithelial component if present is typically benign in nature

Divided into low and high grade depending on the degree of cytologic atypia

PSS, low grade, has low-to-moderate stromal cellularity, minimal cytologic atypia, mitosis <2/10 high-power field (HPF), and lacks necrosis

PSS, high grade, has moderate-to-high cellularity, nuclear pleomorphism, mitosis >5/10 HPF, and frequent necrosis

Immunohistochemical features

Both STUMP and PSS typically express CD34 and vimentin

Progesterone receptor is frequently present while estrogen receptor is infrequently expressed

Desmin, HHF-35, and smooth muscle actin are often positive in STUMP but negative in PSS

In a subset of cases, pancytokeratin and CAM5.2 stains are focally expressed

Differential diagnosis (*see* Fig. 11.7)

In transurethral resections, prominent stromal hyperplasia (BPH) may get confused with STUMP. Presence of multinodularity, lack of intermingling glands, uniform spindle cells, prominent blood vessels, and presence of chronic inflammatory cells favor stromal BPH

Past history of prostate adenocarcinoma and the presence of malignant glands suggest the diagnosis of sarcomatoid carcinoma (*see* Fig. 6.12)

C-kit or ALK-1 immunoreactivity suggests a specific diagnosis of GIST or inflammatory myofibroblastic tumor, respectively

Definitive diagnosis in small needle biopsy may not be feasible and may need an excision for definitive classification

Clinical presentation and significance

PSS occurs with an age range of 25–86 years and approximately half of the cases affect patients <50 years

Patients usually present with obstructive urinary symptoms, hematuria, and abnormal digital rectal examination (DRE)

Rectal pain and palpable mass are present in minority of cases

STUMPs are clinically heterogeneous in behavior but usually behave in an indolent manner; are typically confined to the prostate; rare cases progress to stromal sarcoma; therefore should be considered to have an unpredictable malignant potential

PSS may extend out of the prostate and may metastasize to distant sites, such as bone, lung, abdomen, and retroperitoneum

11.3 Clinical, Morphologic, and Immunohistochemical Features Suggestive of Prostate Origin of the Spindle Cell Lesions

Table 11.3 Clinical, morphologic, and immunohistochemical features suggestive of prostate origin of the spindle cell lesions

Elevated serum prostate-specific antigen level and/or abnormal DRE
Prior history of prostatic adenocarcinoma
Admixture of spindle cell component and benign or malignant prostate glands
Expression of both CD34 and progesterone receptors

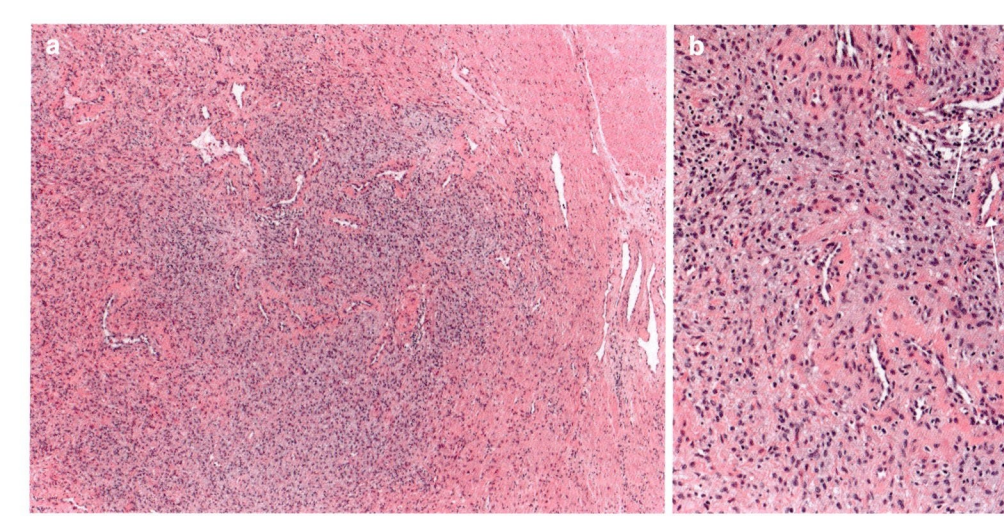

Fig. 11.1 Stromal hyperplasia. (**a–b**) At low magnification, stromal hyperplasia is characterized by nodular proliferation of uniform spindle cells usually without admixed prostate glands (**a**). At higher magnification, spindle cells are bland, uniform, and lack cytologic atypia and/or mitotic activity. Scattered inflammatory cells and prominent blood vessels with thick hyalinized wall (*arrows*) are also evident (**b**)

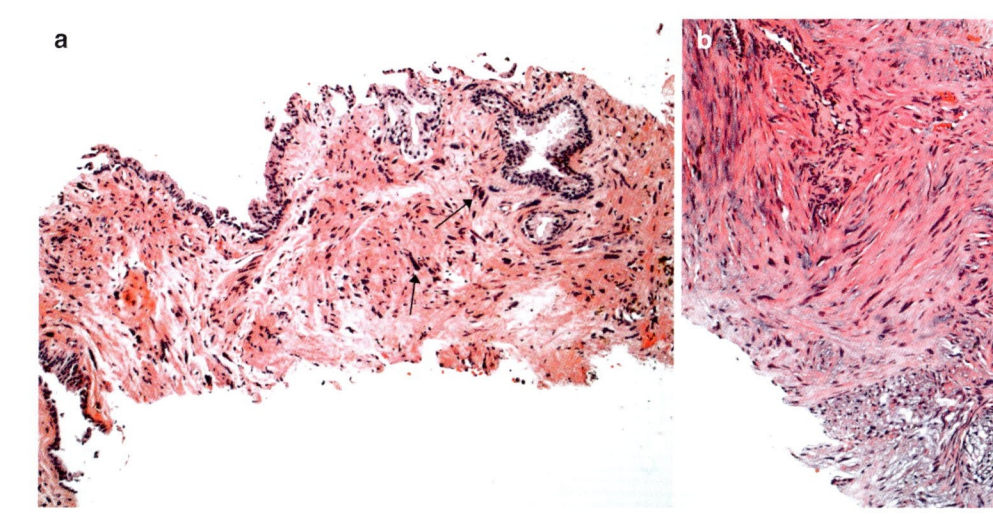

Fig. 11.2 STUMP. (**a–d**) Classic pattern is characterized by proliferation of spindle cells admixed with benign prostate glands. Note the presence of scattered pleomorphic atypical cells (*arrows*) (**a**) and focal prominent myxoid changes (**b**). Another example showing stromal and glandular proliferation reminiscent of phyllodes tumor of the breast (**c**). Hypercellular stroma pattern demonstrating atypical stromal proliferation (*arrows*) without admixed prostate glands. Note atypia is degenerative in nature without any mitotic activity (**d**)

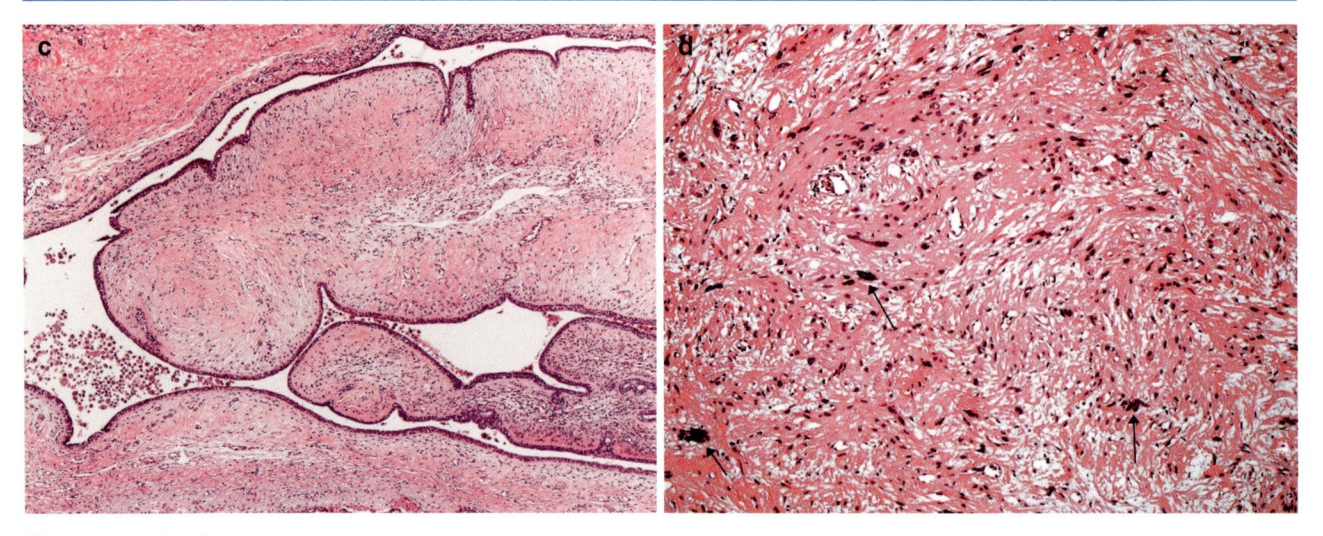

Fig. 11.2 (continued)

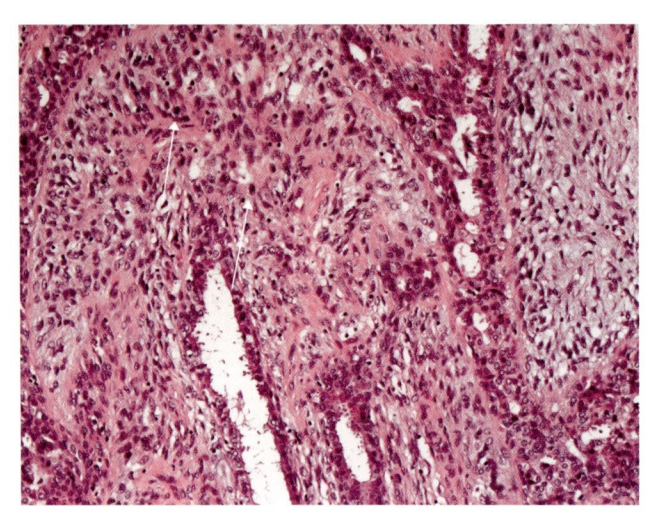

Fig. 11.3 PSS. In contrast to STUMP, PSS demonstrates high cellularity and obvious cytologic atypia with frequent mitoses (*arrows*). In this example, malignant phyllodes-like stromal sarcoma demonstrate hypercellular, atypical stromal cells with increased mitotic activity. The leaf-like elements are lined by benign prostatic epithelium, a helpful feature to differentiate it from carcinosarcoma (sarcomatoid carcinoma) of the prostate

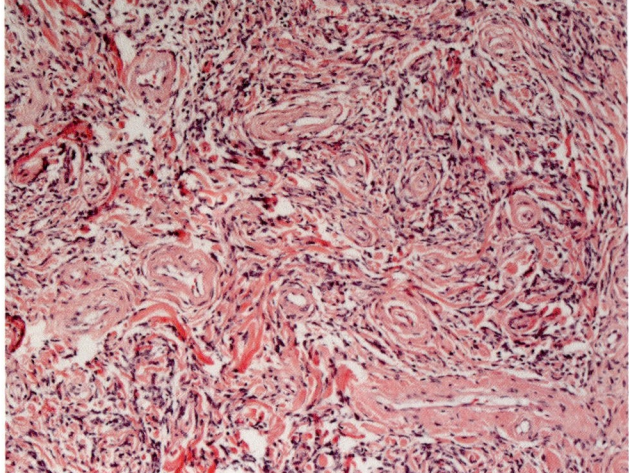

Fig. 11.4 Solitary fibrous tumor involving the prostate gland demonstrates proliferation of bland spindle cells with a "pattern-less" pattern of stroma that is collagenized. Lack of admixed prostate glands and prominent collagen deposition in the stroma distinguishes it from a prostate stromal tumor. Immunohistochemical features are usually not helpful in this distinction as solitary fibrous tumors typically express CD34 and often are also positive for progesterone receptor

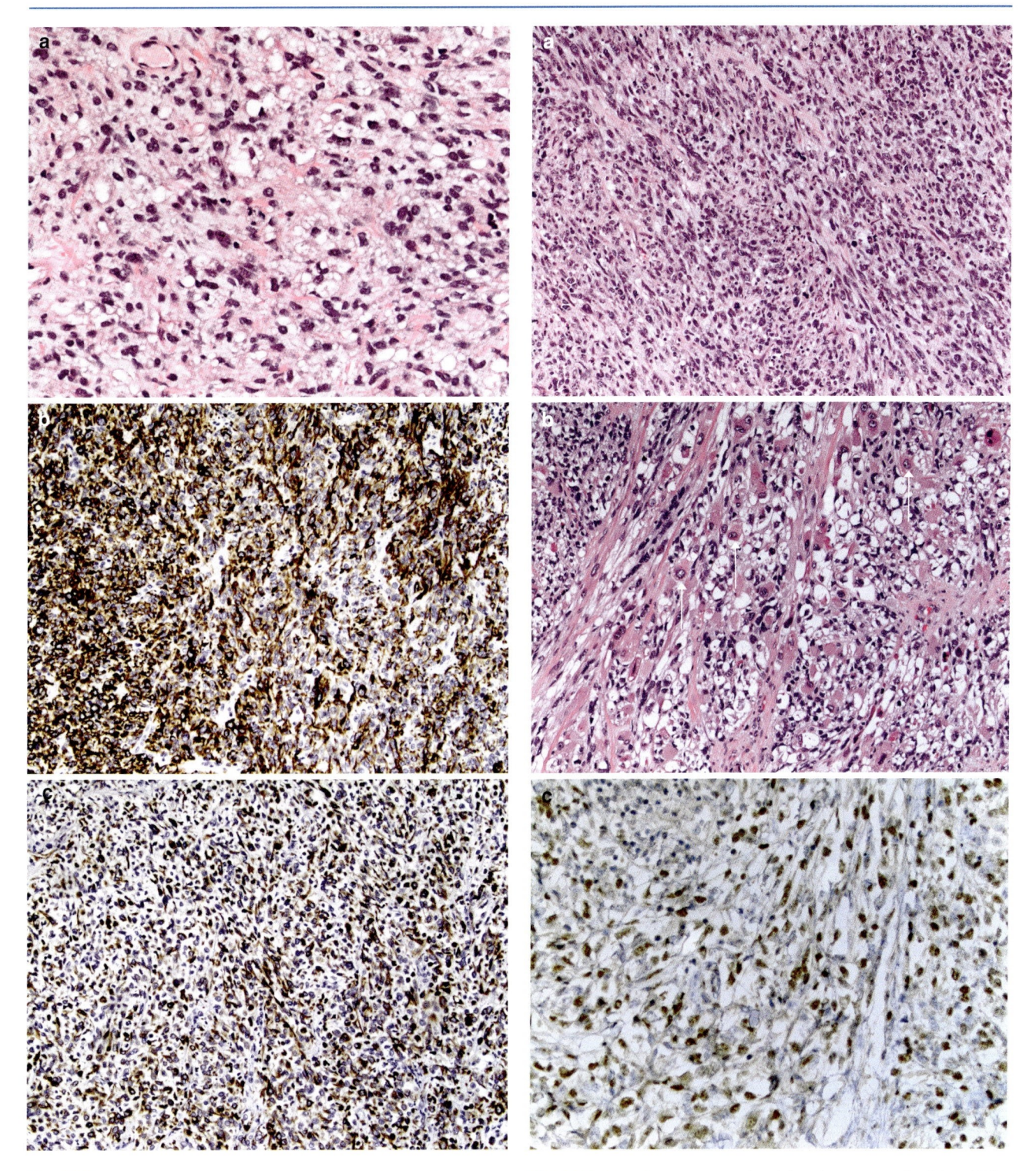

Fig. 11.5 High-grade spindle cell neoplasm involving the prostate gland, diagnosed as high-grade leiomyosarcoma. (**a–c**) The transurethral resection of the prostate (TURP) specimen from a 58-year-old man demonstrated diffuse proliferation of high-grade spindle and epithelioid cells in a haphazard pattern. Some nuclei have a cigar shape and demonstrate frequent atypical mitoses. The differential diagnosis included PSS, sarcomatoid carcinoma, and leiomyosarcoma. Tumor cells were diffusely and strongly positive for several muscle markers including desmin (**b**), calponin, and muscle-specific actin (*not shown*). The tumor cells also demonstrated focal aberrant reactivity for pan cytokeratin (**c**). The diagnosis of high-grade leiomyosarcoma was made

Fig. 11.6 Rhabdomyosarcoma involving the prostate gland. (**a–c**) The prostate gland is replaced by a high-grade undifferentiated sarcoma with numerous atypical mitoses and cellular pleomorphism (**a**). Another area demonstrated characteristic rhabdomyoblasts (*arrow*) with abundant eosinophilic cytoplasm (**b**). Both myogenin (**c**) and desmin were strongly positive, supporting the diagnosis of rhabdomyosarcoma

11.4 Diagnostic Approach to Spindle Cell Lesions of the Prostate

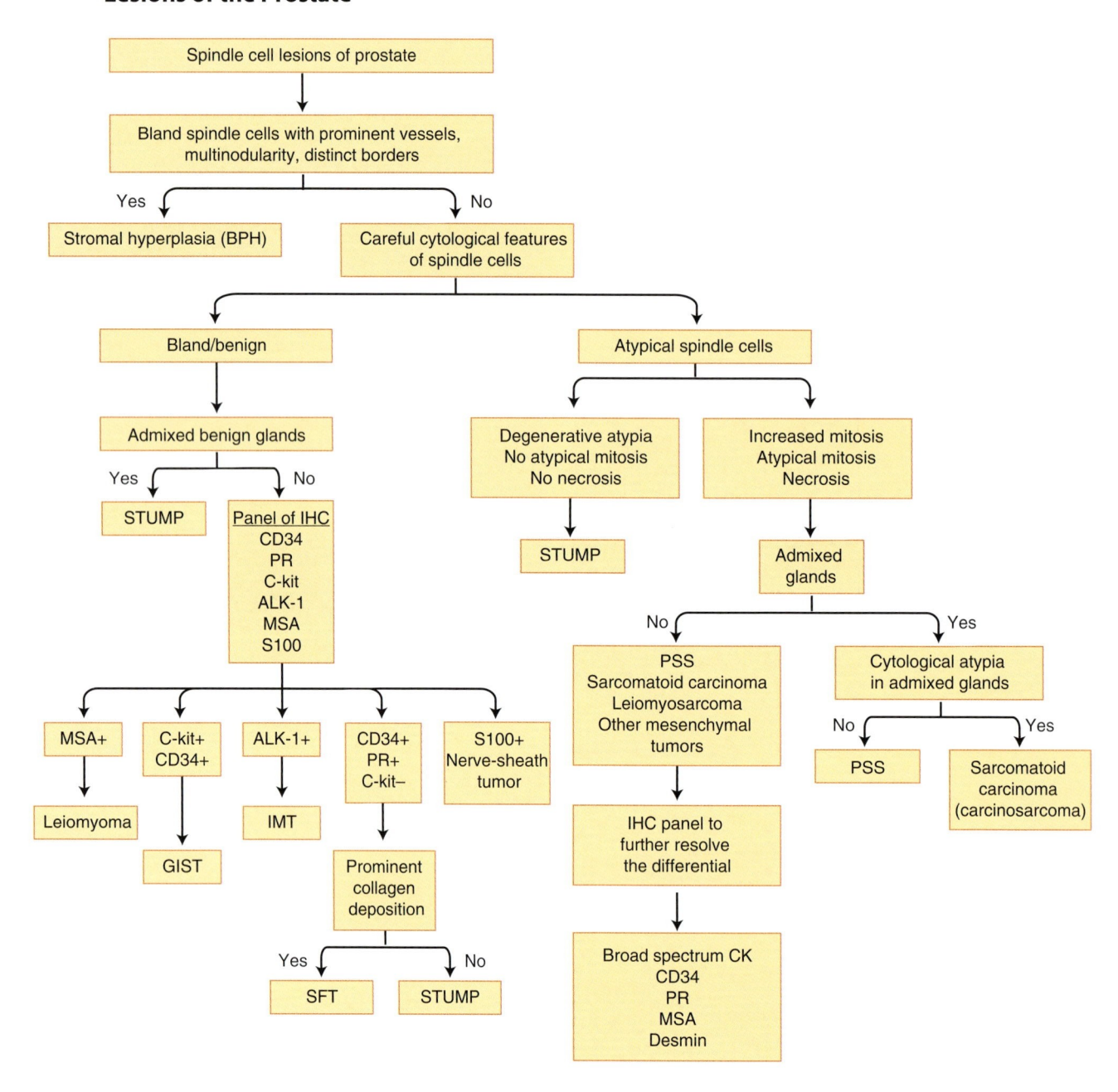

Fig. 11.7 Diagnostic approach to spindle cell lesions of the prostate

11.5 Immunohistochemical Characteristics of Select Spindle Cell Lesions of the Prostate

Table 11.4 Immunohistochemical characteristics of select spindle cell lesions of prostate [1–5, 9, 15, 16]

	CD34	PR	ER	C-kit	ALK-1	SMA	Desmin	Myogenin
STUMP	+	+	±	−	−	±	±	−
Stromal sarcoma	+	+	±	−	−	−	−	−
IMT	−	−	−	±	+	+	+	−
SFT	+	±	−	−	−	−	−	−
GIST	+	−	−	+	−	±	±	−
Leiomyosarcoma	−	±	±	−	−	+	+	−
Rhabdomyosarcoma	−	−	−	−	−	+	+	+

Adapted from Hansel et al. [3]

± variable expression, *ER* estrogen receptor, *GIST* gastrointestinal stromal tumor, *IMT* inflammatory myofibroblastic tumor, *PR* progesterone receptor, *SFT* solitary fibrous tumor, *SMA* smooth muscle actin, *STUMP* stromal tumors of uncertain malignant potential

References

1. Bostwick DG, Hossain D, Qian J et al (2004) Phyllodes tumor of the prostate: long-term followup study of 23 cases. J Urol 172:894–899
2. Grasso M, Blanco S, Franzoso F et al (2002) Solitary fibrous tumor of the prostate. J Urol 168:1100
3. Hansel DE, Herawi M, Montgomery E, Epstein JI (2007) Spindle cell lesions of the adult prostate. Mod Pathol 20:148–158
4. Herawi M, Epstein JI (2006) Specialized stromal tumors of the prostate: a clinicopathologic study of 50 cases. Am J Surg Pathol 30:694–704
5. Herawi M, Montgomery EA, Epstein JI (2006) Gastrointestinal stromal tumors (GISTs) on prostate needle biopsy: a clinicopathologic study of 8 cases. Am J Surg Pathol 30:1389–1395
6. Hossain D, Meiers I, Qian J et al (2008) Prostatic stromal hyperplasia with atypia: follow-up study of 18 cases. Arch Pathol Lab Med 132:1729–1733
7. Attah EB, Powell ME (1977) Atypical stromal hyperplasia of the prostate gland. Am J Clin Pathol 67:324–327
8. Egevad L, Carbin BE, Castellanos E et al (2008) Atypical stromal hyperplasia of the prostate. Scand J Urol Nephrol 42:484–487
9. Gaudin PB, Rosai J, Epstein JI (1998) Sarcomas and related proliferative lesions of specialized prostatic stroma: a clinicopathologic study of 22 cases. Am J Surg Pathol 22:148–162
10. Kerley SW, Pierce P, Thomas J (1992) Giant cystosarcoma phyllodes of the prostate associated with adenocarcinoma. Arch Pathol Lab Med 116:195–197
11. Kevwitch MK, Walloch JL, Waters WB, Flanigan RC (1993) Prostatic cystic epithelial-stromal tumors: a report of 2 new cases. J Urol 149:860–864
12. Lam KC, Yeo W (2002) Chemotherapy induced complete remission in malignant phyllodes tumor of the prostate metastasizing to the lung. J Urol 168:1104–1105
13. Leong SS, Vogt PJ, Yu GS (1988) Atypical stromal smooth muscle hyperplasia of prostate. Urology 31:163–167
14. Löpez-Beltran A, Gaeta JF, Huben R, Croghan GA (1990) Malignant phyllodes tumor of prostate. Urology 35:164–167
15. Schapmans S, Van Leuven L, Cortvriend J et al (2000) Phyllodes tumor of the prostate. A case report and review of the literature. Eur Urol 38:649–653
16. Sexton WJ, Lance RE, Reyes AO et al (2001) Adult prostate sarcoma: the MD Anderson Cancer Center Experience. J Urol 166:521–525
17. Tijare JR, Shrikhande AV, Shrikhande VV (1999) Phyllodes type of atypical prostatic hyperplasia. J Urol 162:803–804
18. Watanabe M, Yamada Y, Kato H et al (2002) Malignant phyllodes tumor of the prostate: retrospective review of specimens obtained by sequential transurethral resection. Pathol Int 52:777–783
19. Young JF, Jensen PE, Wiley CA (1992) Malignant phyllodes tumor of the prostate. A case report with immunohistochemical and ultrastructural studies. Arch Pathol Lab Med 116:296–299

Treatment Effect in Benign and Malignant Prostate Tissue

12

Prostate lesions can be managed by several surgical and nonsurgical modalities, including surgical resection and, ablation by physical methods such as cryo- and thermal ablation (*see* Table 12.1). Treatment can cause significant histological changes in both benign and malignant prostate tissue [1]. Such changes may pose a significant challenge in interpretation, particularly in needle biopsy specimens. In addition, prostate cancer with treatment effect should not be assigned a Gleason grade. History of such treatment, however, is not always provided by clinicians. Therefore, pathologists should be aware of the histological changes associated with treatment in benign and malignant prostate tissue.

12.1 Treatment Modalities for Prostate Lesions

Table 12.1 Treatment modalities for prostate lesions

Treatment modality	Clinical indication
Active surveillance	Men with very low-risk prostate cancer (PCa) and life expectancy < 20 years or men with low-risk PCa and life expectancy < 10 years
Radical prostatectomy	Clinically organ-confined PCa
Androgen deprivation (luteinizing hormone-releasing hormone [LHRH] antagonists and anti-androgens)	In conjunction with definitive radiation therapy for high-risk, clinically localized, or locally advanced PCa; metastatic PCa
5-α–reductase inhibitors	Benign prostatic hypertrophy
Radiation (external beam, brachytherapy)	Clinically localized prostate cancer
Cryotherapy	Less well-established alternative to prostatectomy and radiation; may be used as salvage therapy for failed radiation or focal therapy
Hyperthermia (laser, microwave)	Benign prostatic hypertrophy; less well-established alternative to prostatectomy and radiation for localized PCa

12.2 Androgen Pathway and Anti-androgen Therapy in Prostate Lesions

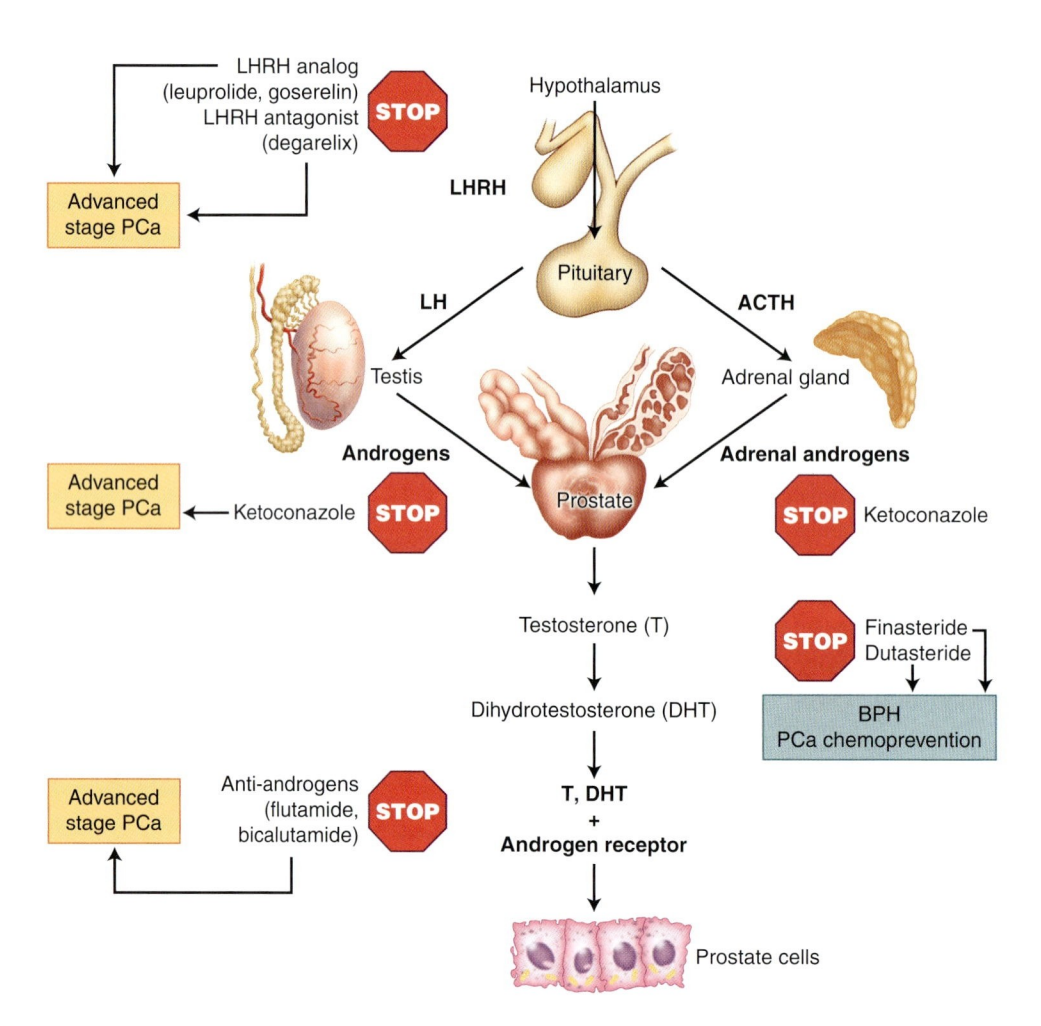

Fig. 12.1 Androgen pathway and androgen-deprivation therapy in prostate cancer. Androgens play critical roles in the development and function of the normal prostate gland and in prostate carcinogenesis. Agents that block androgen production (LHRH agonists [leuprolide and goserelin] and antagonists [degarelix], and ketoconazole) and androgen receptors (flutamide and bicalutamide) are prescribed for advanced stage prostate cancer. A combination of LHRH agonists and anti-androgens is a very potent inhibitor of androgen pathways and can often achieve castrate levels of serum testosterone, and significant histological changes in both benign and malignant prostate tissue [2]. 5-α–reductase inhibitors (finasteride and dutasteride) block the conversion of testosterone to more potent dihydrotestosterone. They are prescribed for benign prostatic hypertrophy and recently are used in prostate cancer prevention trial. However, testosterone is still present; therefore, total androgen withdrawal is not achieved. As a result, 5-α–reductase inhibitors causes minimum to no histological changes in prostate tissue [3, 4]

12.3 Histologic Changes Following Androgen-deprivation Therapy in Benign and Malignant Prostate Tissue

Table 12.2 Histologic changes following androgen-deprivation therapy in benign and malignant prostate tissue

Benign prostatic tissue (*See* Fig. 12.2 and 12.3)
   Secretory cells
      Decreased gland/stroma ratio
      Glandular atrophy
      Cytoplasmic vacuolation and clearing
      Small and dense nuclei
   Basal cells
      Basal cell hyperplasia
      Urothelial and squamous metaplasia
   Stroma
      Stromal prominence
      Edema and fibrosis
      Lymphohistiocytic infiltration

Malignant prostatic tissue (*See* Fig. 12.4–12.10)
   Architecture
      Loss of glandular architecture simulating pattern 4/5
      Single cells resembling histiocytes
      Mucinous degeneration with formation of mucin lake
   Cytoplasm
      Atrophic changes mimicking benign atrophy
      Cytoplasmic clearing and vacuolation
   Nuclei
      Shrunken or pyknotic

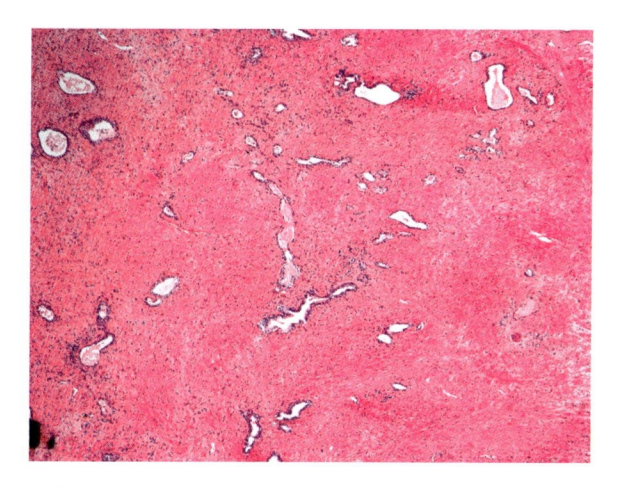

Fig. 12.2 Benign prostate tissue after androgen deprivation: glandular atrophy. Benign glands become diffusely atrophic, although they still maintain their size and lobulated architecture. As a result, stroma is prominent. It also shows fibrosis and patchy lymphohistiocytic inflammatory infiltration

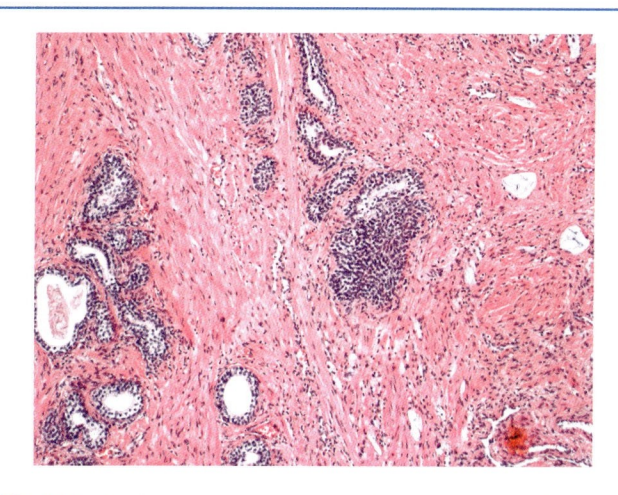

Fig. 12.3 Benign prostate tissue after androgen deprivation: basal cell hyperplasia. Benign glands show prominent basal cell hyperplasia and may undergo urothelial and squamous metaplasia. Secretory cells are atrophic with reduced cell height. The stroma shows fibrosis and mixed inflammatory infiltrates. Also notice cancer glands (*right*) disintegrate into single cells or small clusters

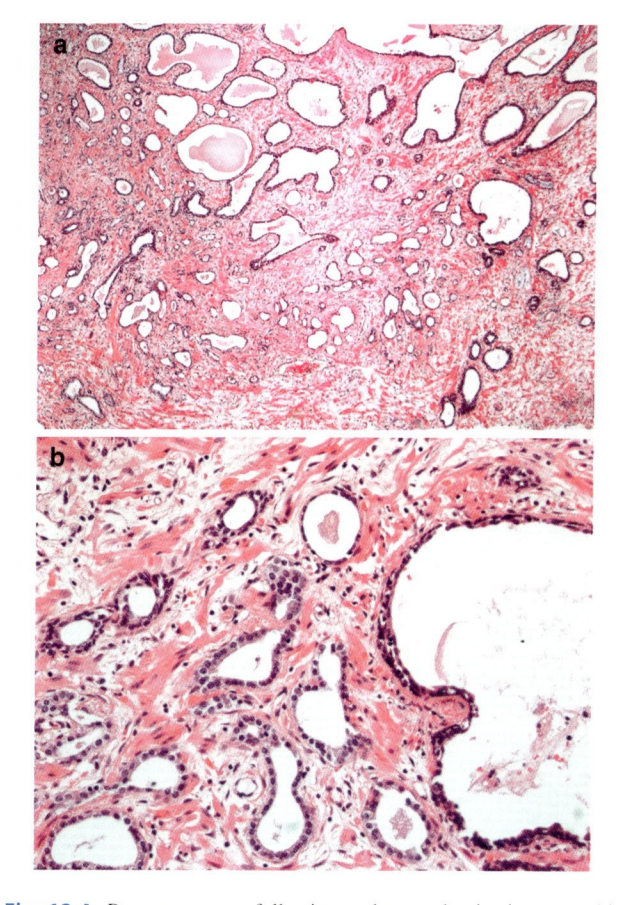

Fig. 12.4 Prostate cancer following androgen deprivation: atrophic changes. Cancer glands become atrophic (*lower half*). They intermingle with larger atrophic benign glands (*upper half*) and are indistinguishable from the latter at the low magnification (**a**). They are small and crowded, however, and exhibit infiltrative growth between the benign glands, a telltale sign of cancer. At high magnification, some cancer cells, although atrophic, still have prominent nucleoli (**b**)

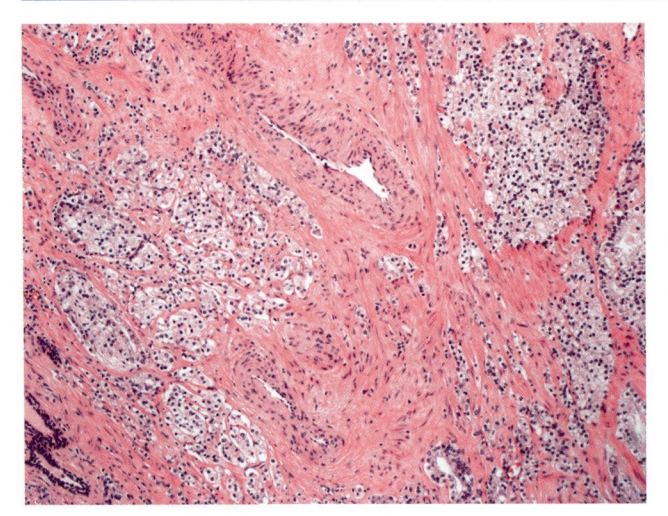

Fig. 12.5 Prostate cancer following androgen deprivation: loss of glandular architecture. This is the most common finding after androgen deprivation. Cancer cells form single cells, single-file, small and large irregular nests

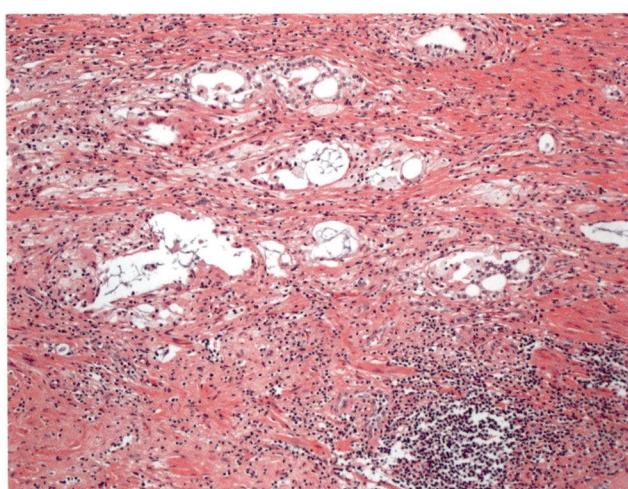

Fig. 12.7 Prostate cancer following androgen deprivation: mucinous degeneration. Cancer glands disintegrate and form "mucin lake" in which wisps of blue mucin and occasional cancer cells are seen. Sometimes, clear acellular space is seen

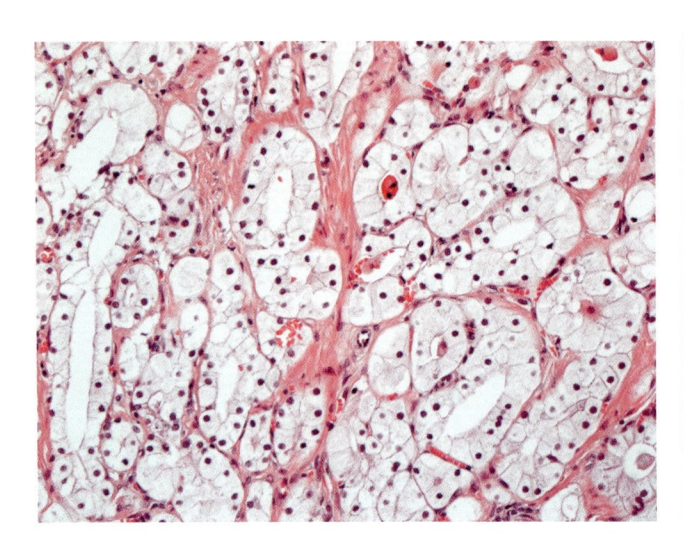

Fig. 12.6 Prostate cancer following androgen deprivation: "bland cytology." Cancer cells have abundant clear cytoplasm and small, dense nuclei without prominent nucleoli

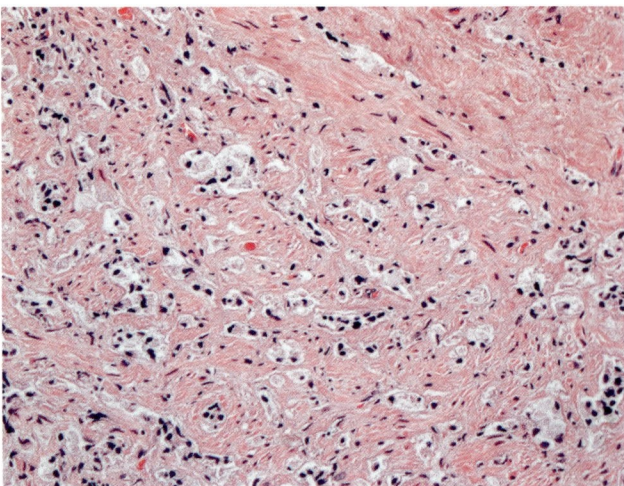

Fig. 12.8 Prostate cancer following androgen deprivation: "histiocyte-like." Single or small cluster of cancer cells have abundant xanthomatous cytoplasm and pyknotic nuclei, resembling foamy histiocytes

12.4 Histological Changes Associated with Radiation Therapy

12.4.1 Histological Changes Following Radiation Therapy in Benign and Malignant Prostate Tissue

Table 12.3 Histological changes following radiation therapy in benign and malignant prostate tissue

	Benign (*See* Fig. 12.11–12.13)	Cancer (*See* Fig. 12.14–12.16)
Architecture	Lobulated architecture maintained	Atrophic changes
	Individual glands with marked distortion of glandular contour	Cancer glands disintegrating into single or small cluster of cells
	Glands lined with multilayered cells	
	Basal and squamous metaplasia common	
Cytological and nuclear features	Atrophic cytoplasm	Abundant vacuolated, clear, or foamy cytoplasm
	Scattered, markedly atypical nuclei with degenerative atypia	Small, pyknotic nuclei
Stroma	Fibrosis	
	Vascular changes (intimal thickening and medial fibrosis) uncommon	

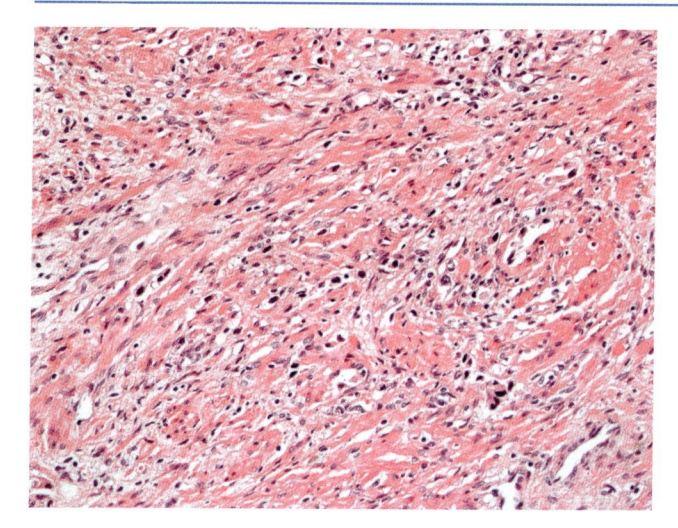

Fig. 12.9 Prostate cancer following androgen deprivation: individual cells. Individual cancer cells, mixed with other inflammatory cells and embedded in a fibrotic stroma, are easy to overlook. At high magnification, some nuclei are hyperchromatic and atypical. Immunostains for pancytokeratin and prostate-specific antigen (PSA) markers are often required to identify the cancer cells

12.4.2 Significance of Postradiotherapy Prostate Biopsy

Table 12.4 Significance of postradiotherapy prostate biopsy

Biopsy timing: 30–36 months after radiotherapy (30% of men with positive biopsy at 12 months after radiotherapy showed no evidence of disease at 30 months)

Outcomes of biopsies harboring cancer with radiation effect:
    30% no evidence of disease
    34% biopsy continues to show cancer with radiation effect
    36% local and distant metastasis

Impact of postradiotherapy biopsy on clinical outcomes:
    Degree of radiation effect in cancer does not predict outcomes
    Biopsy status at 24–36 months, together with posttreatment nadir, predicts outcomes

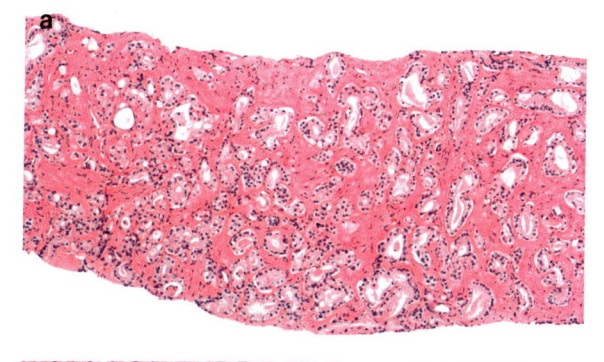

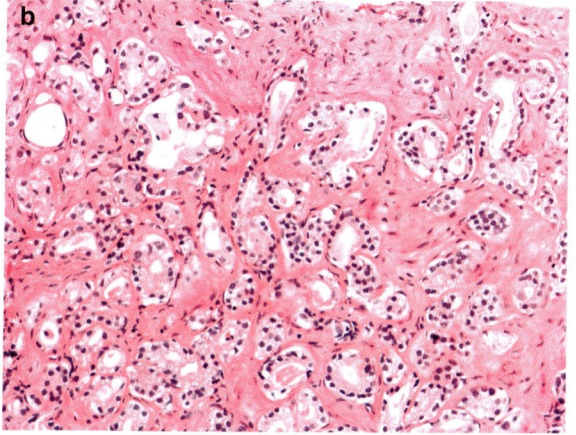

Fig. 12.10 Prostate cancer after finasteride treatment. Cancer glands show minimum histological changes (**a**). Several glands have slightly atrophic cytoplasm, small and dark nuclei without prominent nucleoli (**b**). Recently, the Prostate Cancer Prevention Trial (PCPT) reported a decreased overall incidence of prostate cancer but an increase in the incidence of high-grade prostate cancer with finasteride. It is thought that finasteride might have contributed to the increase in high-grade cancer by reducing the prostate volume and selective inhibition of low-grade cancer, rather than effects on tumor morphology [5]

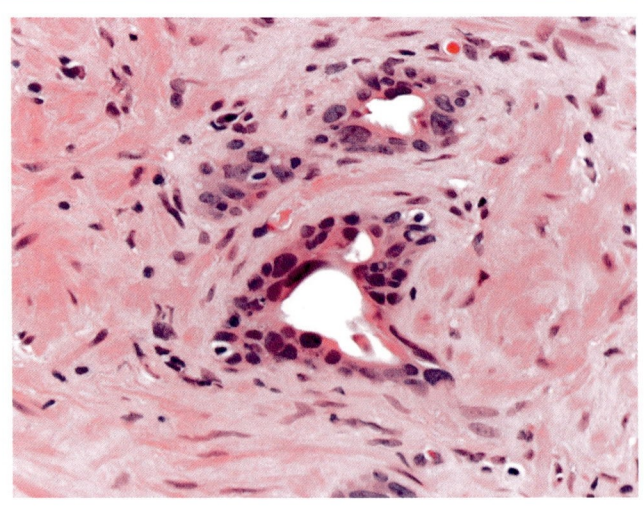

Fig. 12.12 Benign glands showing radiation atypia. The gland has an irregular contour and is lined with multiple layers of cells. The cytoplasm is eosinophilic rather than being clear. The nuclei are piled up with degenerative appearance. There are scattered, enlarged, and hyperchromatic nuclei

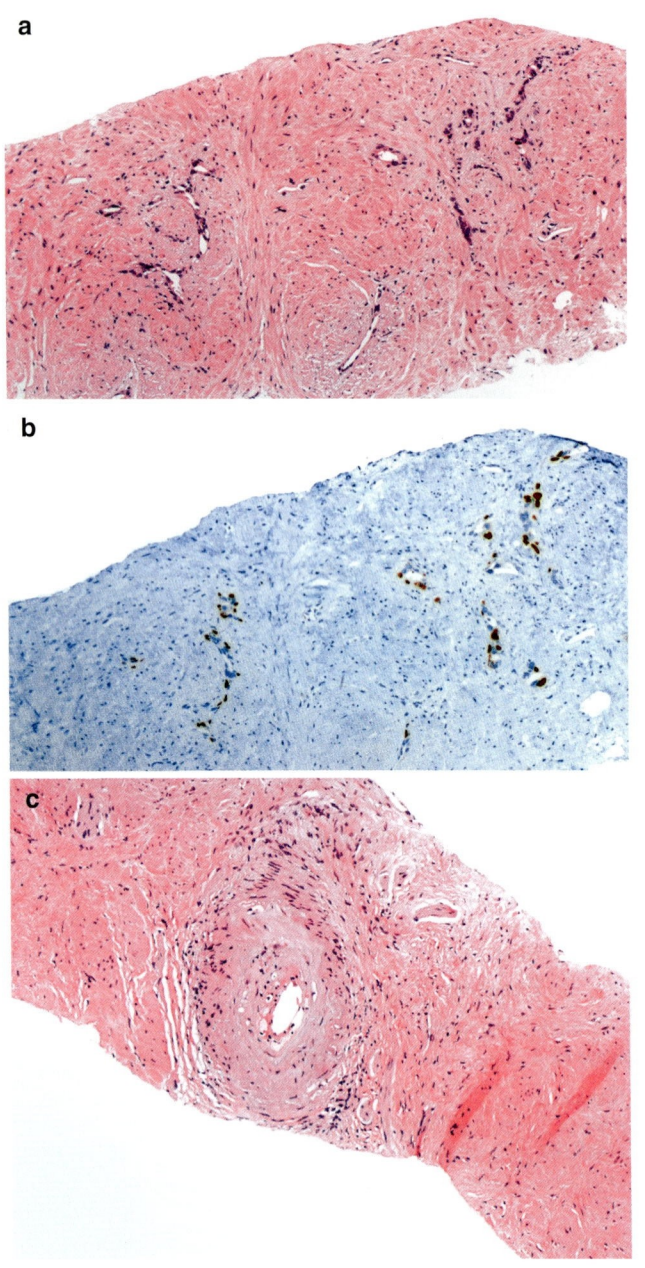

Fig. 12.11 Benign prostatic tissue showing radiation atypia. Benign glands are markedly atrophic but still maintain their lobular architecture (**a**). Glands have a highly irregular contour and are lined predominantly with basal cells confirmed by the immunohistochemical stain for p63 (**b**). The stroma is prominent. Radiation-induced vascular changes, including intimal thickening with atheroma-like changes and medial fibrosis (**c**), can be seen. The degree of radiation-induced changes varies with the dose and duration and the interval between treatments. Such a biopsy should be signed out as "benign prostatic tissue with radiation atypia" [6, 7]

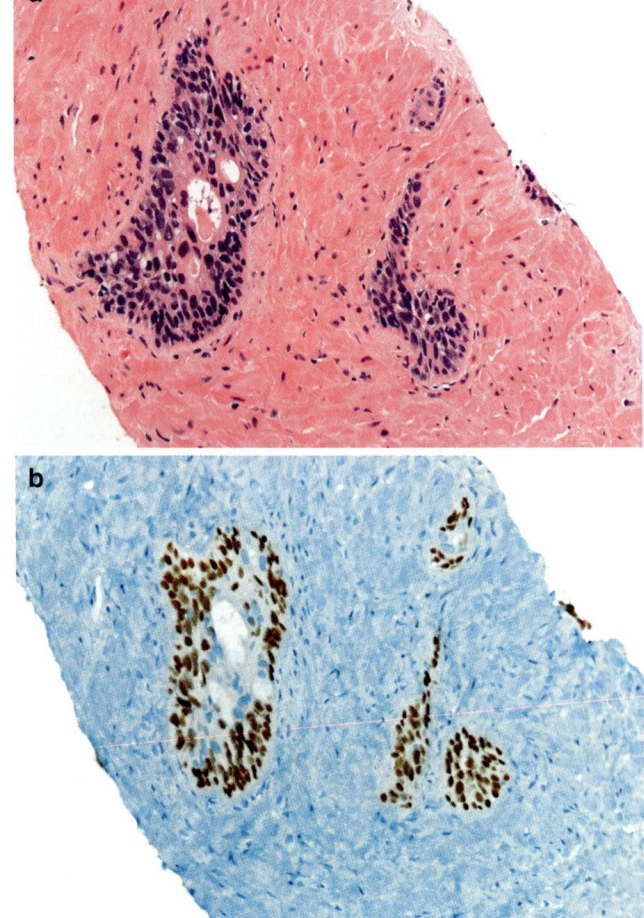

Fig. 12.13 Benign glands showing radiation atypia with basal cell hyperplasia (**a**) confirmed by the immunostain for p63 (**b**). Squamous cell metaplasia is also commonly seen

12.4 Histological Changes Associated with Radiation Therapy

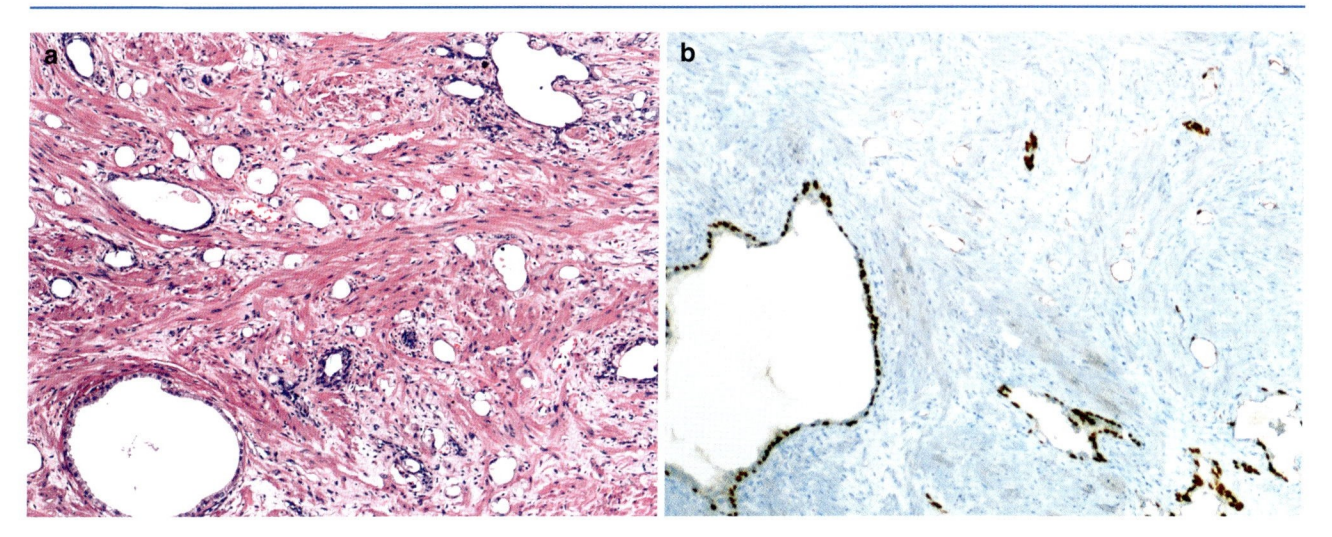

Fig. 12.14 Prostate cancer glands with radiation effect. The cancer glands show atrophic cytoplasm and pyknotic nuclei (**a**) indistinguishable from benign atrophy. However, they exhibit characteristic "infiltrative growth pattern." They are negative for p63 but positive for α-methylacyl-CoA racemase (AMACR) (**b**). It is still controversial whether it is necessary to perform needle biopsy to document histological presence of cancer for rising PSA following radiation therapy. However, it is generally agreed upon that a biopsy should be performed to distinguish local recurrence from distant metastases and to have a histological confirmation before a salvage prostatectomy

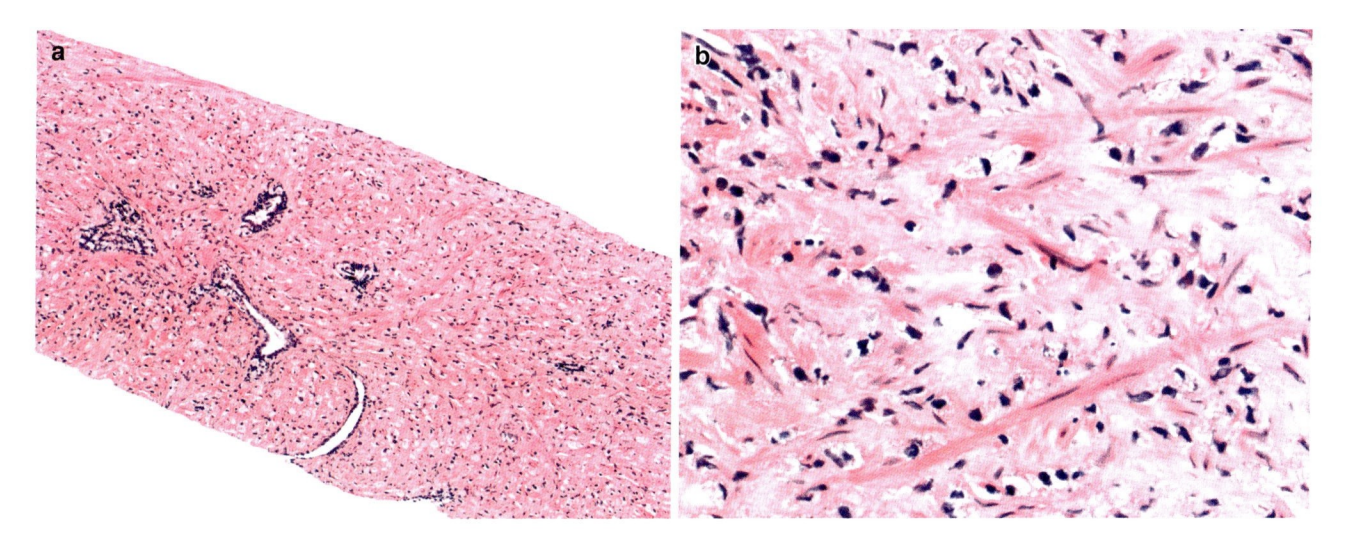

Fig. 12.15 Prostate cancer with radiation effect. Cancer demonstrates single or cords of cells (**a**) with voluminous foamy cytoplasm and pyknotic nuclei (**b**). Notice the larger benign glands with radiation atypia in (**a**). Cancer with radiation effect should not be assigned a Gleason grade

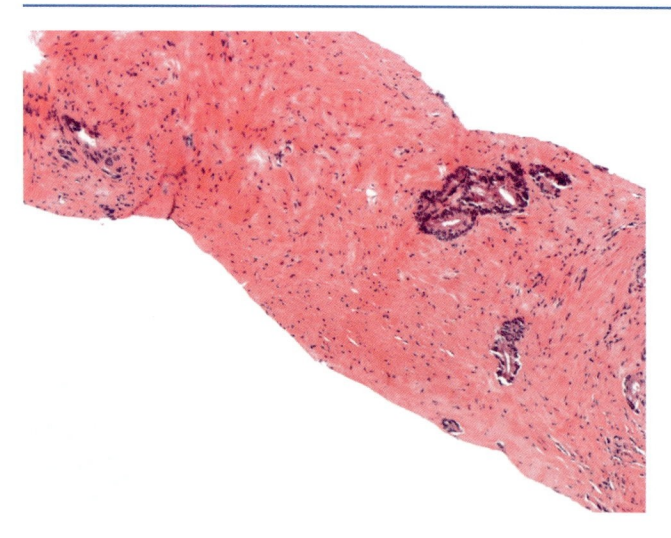

Fig. 12.16 Prostate cancer showing minimum or no radiation effect after treatment. Note that a benign gland (*upper left*) demonstrates radiation effect. Gleason grade can be assigned for cancer without significant radiation effect

12.5 Histological Changes Associated with Cryotherapy

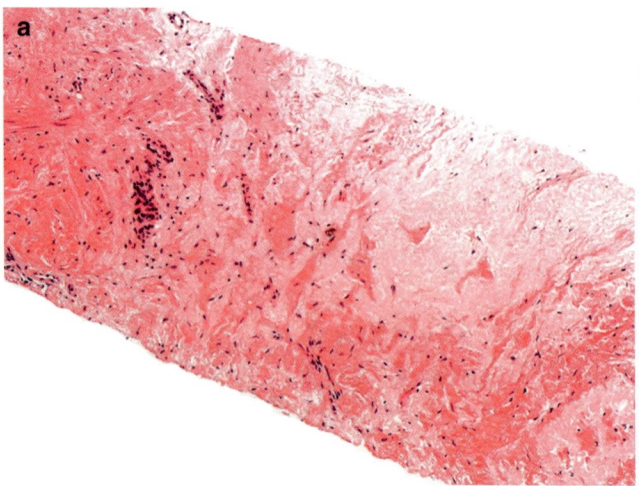

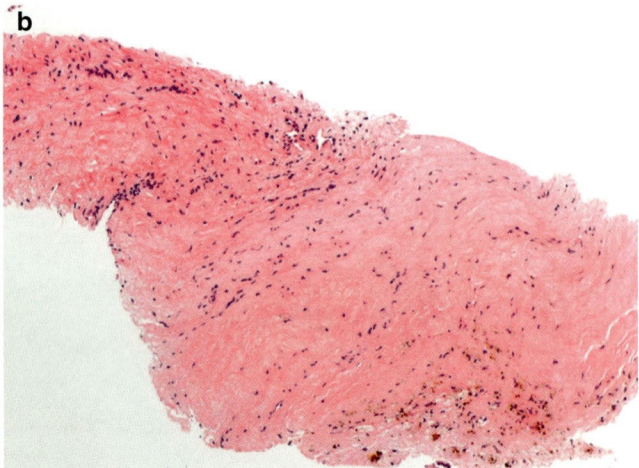

Fig. 12.17 Histological changes in benign prostate tissue after cryoablation. Cryoablation utilizes multiple cryoprobes filled with circulating liquid nitrogen to freeze and destroy prostate tissue. Following cryoablation, the benign prostate tissue shows features of tissue damage and repair, including marked reduction of glandular tissue (**a**) and prominent stroma with myxoid degeneration (**a**), hemorrhage, hemosiderin deposition (**b**), and at later stages, fibrosis and chronic inflammation. Residual viable glands show regenerative changes and basal cell hyperplasia and squamous cell metaplasia. Coagulative necrosis may be seen within several weeks and months after the treatment [8]

12.6 Histological Changes Associated with Hyperthermia

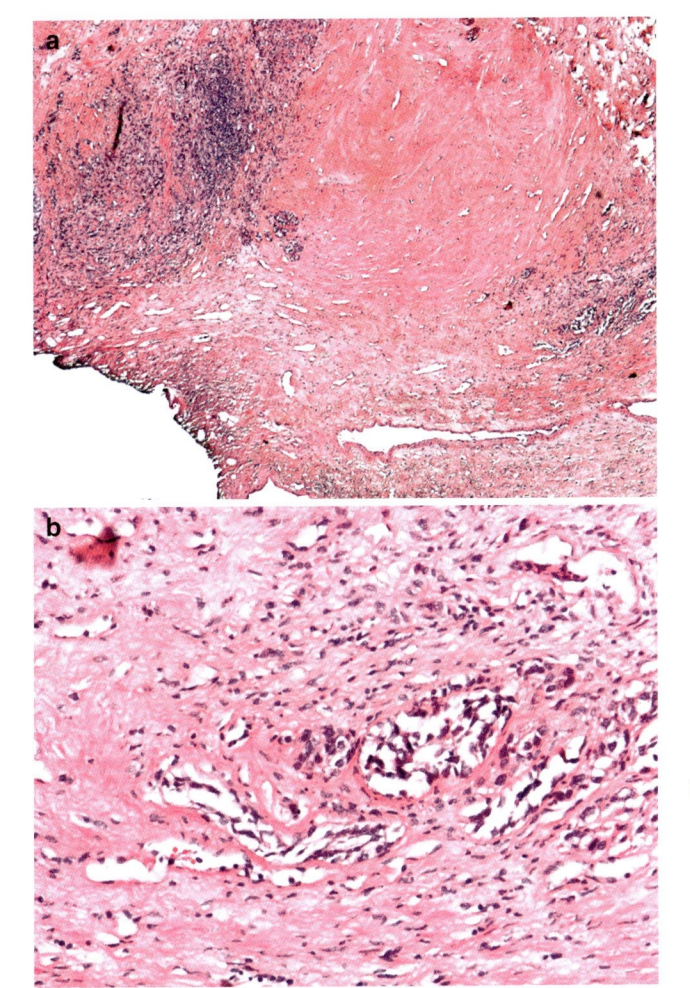

Fig. 12.18 Transurethral resection of prostate (TURP) that was previously treated with laser ablation. The specimen contains a fibrotic area surrounded by inflammation (**a**). The glands on the periphery show hyperthermia-induced changes including cytoplasmic vacuolation and pyknotic nuclei (**b**). Hyperthermia uses high temperature generated by various sources (high-intensity focused ultrasound, microwave, and laser) to destroy prostate tissue. It produces circumscribed hemorrhagic and coagulative necrosis that later organizes with granulation tissue and fibrosis. Residual prostate glands often are atrophic, with basal cell predominance [9, 10]

References

1. Petraki CD, Sfikas CP (2007) Histopathological changes induced by therapies in the benign prostate and prostate adenocarcinoma. Histol Histopathol 22:107–118
2. Tetu B (2008) Morphological changes induced by androgen blockade in normal prostate and prostatic carcinoma. Best Pract Res Clin Endocrinol Metab 22:271–283
3. Gleave M, Qian J, Andreou C et al (2006) The effects of the dual 5alpha-reductase inhibitor dutasteride on localized prostate cancer – results from a 4-month pre-radical prostatectomy study. Prostate 66:1674–1685
4. Yang XJ, Lecksell K, Short K (1999) Does long-term finasteride therapy affect the histologic features of benign prostatic tissue and prostate cancer on needle biopsy? PLESS Study Group. Proscar Long-Term Efficacy and Safety Study. Urology 53:696–700
5. Lucia MS, Epstein JI, Goodman PJ et al (2007) Finasteride and high-grade prostate cancer in the Prostate Cancer Prevention Trial. J Natl Cancer Inst 99:1375–1383
6. Cheng L, Cheville JC, Bostwick DG (1999) Diagnosis of prostate cancer in needle biopsies after radiation therapy. Am J Surg Pathol 23:1173–1183
7. Magi-Galluzzi C, Sanderson H, Epstein JI (2003) Atypia in nonneoplastic prostate glands after radiotherapy for prostate cancer: duration of atypia and relation to type of radiotherapy. Am J Surg Pathol 27:206–212
8. Borkowski P, Robinson MJ, Poppiti RJ Jr, Nash SC (1996) Histologic findings in postcryosurgical prostatic biopsies. Mod Pathol 9:807–811
9. Biermann K, Montironi R, Lopez-Beltran A et al (2010) Histopathological findings after treatment of prostate cancer using high-intensity focused ultrasound (HIFU). Prostate 70:1196–1200
10. Van Leenders GJ, Beerlage HP, Ruijter ET et al (2000) Histopathological changes associated with high intensity focused ultrasound (HIFU) treatment for localised adenocarcinoma of the prostate. J Clin Pathol 53:391–394

Molecular Biology of Prostate Cancer and Emerging Diagnostic and Prognostic Biomarkers

Prostate cancer, like other cancers, develops as the result of multiple, complex molecular events of initiation, unregulated growth, invasion, and metastasis. These complex molecular events include both loss of specific genomic sequences that lead to inactivation of tumor suppressor genes and gain of specific chromosome regions that are associated with activation of oncogenes. In prostate carcinogenesis, androgen receptor is believed to play a central role. The most common chromosomal aberrations demonstrated in prostatic intraepithelial neoplasia (PIN) and carcinoma are *TMPRSS2:ETS* gene fusions, *PTEN* deletion, gain of chromosome 7 (particularly 7q31), loss of 8p and gain of 8q, and loss of 10q, 16q, and 18q.

Although prostate-specific antigen (PSA) testing has led to a dramatic increase in prostate cancer detection, PSA has substantial drawbacks. As PSA is also produced by benign prostate glands, PSA is often elevated in benign conditions, such as benign prostatic hyperplasia (BPH) and prostatitis, accounting for the poor specificity of only 20% at a sensitivity of 80% [1]. To improve the specificity of PSA, derivative measurements such as percentage-free PSA, age-specific PSA, and PSA velocity have been proposed, but these measurements have drawbacks similar to total PSA. Furthermore, more than 15% of patients with PSA level less than 4 ng/mL had biopsy-proven cancer [1]. Detection of clinically insignificant disease is another important issue [2, 3]. Together, these data emphasize the need for biomarkers that can supplement PSA as a diagnostic test, reduce the number of unnecessary biopsies, and distinguish indolent from clinically significant prostate cancer. Despite extensive research, very few biomarkers have come into routine clinical practice. Lack of vigorous prospective-blinded studies to validate biomarkers is one of the important reasons for poor clinical acceptance. In addition, biomarker development and validation are affected by many compounding factors, including specimen collection and assay platforms.

This chapter summarizes the types of PSA measurements utilized in routine clinical practice, current understanding of molecular prostate carcinogenesis, and the potential application of some of the most promising biomarkers in the diagnosis and management of prostate cancer. For many of these proposed biomarkers, additional studies are needed to validate their clinical utility.

13.1 Types of Prostate-Specific Antigen (PSA) Measurements in Clinical Practice

Table 13.1 Types of prostate-specific antigen (PSA) measurements in clinical practice

PSA measurement	Normal range	Definition and significance
Total PSA	<4 ng/mL	Free + bound PSA
Free PSA, %	> 25% 10–25% (intermediate range)	Patients with a lower percentage of free PSA have a higher risk of prostate cancer; used for PSA levels of 4–10 ng/mL
PSA velocity	If baseline PSA is <4 ng/mL, increase of ≥0.35 ng/mL is suspicious If baseline PSA is 4–10 ng/mL, increase of ≥0.75 ng/mL is suspicious	A higher rate of PSA increase is more suspicious for malignancy than a single PSA measurement; used in patients with PSA levels of 4–10 ng/mL; not recommended by the American Cancer Society
Age-related PSA	40–49 years; ≤2.5 ng/mL 50–59 years; ≤3.5 ng/mL 60–69 years; ≤4.5 ng/mL 70–79 years; ≤6.5 ng/mL	Useful in younger men who generally have lower baseline PSA levels
PSA density	40–49 years; ≤0.10 ng/mL 50–59 years; ≤0.12 ng/mL 60–69 years; ≤0.14 ng/mL 70–79 years; ≤0.16 ng/mL	Calculated by dividing the total serum PSA level by the estimated gland volume (determined by transrectal ultrasonography measurement). An adjustment is required for men with a larger prostate volume, especially due to conditions such as BPH

13.2 Multistep Model of Prostate Cancer Progression

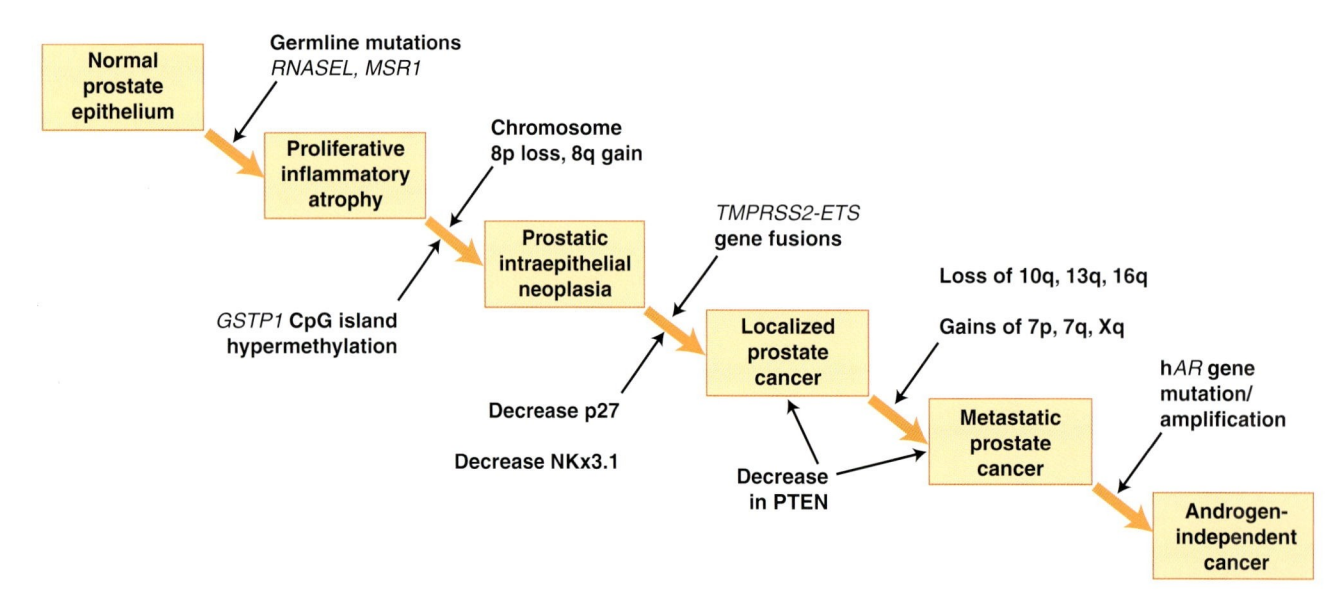

Fig. 13.1 Multistep model of prostate cancer progression [4]. Prostate cancer development is a multistep process involving complex molecular events. Distinct sets of key genes and proteins promote progression from the putative precursor lesion, termed *high-grade prostatic intraepithelial neoplasia* (HGPIN), or, alternately, from proliferative inflammatory atrophy, to hormone-naïve clinically localized cancer, to metastatic prostate cancer, and finally to androgen-independent (AI) metastatic disease that is invariably fatal. Normal prostate cells accumulate genetic abnormalities over time, resulting in a dysregulated growth, differentiation, and function. In addition to genetic changes, inflammation is also believed to play an important role in prostate carcinogenesis (*Adapted from* Nelson et al. [4])

13.3 Emerging Biomarkers for the Diagnosis and Prognosis of Prostate Cancer

Table 13.2 Emerging biomarkers for the diagnosis and prognosis of prostate cancer

Biomarker	Biology	Clinical applications
PSA derivatives [5–8]	Various forms of PSA in blood, including free PSA (fPSA) and complex PSA (cPSA)	Substantially altered metabolic activity of PSA derivatives in the occurrence and development of prostate cancer
	fPSA includes nicked PSA, intact PSA, and ProPSA, whereas cPSA mostly refers to PSA bound to α1 antichymotrypsin (PSA-ACT) and less frequently PSA bound to α$_2$-macroglobulin (PSA-A2M) and α1 protease inhibitor (PSA-API)	Within the PSA range of 2–10 ng/mL, PSA derivative measurement may aid in an improved early detection of prostate cancer
	ProPSA is a proenzyme without catalytic activity and is formed when a leader sequence at the end of the amino acid chain is cleaved. ProPSA with leader peptides are further named as [−2], [−4], [−5], and [−7] ProPSA depending on cleavage by human kallikrein 2(hk2)	Overall significance in the early detection of prostate cancer need to be validated
	Benign PSA (BPSA) is formed when the internal peptide bonds between 145 and 146 amino acids and between 182 and 183 amino acids are ruptured. It mainly correlates with the volume of the transition zone of prostate	
Prostate cancer antigen 3 (*PCA 3*)-DD3 (Progensa, Gen-probe) [9–11]	*PCA3* gene, located on chromosome 9 (9q21-22), produces *PCA3* RNA with no resultant protein	*PCA3* RNA can be detected in the urine and prostatic fluid collected following attentive digital rectal examination for prostate cancer (each lobe passed 3 times)
	PCA3 RNA specific for prostate cancer	The *PCA3* assay result is reported as a *PCA3* score, which is a quantitative ratio of *PCA3* RNA to PSA RNA, multiplied 1000× to normalize the amount of prostate RNA present in the urine sample
		A *PCA3* score ≥35 is considered to be positive
	PCA3 RNA levels are independent of prostate volume and serum PSA, but may be higher in patients with larger, more aggressive tumors	Higher *PCA3* score correlates with higher probability of a prostate cancer
	PCA3 is a more specific predictor of prostate cancer than serum PSA and/or percent-free PSA	Currently, *PCA3* is largely utilized as an adjunct to serum PSA for cancer risk stratification of patients undergoing repeat prostate biopsy
	A *PCA3* cutoff score of ≥35 has a sensitivity of 54% and a specificity of 74% compared with a sensitivity of 83% and a specificity of 17% for a serum PSA of 4.0 ng/mL	
Glutathione s-transferase π 1 (*GSTP1*) [12, 13]	Most common epigenetic change in prostate cancer	Using methylation-specific polymerase chain reaction (PCR) assay, detection of the methylation of *GSTP1* promoter region is utilized as a tissue-based diagnostic marker to differentiate PIN and cancer from benign prostate tissue including BPH
	The *GSTP1* gene methylation silences the gene	
	GSTP1 gene methylation deprives normal cells of protection against damage by oxidation and electrophilic substances and subsequent malignant transformation	Absent or decreased *GSTP1* activity in cancerous tissue has also been suggested as a potential prognostic marker
	GSTP1 expression is rarely detected in prostate cancers	
	Methylation of the *GSTP1* is present in PIN and cancer but not in benign glands	

(continued)

Table 13.2 (continued)

Biomarker	Biology	Clinical applications
α-Methylacyl-CoA racemase (AMACR) [14–17]	AMACR is an enzyme that participates in the β-oxidation of branched chain fatty acids	AMACR is first prostate cancer tissue biomarker that, combined with basal cell markers, is now routinely utilized to resolve the diagnosis of "atypia" or to confirm the diagnosis of small volume cancer in needle biopsies
	Consistent overexpression of AMACR in prostate cancer compared to benign prostate tissues	Average sensitivity of prostate cancer detection in needle biopsies is in the range of 70–80% with lower sensitivity in certain morphologic variants including foamy, pseudohyperplastic, and atrophic variants of prostate cancer
	Both monoclonal and polyclonal antibodies to AMACR are developed. P504S is the commercially available monoclonal antibody to AMACR	AMACR is not entirely specific for prostate cancer detection. The majority of high-grade PIN, nephrogenic adenoma and a subset of partial atrophy, adenosis lesions, and even benign glands may demonstrate AMACR expression
	AMACR is not prostate cancer–specific; other cancer types that express AMACR include, most notably, colorectal cancers and renal cell carcinoma, papillary type	
	AMACR expression is cytoplasmic, granular, and apical in distribution; expression is frequently heterogeneous	
TMPRSS2:ETS fusion genes [18–33]	TMPRSS2 is an androgen-controlled prostate-specific transmembrane serine protease and is expressed in both benign and malignant prostate tissues	TMPRSS2:ETS gene fusions have potential applications both in the diagnosis and prognosis of prostate cancer
	The ETS genes are a family of oncogenic transcription factors	TMPRSS2:ETS gene fusions provide a highly specific candidate biomarker that can be detected in tissue, urine, and potentially from blood
	Recurrent gene fusions involving the 3′ ETS transcription factor gene family members ERG (21q22.2), ETV1 (7p22.2), ETV4 (17q21), or ETV5 (3q28) fused to 5′ partner TMPRSS2 gene (21q22.3) have been identified in the majority (~60%) of prostate cancers (see Table 13.3)	TMPRSS2:ETS gene fusions can be detected by using ERG antibody immunohistochemistry (see Table 4.4 and Fig. 4.12), break-apart fluorescence in situ hybridization (FISH) probes (see Fig. 13.2), and PCR methods
	TMPRSS2:ERG fusion is the most prevalent, occurring in approximately 50% of localized prostate cancers and 30% of androgen-independent metastatic prostate cancers	TMPRSS2:ERG gene fusions, most notably interstitial deletions and duplication of deleted copy, have been suggested to be associated with poor outcomes; however, overall significance and evidence of TMPRSS2:ERG gene fusions in prostate cancer outcomes remain controversial
	AS TMPRSS2 and ERG are located only ~3 Mb apart on chromosome 21, gene fusions between two partners occur through genomic loss (interstitial deletion) or nonhomologous translocation (insertion) between two chromosomes 21 (see Fig. 13.2)	Prognostic significance improves when the class of TMPRSS2:ERG gene fusions is combined with PTEN deletions (see below)
	The TMPRSS2:ETS fusion gene enables the ETS gene to be activated by the promoter of the androgen-controlled TMPRSS2 gene and to cooperate with other genes, most notably PTEN in initiation and progression of prostate carcinogenesis (see Fig. 13.4)	
	TMPRSS2:ETS gene fusions are restricted to prostate cancer and small fraction (~18%) of HGPIN lesions intermingled with adjacent cancer demonstrating identical gene fusions, suggesting that they are involved in early prostate carcinogenesis	
	TMPRSS2:ETS gene fusions maintain fidelity during prostate carcinogenesis (i.e. progression from HGPIN to metastatic prostate cancer pathway) (see Fig. 13.4)	

13.3 Emerging Biomarkers for the Diagnosis and Prognosis of Prostate Cancer 161

Phosphate and tensin homolog deleted on chromosome 10 (*PTEN*) [34–37]	*PTEN* is a key tumor suppressor gene in prostate cancer	*PTEN* genomic deletion and absence of PTEN protein expression are associated with unfavorable clinical outcome
	Loss of *PTEN* function results in increased PIP3 (phosphatidylinositol [3–5]- triphosphate) levels and subsequent Akt phosphorylation and modulation of its downstream molecular oncogenic processes	Status of *PTEN* deletion along with *ERG* rearrangement status has been proposed as a genomic grade to supplement the Gleason grade and clinical parameters for prostate cancer outcome
	PTEN inactivation plays an important role in prostate cancer during progression to androgen independence	Poor genomic grade defined as both *PTEN* deletion and *TMPRSS2:ERG* gene fusions, intermediate genomic grade with either *PTEN* deletion or *TMPRSS2:ERG* fusion and favorable genomic grade as neither rearrangements present
	PTEN deletion correlates with prostate cancer progression, with lowest frequency in HGPIN and highest in metastatic prostate cancers	
	PTEN deletion and *ERG* rearrangement may cooperate, but likely contribute to different stages of prostate cancer progression (*see* Fig. 13.4)	
	Collective data suggest *PTEN* deletion is a late genetic event, possibly a "second hit" after *ERG* rearrangement	
Hereditary prostate cancer 1 (*HPC1*) [38, 39]	*HPC1* is a susceptibility gene of prostate cancer, located on chromosome 1(1q24-25)	Mutation or deletion of *RNASEL* is potentially associated with increased risk of developing prostate cancer and has been proposed as a candidate susceptibility gene for prostate cancer development
	Site of *RNASEL* gene (1q25), a candidate allele for *HPC1*	
	RNASEL plays antiviral and antiproliferative activities mediated by 2-5A pathway, which, alternatively is regulated by interferon; mutation of *RNASEL* results in significantly reduced antiproliferative activity	
	HPC1 is likely involved in initiation of hereditary prostate cancer	
Early prostate cancer antigen (EPCA) [40, 41]	EPCA is a nuclear matrix protein that maintains nuclear shape and function	EPCA can be detected using anti-EPCA antibody immunohistochemistry and enzyme-linked immunosorbent assay (ELISA) technique
	Change in nuclear matrix proteins may be an early event in tumorigenesis expression	Positive EPCA staining in patients with negative biopsy is associated with development of prostate cancer within 5 years
	Altered EPCA expression probably precedes microscopic pathology changes and is thus a potential tumor marker that may be an early indicator of cancer	Sensitivity and specificity in range of 92%–94% for prostate cancer detection in early studies
		Additional validation studies are needed to fully characterize its application in prostate cancer management
Golgi phosphoprotein 2 (GOLPH2) [42]	Also known as GOLM1 or GP73, is type II Golgi membrane protein	Overexpression of GOLPH2 mRNA can be detected by PCR in tissues and urine samples after digital rectal examination
	Overexpressed in prostate cancer compared to benign prostate tissue	Potential role in the setting of a multiplex diagnostic biomarkers to improve the early detection of prostate cancer (*see multiple biomarker section below*)
Sarcosine [43]	A metabolite that can be measured from body fluids	High levels of sarcosine is associated with poor prognosis and outcome in prostate cancer
	Sarcosine levels correlate with prostate cancer progression and highest levels are detected in metastatic prostate cancer, followed by localized prostate cancers compared to adjacent benign prostate tissue	Proposed as a potential marker of aggressive prostate cancer

(continued)

Table 13.2 (continued)

Biomarker	Biology	Clinical applications
SPINK1 (serine peptidase inhibitor, Kazal type 1) [44]	SPINK1 outlier expression seen exclusively in a subset of ETS rearrangement – negative (~10%) prostate cancers	SPINK1 is associated with prostate cancer aggressiveness and can be detected noninvasively in urine using RT-PCR-based methods
	SPINK1 expression and ETS gene fusion status mutually exclusive	SPINK1 is a biomarker specific for subset of aggressive ETS-negative prostate cancers
	SPINK1 has a functional role in ETS rearrangement – negative prostate cancers	The role of SPINK1 as a biomarker can be improved when combined or multiplexed with other putative biomarkers (see multiple biomarker section below)
Prostate-specific membrane antigen (PSMA) and prostate cell surface antigen (PCSA) [45]	PSMA is a type II integral membrane glycoprotein that is highly expressed in the prostate epithelium	PSMA has been utilized as a therapeutic target by using anti-PSMA dendritic cells or PSMA antibody conjugated radioactive isotopes
	It is also expressed in low quantity in small intestine, brain, kidney, liver, spleen, colon, and the capillary endothelium of variety of tumors	PCSA has been utilized as a treatment target and has been correlated with poor prognostic factors such as high Gleason grade, advanced stage, and metastasis
	The membrane-bound form is most abundant in prostate tumors	
	PCSA is a cell surface transmembrane glycoprotein of human prostate epithelial cells	
	PCSA is highly specific for prostate	
Detection of prostate cancer-specific biomarker signature from circulating microvesicles	Circulating microvesicles or exosomes secreted from prostate cancer contain concentrated tissue- and tumor-associated biomarkers (microRNAs, mRNAs, and proteins) and promise to be an important platform to analyze biomarkers in body fluids	Circulating microvesicles can be enriched and used to construct the biomarker "signature" for early diagnosis
Enhancer of zeste homolog 2 (EZH2) [46]	A member of the polycomb gene family	EZH2 is highly overexpressed in metastatic hormone refractory prostate cancer
	Transcriptional repressor known to be active early in embryogenesis	Localized prostate cancers with E2H2 protein overexpression have a higher risk of developing biochemical recurrence following radical prostatectomy
	Expression decreases as cells differentiate	
p27 [47, 48]	A cyclin-dependent kinase inhibitor 1B(p27, KiP1) and is located on 12p13	Quantitative immunohistochemistry analysis of p27 has been suggested as a prognostic biomarker
	p27 expression is downregulated with prostate cancer progression	Lack of or reduced expression of p27 has been correlated with aggressive cancer and poor outcome
Multiple tumor biomarkers [49, 50]	Combination of various biomarkers representing different stages and molecular pathways in prostate cancer development complement each other and improve the accuracy of prostate cancer detection and prognostication	Concomitant detection of TMPRSS2:ERG fusion gene, PCA3, SPINK1, and GOLPH2 in urine sediments improves prostate cancer detection more than using PSA or PCA3 marker alone

13.4 Genes Involved in the Chromosomal Translocations in Prostate Cancer

Table 13.3 Genes involved in the chromosomal translocations in prostate cancer [51]

5′ Partner	3′ Partner	Frequency, %
TMPRSS2	ERG	~40–70
TMPRSS2	ETV1	~2–30
TMPRSS2	ETV4	~2–5
TMPRSS2	ETV5	<1
HERV_K_22q11.23	ETV1	<1
SLC45A3	ETV1	<1
C15orf21	ETV1	<1
HNRPA2B1	ETV1	<1
KLK2	ETV4	<1
CANT1	ETV4	<1
SLC45A3	ETV5	<1

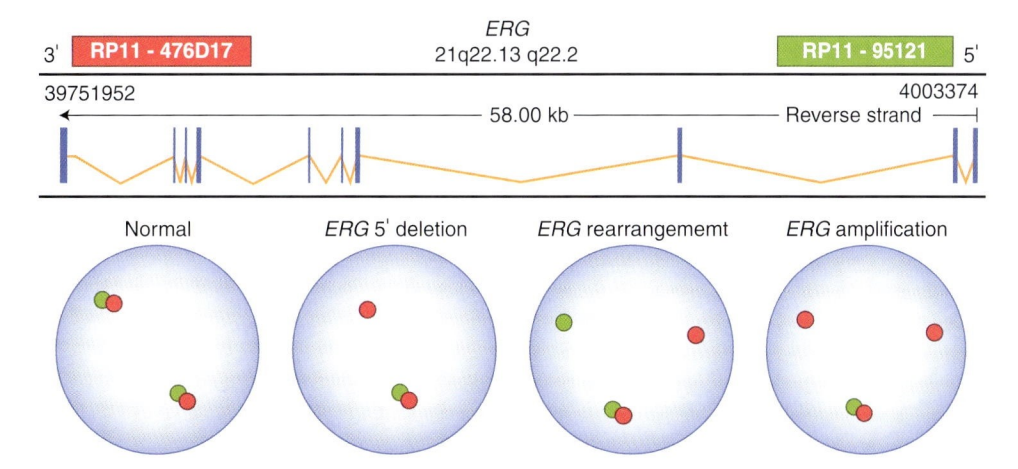

Fig. 13.2 *ERG* break-apart FISH probes to detect common *ERG* rearrangements in prostate cancer. *TMPRSS2:ERG* rearrangement is the most common class of *ETS* gene fusions in prostate cancer. As these two genes are located only approximately 3 Mb apart on chromosome 21, gene fusions between these two partners occur through either interstitial deletion or nonhomologous translocation (insertion). Due to their close proximity, a break-apart strategy (centromeric [*red*] and telomeric probes [*green*]) as shown in the diagram is employed to detect these gene fusions. Probes are synthesized using bacterial artificial chromosome (BAC) clones with its presence verified using metaphase spread of peripheral lymphocytes. *ERG* dual color probes show signal patterns for normal, 5′ deletion, rearrangement (translocation by insertion), and amplification of rearranged chromosomes. Normal cells are expected to demonstrate colocalization of both signals (probes). *Red and green bars* (*top*) indicate the BAC clones used and the number in the blue bar indicates the genomic location of *ERG* gene on chromosome 21 (*Reproduced from* Han et al [52])

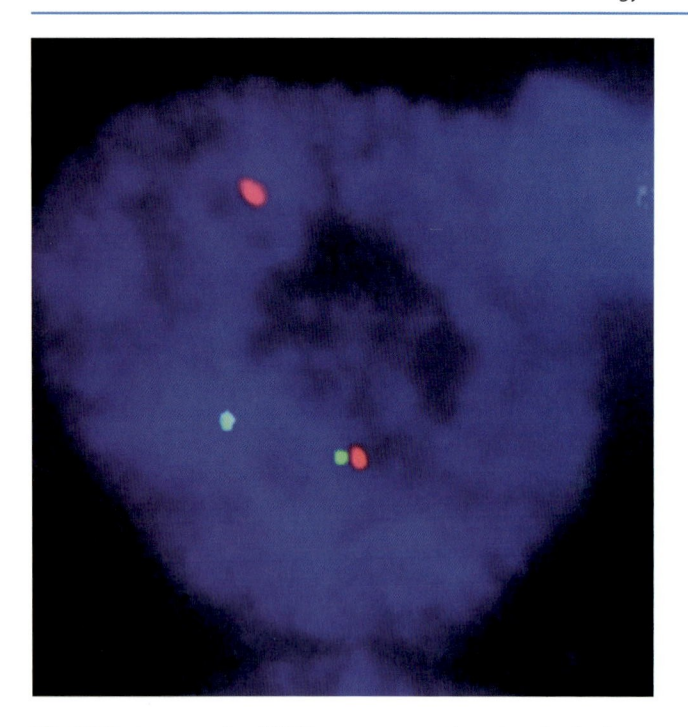

Fig. 13.3 An example of *ERG* rearrangement (translocation by insertion) in prostate cancer cell demonstrated by FISH technique using dual color 3′ and 5′ *ERG* break-apart probes. In this case, one pair of *ERG* demonstrates colocalization of 5′ (*green*) and 3′ (*red*) probes while the other pair demonstrates separation of both probes, suggesting *ERG* rearrangement by translocation mechanism. In normal cells, both *ERG* pairs show colocalization of 3′ and 5′ probes (*see* Fig. 13.2). To confirm the presence of *ERG* rearrangement (translocation by insertion mechanism), the majority of cancer cells should demonstrate separation of at least one pair of 3′ and 5′ *ERG* probes (*Image courtesy of* Dr. Rohit Mehra, The University of Michigan, Ann Arbor, MI)

Fig. 13.4 A model of molecular basis of prostate cancer (PCa) progression demonstrating potential role of *ETS* gene fusions [51]. Distinct sets of molecular events, through mutation, deletion, or amplifications likely dictate progression from benign gland, to the putative precursor lesion, termed HGPIN, to androgen-responsive (AR) clinically localized cancer, and finally to androgen-independent (AI) metastatic disease. This model of progression may occur through two distinct pathways, either in collaboration with *ETS* gene fusions (*red line*) or alternatively without ETS gene fusions (*blue line*). In this schematic, the *TMPRSS2* 5′ promoter acts as an "on-switch" in the presence of androgens, activating the *ETS* transcription factors. Emerging data strongly suggest that *TMPRSS2:ETS* fusion is an early event observed as early as in HGPIN lesion stage (~20%) in the prostate cancer progression process. HGPIN lesions expressing *TMPRSS2:ETS* rearrangements are invariably associated with adjacent invasive cancer, suggesting that they are a subset of true neoplastic precursors for *TMPRSS2:ETS* positive prostate cancer. Clinically localized prostate cancer is typically a multifocal disease, with heterogeneous rearrangement for *TMPRSS2:ETS* fusions between different tumor foci. In this schema of multifocal disease, a primary focus rearranged for *TMPRSS2:ETS* may progress and become capable of dissemination and give rise to metastatic disease. All metastatic foci retain similar *TMPRSS2:ETS* rearrangement like the primary focus, indicating that *ETS* rearrangement occurs before progression to metastatic disease, and metastatic disease arises through the clonal expansion of a single focus of primary prostate cancer capable of dissemination. Alternatively, if prostate cancer progresses without *TMPRSS2:ETS* gene fusion pathway, metastatic disease also invariably lacks this rearrangement (*Reproduced from* Shah RB and Chinniyan AM [51])

13.5 A Model of Molecular Basis of Prostate Cancer Progression Demonstrating Potential Role of *ETS* Gene Fusions

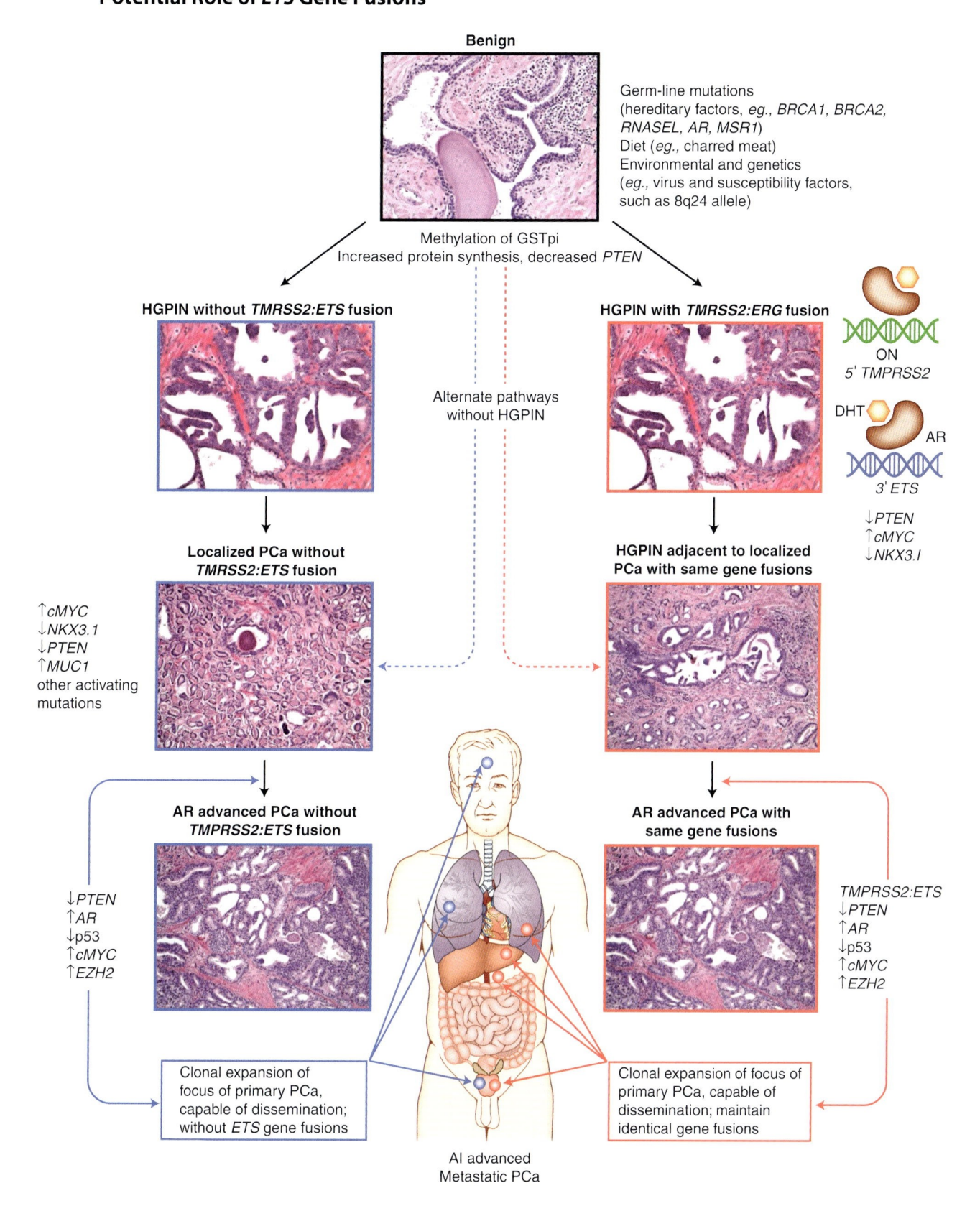

Benign

Germ-line mutations (hereditary factors, *eg.*, *BRCA1*, *BRCA2*, *RNASEL*, *AR*, *MSR1*)
Diet (*eg.*, charred meat)
Environmental and genetics (*eg.*, virus and susceptibility factors, such as 8q24 allele)

Methylation of GSTpi
Increased protein synthesis, decreased *PTEN*

HGPIN without *TMRSS2:ETS* fusion

HGPIN with *TMRSS2:ERG* fusion

ON
5' TMPRSS2

DHT
AR
3' ETS

↓PTEN
↑cMYC
↓NKX3.1

Alternate pathways without HGPIN

Localized PCa without *TMRSS2:ETS* fusion

↑cMYC
↓NKX3.1
↓PTEN
↑MUC1
other activating mutations

HGPIN adjacent to localized PCa with same gene fusions

AR advanced PCa without *TMPRSS2:ETS* fusion

↓PTEN
↑AR
↓p53
↑cMYC
↑EZH2

AR advanced PCa with same gene fusions

TMPRSS2:ETS
↓PTEN
↑AR
↓p53
↑cMYC
↑EZH2

Clonal expansion of focus of primary PCa, capable of dissemination; without *ETS* gene fusions

Clonal expansion of focus of primary PCa, capable of dissemination; maintain identical gene fusions

AI advanced Metastatic PCa

References

1. Thompson IM, Pauler DK, Goodman PJ et al (2004) Prevalence of prostate cancer among men with a prostate-specific antigen level < or =4.0 ng per milliliter. N Engl J Med 350:2239–2246
2. Andriole GL, Crawford ED, Grubb RL 3rd et al (2009) Mortality results from a randomized prostate-cancer screening trial. N Engl J Med 360:1310–1319
3. Schröder FH, Hugosson J, Roobol MJ et al (2009) Screening and prostate-cancer mortality in a randomized European study. N Engl J Med 360:1320–1328
4. Nelson WG, Carter HG, DeWeese TL, Eisenberger MA (2008) Prostate cancer. In: Abeloff MD, Armitage JO, Niederhuber JE et al (eds) Abeloff's clinical oncology, 4th edn. Churchill Livingstone/Elsevier, Philadelphia, pp 1653–1699
5. Bratslavsky G, Fisher HA, Kaufman RP Jr et al (2008) PSA-related markers in the detection of prostate cancer and high-grade disease in the contemporary era with extended biopsy. Urol Oncol 26: 166–170
6. Roddam AW, Duffy MJ, Hamdy FC et al (2005) Use of prostate-specific antigen (PSA) isoforms for the detection of prostate cancer in men with a PSA level of 2–10 ng/ml: systematic review and meta-analysis. Eur Urol 48:386–399; discussion 398–389
7. Sokoll LJ, Wang Y, Feng Z et al (2008) [−2]proenzyme prostate specific antigen for prostate cancer detection: a national cancer institute early detection research network validation study. J Urol 180:539–543; discussion 543
8. Khan MA, Sokoll LJ, Chan DW et al (2004) Clinical utility of proPSA and "benign" PSA when percent free PSA is less than 15%. Urology 64:1160–1164
9. Hessels D, Klein Gunnewiek JM, van Oort I et al (2003) DD3(PCA3)-based molecular urine analysis for the diagnosis of prostate cancer. Eur Urol 44:8–15; discussion 15–16
10. van Gils MP, Hessels D, van Hooij O et al (2007) The time-resolved fluorescence-based PCA3 test on urinary sediments after digital rectal examination; a Dutch multicenter validation of the diagnostic performance. Clin Cancer Res 13:939–943
11. Wang R, Chinnaiyan AM, Dunn RL et al (2009) Rational approach to implementation of prostate cancer antigen 3 into clinical care. Cancer 115:3879–3886
12. Ellinger J, Bastian PJ, Jurgan T et al (2008) CpG island hypermethylation at multiple gene sites in diagnosis and prognosis of prostate cancer. Urology 71:161–167
13. Meiers I, Shanks JH, Bostwick DG (2007) Glutathione S-transferase pi (GSTP1) hypermethylation in prostate cancer: review 2007. Pathology 39:299–304
14. Kunju LP, Chinnaiyan AM, Shah RB (2005) Comparison of monoclonal antibody (P504S) and polyclonal antibody to alpha methyla-cyl-CoA racemase (AMACR) in the work-up of prostate cancer. Histopathology 47:587–596
15. Kunju LP, Rubin MA, Chinnaiyan AM, Shah RB (2003) Diagnostic usefulness of monoclonal antibody P504S in the workup of atypical prostatic glandular proliferations. Am J Clin Pathol 120:737–745
16. Luo J, Zha S, Gage WR et al (2002) Alpha-methylacyl-CoA racemase: a new molecular marker for prostate cancer. Cancer Res 62:2220–2226
17. Rubin MA, Bismar TA, Andrén O et al (2005) Decreased alpha-methylacyl CoA racemase expression in localized prostate cancer is associated with an increased rate of biochemical recurrence and cancer-specific death. Cancer Epidemiol Biomarkers Prev 14: 1424–1432
18. Attard G, Clark J, Ambroisine L et al (2008) Duplication of the fusion of TMPRSS2 to ERG sequences identifies fatal human prostate cancer. Oncogene 27:253–263
19. Demichelis F, Fall K, Perner S et al (2007) TMPRSS2:ERG gene fusion associated with lethal prostate cancer in a watchful waiting cohort. Oncogene 26:4596–4599
20. Gopalan A, Leversha MA, Satagopan JM et al (2009) TMPRSS2-ERG gene fusion is not associated with outcome in patients treated by prostatectomy. Cancer Res 69:1400–1406
21. Helgeson BE, Tomlins SA, Shah N et al (2008) Characterization of TMPRSS2:ETV5 and SLC45A3:ETV5 gene fusions in prostate cancer. Cancer Res 68:73–80
22. Laxman B, Tomlins SA, Mehra R et al (2006) Noninvasive detection of TMPRSS2:ERG fusion transcripts in the urine of men with prostate cancer. Neoplasia 8:885–888
23. Mao X, Shaw G, James SY et al (2008) Detection of TMPRSS2:ERG fusion gene in circulating prostate cancer cells. Asian J Androl 10:467–473
24. Mehra R, Han B, Tomlins SA et al (2007) Heterogeneity of TMPRSS2 gene rearrangements in multifocal prostate adenocarcinoma: molecular evidence for an independent group of diseases. Cancer Res 67:7991–7995
25. Mehra R, Tomlins SA, Shen R et al (2007) Comprehensive assessment of TMPRSS2 and ETS family gene aberrations in clinically localized prostate cancer. Mod Pathol 20:538–544
26. Mehra R, Tomlins SA, Yu J et al (2008) Characterization of TMPRSS2-ETS gene aberrations in androgen-independent metastatic prostate cancer. Cancer Res 68:3584–3590
27. Mosquera JM, Perner S, Genega EM et al (2008) Characterization of TMPRSS2-ERG fusion high-grade prostatic intraepithelial neoplasia and potential clinical implications. Clin Cancer Res 14: 3380–3385
28. Perner S, Demichelis F, Beroukhim R et al (2006) TMPRSS2:ERG fusion-associated deletions provide insight into the heterogeneity of prostate cancer. Cancer Res 66:8337–8841
29. Perner S, Mosquera JM, Demichelis F et al (2007) TMPRSS2-ERG fusion prostate cancer: an early molecular event associated with invasion. Am J Surg Pathol 31:882–888
30. Shah RB, Mehra R, Chinnaiyan AM et al (2004) Androgen-independent prostate cancer is a heterogeneous group of diseases: lessons from a rapid autopsy program. Cancer Res 64:9209–9216
31. Tomlins SA, Laxman B, Dhanasekaran SM et al (2007) Distinct classes of chromosomal rearrangements create oncogenic ETS gene fusions in prostate cancer. Nature 448:595–599
32. Tomlins SA, Mehra R, Rhodes DR et al (2007) Integrative molecular concept modeling of prostate cancer progression. Nat Genet 39:41–51
33. Tomlins SA, Rhodes DR, Perner S et al (2005) Recurrent fusion of TMPRSS2 and ETS transcription factor genes in prostate cancer. Science 310:644–648
34. Carver BS, Tran J, Gopalan A et al (2009) Aberrant ERG expression cooperates with loss of PTEN to promote cancer progression in the prostate. Nat Genet 41:619–624
35. Han B, Mehra R, Lonigro RJ et al (2009) Fluorescence in situ hybridization study shows association of PTEN deletion with ERG rearrangement during prostate cancer progression. Mod Pathol 22:1083–1093
36. Reid AH, Attard G, Ambroisine L et al (2010) Molecular characterisation of ERG, ETV1 and PTEN gene loci identifies patients at low and high risk of death from prostate cancer. Br J Cancer 102:678–684
37. Yoshimoto M, Joshua AM, Cunha IW et al (2008) Absence of TMPRSS2:ERG fusions and PTEN losses in prostate cancer is associated with a favorable outcome. Mod Pathol 21:1451–1460
38. Carpten J, Nupponen N, Isaacs S et al (2002) Germline mutations in the ribonuclease L gene in families showing linkage with HPC1. Nat Genet 30:181–184
39. Casey G, Neville PJ, Plummer SJ et al (2002) RNASEL Arg462Gln variant is implicated in up to 13% of prostate cancer cases. Nat Genet 32:581–583
40. Dhir R, Vietmeier B, Arlotti J et al (2004) Early identification of individuals with prostate cancer in negative biopsies. J Urol 171:1419–1423

41. Paul B, Dhir R, Landsittel D et al (2005) Detection of prostate cancer with a blood-based assay for early prostate cancer antigen. Cancer Res 65:4097–4100
42. Kristiansen G, Fritzsche FR, Wassermann K et al (2008) GOLPH2 protein expression as a novel tissue biomarker for prostate cancer: implications for tissue-based diagnostics. Br J Cancer 99:939–948
43. Sreekumar A, Poisson LM, Rajendiran TM et al (2009) Metabolomic profiles delineate potential role for sarcosine in prostate cancer progression. Nature 457:910–914
44. Tomlins SA, Rhodes DR, Yu J et al (2008) The role of SPINK1 in ETS rearrangement-negative prostate cancers. Cancer Cell 13:519–528
45. Sardana G, Dowell B, Diamandis EP (2008) Emerging biomarkers for the diagnosis and prognosis of prostate cancer. Clin Chem 54:1951–1960
46. Varambally S, Dhanasekaran SM, Zhou M et al (2002) The polycomb group protein EZH2 is involved in progression of prostate cancer. Nature 419:624–629
47. Cordon-Cardo C, Koff A, Drobnjak M et al (1998) Distinct altered patterns of p27KIP1 gene expression in benign prostatic hyperplasia and prostatic carcinoma. J Natl Cancer Inst 90:1284–1291
48. Yang RM, Naitoh J, Murphy M et al (1998) Low p27 expression predicts poor disease-free survival in patients with prostate cancer. J Urol 159:941–945
49. Hessels D, Smit FP, Verhaegh GW et al (2007) Detection of TMPRSS2-ERG fusion transcripts and prostate cancer antigen 3 in urinary sediments may improve diagnosis of prostate cancer. Clin Cancer Res 13:5103–5108
50. Laxman B, Morris DS, Yu J et al (2008) A first-generation multiplex biomarker analysis of urine for the early detection of prostate cancer. Cancer Res 68:645–649
51. Shah RB, Chinnaiyan AM (2009) The discovery of common recurrent transmembrane protease serine 2 (TMPRSS2)-erythroblastosis virus E26 transforming sequence (ETS) gene fusions in prostate cancer: significance and clinical implications. Adv Anat Pathol 16:145–153
52. Han B, Suleman K, Wang L et al (2010) ETS gene aberrations in atypical cribriform lesions of the prostate: implications for the distinction between intraductal carcinoma of the prostate and cribriform high-grade prostatic intraepithelial neoplasia. Am J Surg Pathol 34:478–485

Biopsy Specimen Handling, Processing, Quality Assurance Program

With widespread use of prostate-specific antigen (PSA) screening, a greater number of prostate biopsies are performed. It is estimated that more than one million prostate biopsies are performed in the United States annually, with each biopsy consisting of an average of 8–10 sample cores, creating an estimated ten million tissue samples. This trend has created a challenge for effective and timely handling and processing of prostate biopsies in histology laboratories, in addition to their accurate interpretation and quality assurance by surgical pathologists. Various laboratory-controlled factors influence the prostate cancer detection rate in contemporary prostate biopsy practice. This chapter addresses ideal practices for the submission, handling, and processing of prostate biopsies, as well as commonly applied quality assurance programs known to improve overall practice.

Fig. 14.1 A prostate biopsy slide with all the tissue cores placed in the same block. When multiple cores are in the same block, all the tissue cores may not be embedded at the same plane; therefore, some cores may not be sectioned and be missing at certain levels. This practice has been shown to be less than optimal, and is more likely to result in equivocal pathology reports and missing small foci of cancer [1, 2]. For optimal results, no more than two to three tissue cores should be embedded in the same block

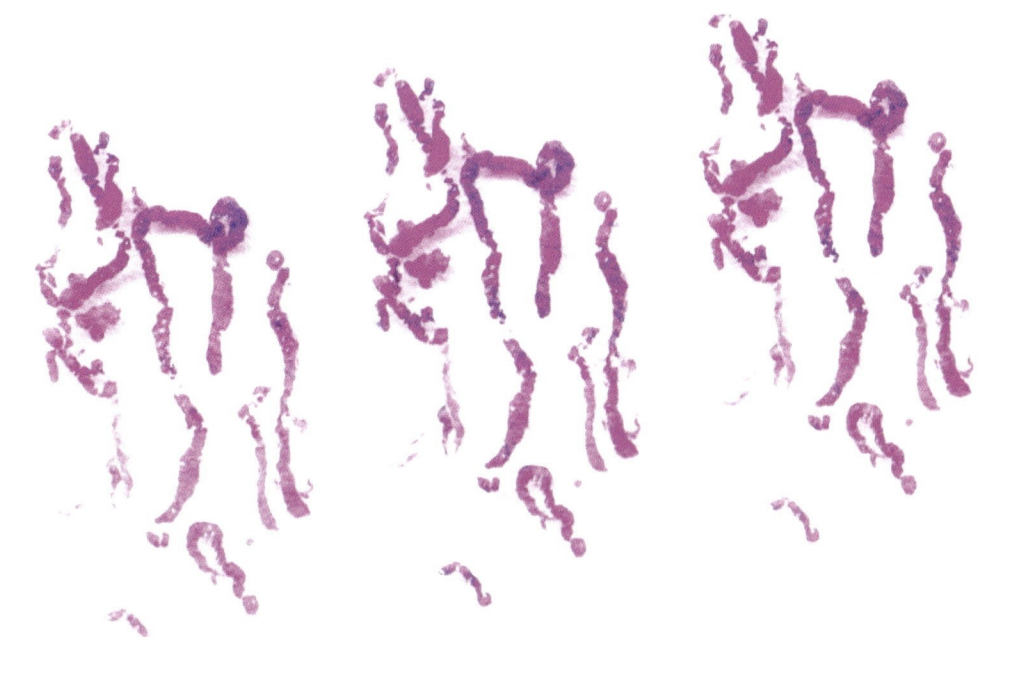

R.B. Shah, M. Zhou, *Prostate Biopsy Interpretation: An Illustrated Guide*,
DOI 10.1007/978-3-642-21369-4_14, © Springer-Verlag Berlin Heidelberg 2012

14.1 Best Practices for Submission, Handling, and Processing of Prostate Biopsies

Table 14.1 Best practices for submission, handling, and processing of prostate biopsies [1–11]

Submission

Submit cores from different site separately to preserve site (location of the biopsy) information

(A) Reduce equivocal pathology reports (e.g., reduce potential diagnostic pitfalls associated with specific anatomic site, such as misinterpreting central zone glands as high-grade prostatic intraepithelial neoplasia [HGPIN] in the biopsy from the base)

(B) Help design a focused rebiopsy sampling strategy for patients with "atypia" diagnosis

(C) Improve preoperative biopsy prediction of radical prostatectomy Gleason grade

(D) Help determine cancer distribution for planning radiotherapy field (e.g., placing seed implants for brachytherapy)

(E) Help with additional tissue sectioning in cases with no cancer in radical prostatectomy

Handling

Place a maximum of 2–3 cores in each block, even if multiple cores are obtained from one specific site.

(A) Minimize the tissue core fragmentation

(B) Maximize the surface area to be examined by keeping tissue flat for embedding

Processing

Prepare multiple levels (see Fig. 14.3)

(A) Allow optimal representation of small foci of atypical glands/cancer

Prepare intervening unstained levels for possible immunohistochemical work-up (see Figs. 14.2 and 14.3)

(B) Allow optimal representation of small foci of atypical glands for potential immunohistochemical or molecular work-up of prostate cancer

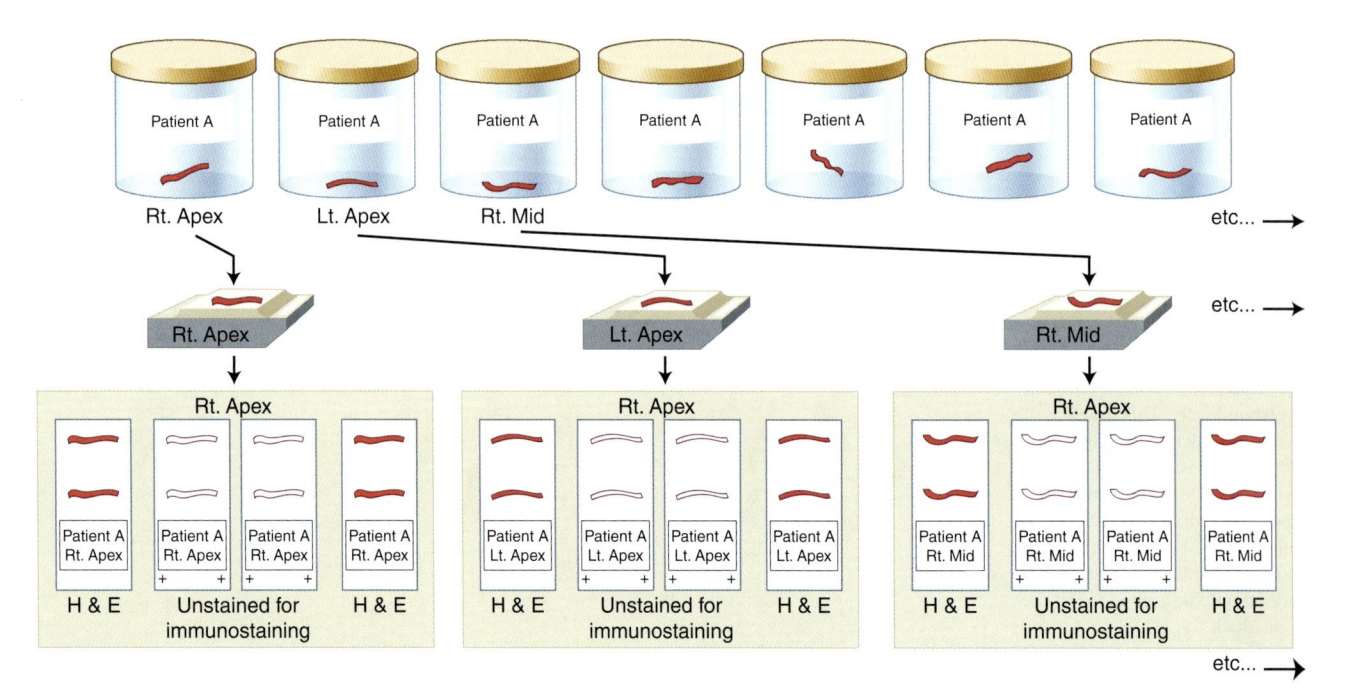

Fig. 14.2 A diagrammatic representation of best practice for submission and laboratory processing of prostate biopsies. For an optimal prostate biopsy interpretation and providing quality pathology parameters, the urologist should submit prostate biopsy core(s) from each anatomic site in separate containers to preserve the location information. The laboratory should submit and process the biopsy core(s) the same way in order to preserve the location information. For each site, multiple levels (minimum three levels) should be examined for hematoxylin–eosin stain (*H&E*); intervening sections should be kept on positive-charged slides for potential immunohistochemistry and molecular work-up. This approach ensures preservation of small focus of cancer or atypical glands that may be lost on subsequent deeper levels. Studies have shown that this practice reduces "equivocal" pathology reports, provides better guidance to urologists for rebiopsy strategy in case of "atypia" diagnosis, and improves preoperative Gleason score prediction [1–4, 6, 7, 9]

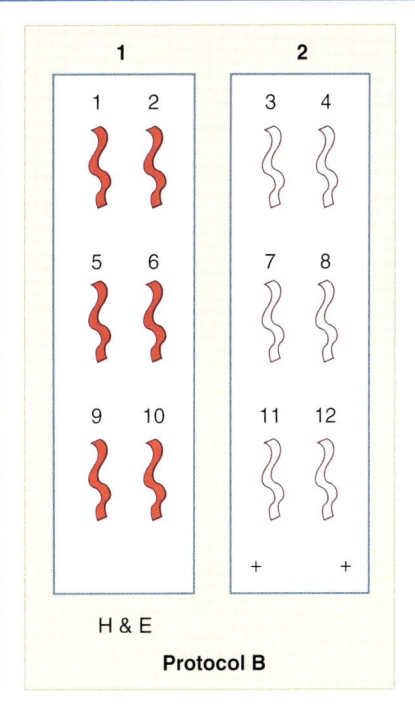

Fig. 14.3 Two prostate biopsy sectioning protocols that provide cost-effective yet optimal biopsy interpretation. Many different prostate biopsy sectioning protocols have been utilized. An ideal protocol provides multiple levels (at least three) of H&E stain for adequate visualization of the needle biopsy cores. Inadequate number of levels may miss atypical foci or cancer. In protocol A, three different slides are utilized for each biopsy block. Slide 1 and 3 are stained for H&E examination and one intervening slide is kept unstained on the charged slide for potential immunohistochemical work-up. In protocol B, two slides are utilized per block, with multiple levels on each slide. Slide 1 is stained for H&E and slide 2 unstained on the charged slide for immunohistochemical work-up. The number on the slide reflects the sequence of level of tissue sectioning during microtomy. In cases in which atypical focus appears only on later levels, additional immediate levels could be obtained for immunohistochemistry work-up and/or H&E stains and may yield additional useful information to resolve the "atypia" diagnosis

14.2 Recommendations for Tissue Submission of Transurethral Resection Specimens

Table 14.2 Recommendation for tissue submission of transurethral prostate resection specimens [10]

Gross specimen and initial pathology findings	Submission recommendations
Tissue chips < 12 g total	Submit entire tissue for examination
Tissue chips > 12 g total	Submit initial 12 g of grossly abnormal tissue (yellow, firm tissue, etc.) and add 1 cassette for every additional 5 g of tissue
Incidental (<5% of tissue chips involved) prostate cancer detected in initial prostate chips (cT1a)	Submission of remaining tissue desirable, especially in younger patients

14.3 Quality Assurance Measures Known to Improve Prostate Biopsy Practice

Table 14.3 Quality assurance measures known to improve prostate biopsy practice [12–20]

Improvement-related factors

Handling, grossing, and embedding of specimen

(A) Avoid processing two prostate biopsy specimens consecutively. Process a different type of specimen between two prostate biopsies

(B) Ink the prostate cores of different patients with different colors (e.g., red ink for patient A, yellow ink for patient B)

Interpretation-related factors

(A) Document "atypia" and "HGPIN" rate

(B) Record Gleason score distribution

(C) Tally distribution of key diagnosis and Gleason score distribution among different pathologists

Quality control audit

(A) Random blinded reevaluation of 5% prostate biopsies

(B) Prospective intradepartmental consultations or re-review of:
"Atypia" diagnosis
Small volume cancer diagnosis (<5% involvement) of biopsy tissue
Benign diagnosis with ≥PSA 10 ng/mL
Young patients (<50 years) with cancer involving < 10% from a single location

(C) Expert second opinion of "equivocal" or "atypia" diagnosis

References

1. Gupta C, Ren JZ, Wojno KJ (2004) Individual submission and embedding of prostate biopsies decreases rates of equivocal pathology reports. Urology 63:83–86
2. Kao J, Upton M, Zhang P, Rosen S (2002) Individual prostate biopsy core embedding facilitates maximal tissue representation. J Urol 168:496–499
3. Green R, Epstein JI (1999) Use of intervening unstained slides for immunohistochemical stains for high molecular weight cytokeratin on prostate needle biopsies. Am J Surg Pathol 23:567–570
4. Renshaw AA (1997) Adequate tissue sampling of prostate core needle biopsies. Am J Clin Pathol 107:26–29
5. Rogatsch H, Moser P, Volgger H (2000) Diagnostic effect of an improved preembedding method of prostate needle biopsy specimens. Hum Pathol 31:1102–1107
6. Allen EA, Kahane H, Epstein JI (1998) Repeat biopsy strategies for men with atypical diagnoses on initial prostate needle biopsy. Urology 52:803–807
7. Brat DJ, Wills ML, Lecksell KL, Epstein JI (1999) How often are diagnostic features missed with less extensive histologic sampling of prostate needle biopsy specimens? Am J Surg Pathol 23: 257–262
8. DiGiuseppe JA, Sauvageot J, Epstein JI (1997) Increasing incidence of minimal residual cancer in radical prostatectomy specimens. Am J Surg Pathol 21:174–178
9. Kunju LP, Daignault S, Wei JT, Shah RB (2009) Multiple prostate cancer cores with different Gleason grades submitted in the same specimen container without specific site designation: should each core be assigned an individual Gleason score? Hum Pathol 40:558–564
10. McDowell PR, Fox WM, Epstein JI (1994) Is submission of remaining tissue necessary when incidental carcinoma of the prostate is found on transurethral resection? Hum Pathol 25:493–497
11. Srodon M, Epstein JI (2002) Central zone histology of the prostate: a mimicker of high-grade prostatic intraepithelial neoplasia. Hum Pathol 33:518–523
12. Cooper K (2006) Errors and error rates in surgical pathology: an Association of Directors of Anatomic and Surgical Pathology survey. Arch Pathol Lab Med 130:607–609
13. Epstein JI, Walsh PC, Sanfilippo F (1996) Clinical and cost impact of second-opinion pathology. Review of prostate biopsies prior to radical prostatectomy. Am J Surg Pathol 20:851–857
14. Frable WJ (2006) Surgical pathology – second reviews, institutional reviews, audits, and correlations: what's out there? Error or diagnostic variation? Arch Pathol Lab Med 130:620–625
15. Nakhleh RE (2006) Error reduction in surgical pathology. Arch Pathol Lab Med 130:630–632
16. Nguyen PL, Schultz D, Renshaw AA (2004) The impact of pathology review on treatment recommendations for patients with adenocarcinoma of the prostate. Urol Oncol 22:295–299
17. Raab SS (2006) Improving patient safety through quality assurance. Arch Pathol Lab Med 130:633–637
18. Raff LJ, Engel G, Beck KR et al (2009) The effectiveness of inking needle core prostate biopsies for preventing patient specimen identification errors: a technique to address Joint Commission patient safety goals in specialty laboratories. Arch Pathol Lab Med 133:295–297
19. Singh PB, Saw NK, Haq A et al (2008) Use of tissue ink to maintain identification of individual cores on needle biopsies of the prostate. J Clin Pathol 61:1055–1057
20. Sirota RL (2006) Defining error in anatomic pathology. Arch Pathol Lab Med 130:604–606

Reporting of Prostate Biopsy

The primary goal of prostate needle biopsy is to diagnose prostate cancer (PCa). Biopsy evaluation also provides a significant quantity of important data, including histological type, Gleason score, and tumor volume and extent, which are all critical for clinicians to prognosticate and manage patients. In keeping with the current trend of standardization of surgical pathology reports [1–3], several pathology organizations periodically issue recommendations for the reporting of prostate cancer in needle biopsy specimens [4]. The information that must be included in prostate biopsy reports is understandably in flux as our understanding of the pathological and molecular characteristics of prostate cancer expands, and diagnosis and treatment of prostate cancer continue to evolve. In addition, the prostate biopsy report should be written in a way that facilitates effective communications between pathologists and clinicians.

15.1 Benign Diagnosis

Table 15.1 Reporting biopsies with benign prostate tissue [4]

Benign prostate glands and stroma (See Fig. 15.1–15.3)
Optional:
Benign mimickers of cancer
Chronic and acute inflammation[a]
Nonspecific granulomatous prostatitis[a]
Atypical adenomatous hyperplasia (adenosis)
Severe atrophy

[a]Acute inflammation may cause prostate-specific antigen (PSA) elevation. Nonspecific granulomatous prostatitis clinically mimics cancer as patients present with indurated prostate gland and elevated serum PSA levels. Therefore, these conditions are recommended to be included in the biopsy report as they may provide an explanation for patients' elevated PSA levels (See Figure 15.3)

15.2 High-Grade Prostatic Intraepithelial Neoplasia and Atypical Glands Suspicious for Cancer

Table 15.2 Reporting biopsies with high-grade prostatic intraepithelial neoplasia (HGPIN) or atypical glands suspicious for cancer (ATYP)

HGPIN[a] or ATYP[b]
Optional:
Extent of HGPIN[c]
    Focality: unifocal vs. multifocal
    Number of involved cores
    Laterality: unilateral or bilateral
Location of ATYP[d]

[a]Low-grade PIN should not be diagnosed and reported in needle biopsies as it is of no clinical significance
[b]Atypical small acinar proliferation (ASAP) is also widely used as an alternative to ATYP by pathologists and clinicians [6]. The cancer risk associated with ATYP is similar to that associated with HGPIN with adjacent atypical glands (PINATYP)
[c]The extent of HGPIN should be mentioned in the biopsy report, as recent studies have found that multifocal HGPIN (involving ≥2 or 3 cores) carries a cancer risk significantly higher than that associated with unifocal HGPIN [7, 8]
[d]Knowing the location of the biopsy core containing ATYP can help urologists choose the re-biopsy strategy. For example, if the biopsy from the right mid contains ATYP, urologists will increase sampling of the right mid in the repeat biopsy

15.3 Adenocarcinoma of the Prostate

Table 15.3 Reporting of prostate biopsies with cancer

Adenocarcinoma of the prostate
Location and distribution of cancer (site of biopsy if specified)[a]
Histological type (see Fig. 15.4)
Gleason grade, including primary and secondary patterns (see Fig. 15.5)[b]
Extent of involvement (tumor volume; see Fig. 15.6)
Local invasion
Extraprostatic extension (tumor in periprostatic adipose tissue) (See Fig. 15.7)
Seminal vesicle (cancer involving specimen directed at and/or containing seminal vesicle) (See Fig. 15.8 and 15.9)
Lymphovascular invasion (report only if identified; see Fig. 15.10)
Therapy-related changes (if clinical history of radiation or hormonal therapy)
Perineural invasion (report only if identified; see Fig. 15.11)
Optional
Extent (focal, multifocal)
Caliber of nerve bundles

[a]Knowing the specific location of biopsy cores containing cancer, therefore the location of cancer within the prostate gland, is important for prognosis, therapy planning, and subsequent repeat biopsy [9–12]. (See Chap. 14 for more details.)

[b]If a biopsy contains a third (tertiary) pattern that is higher than the secondary pattern, it should be included in the final Gleason grade as the "secondary pattern" regardless of its amount. For example, if a cancer in a biopsy is 70% pattern 3, 25% pattern 4, and 5% pattern 5, it should be assigned a Gleason score 3 + 5 = 8, not 3 + 4 = 7

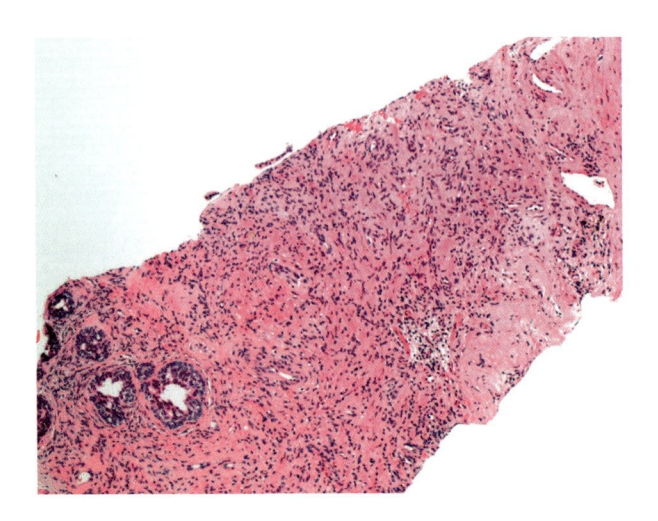

Fig. 15.1 A prostate biopsy core containing a stromal nodule with bland spindle cells, several small vessels with hyalinized wall, and lymphocytic infiltrates. It is recommended not to diagnose such a prostate biopsy as "hyperplastic prostate tissue" or "benign prostatic hyperplasia (BPH)" as transrectal prostate needle biopsy typically does not sample transition zones that BPH most commonly affects. Furthermore, microscopic findings of prostatic hyperplasia in needle biopsy do not correlate with the clinical symptomatology of BPH or the size of the prostate [5]

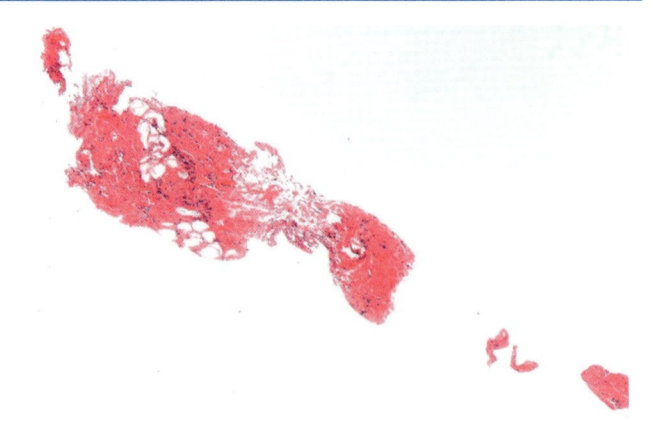

Fig. 15.2 A prostate biopsy core contains scant amount of fibroadipose tissue and no prostate glands. It is signed out as "fibromuscular tissue only; no prostatic glands present." If the biopsy contains a scant amount of tissue or fibromuscular tissue only, it should be mentioned so that the inadequacy of the biopsy material can be brought to the attention of the urologists who performed the biopsy

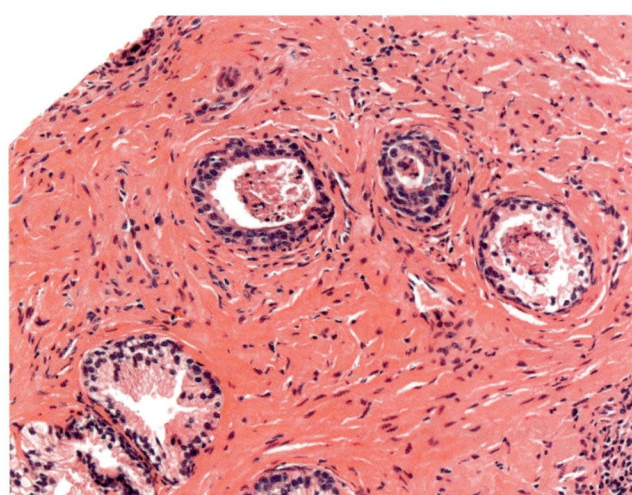

Fig. 15.3 A prostate biopsy contains acute inflammation within the lumens of several glands. This biopsy is signed out as "benign prostatic tissue with focal acute inflammation." Use of the term *prostatitis* is discouraged because prostatitis is a clinical diagnosis and microscopic inflammation does not always indicate a clinical prostatitis

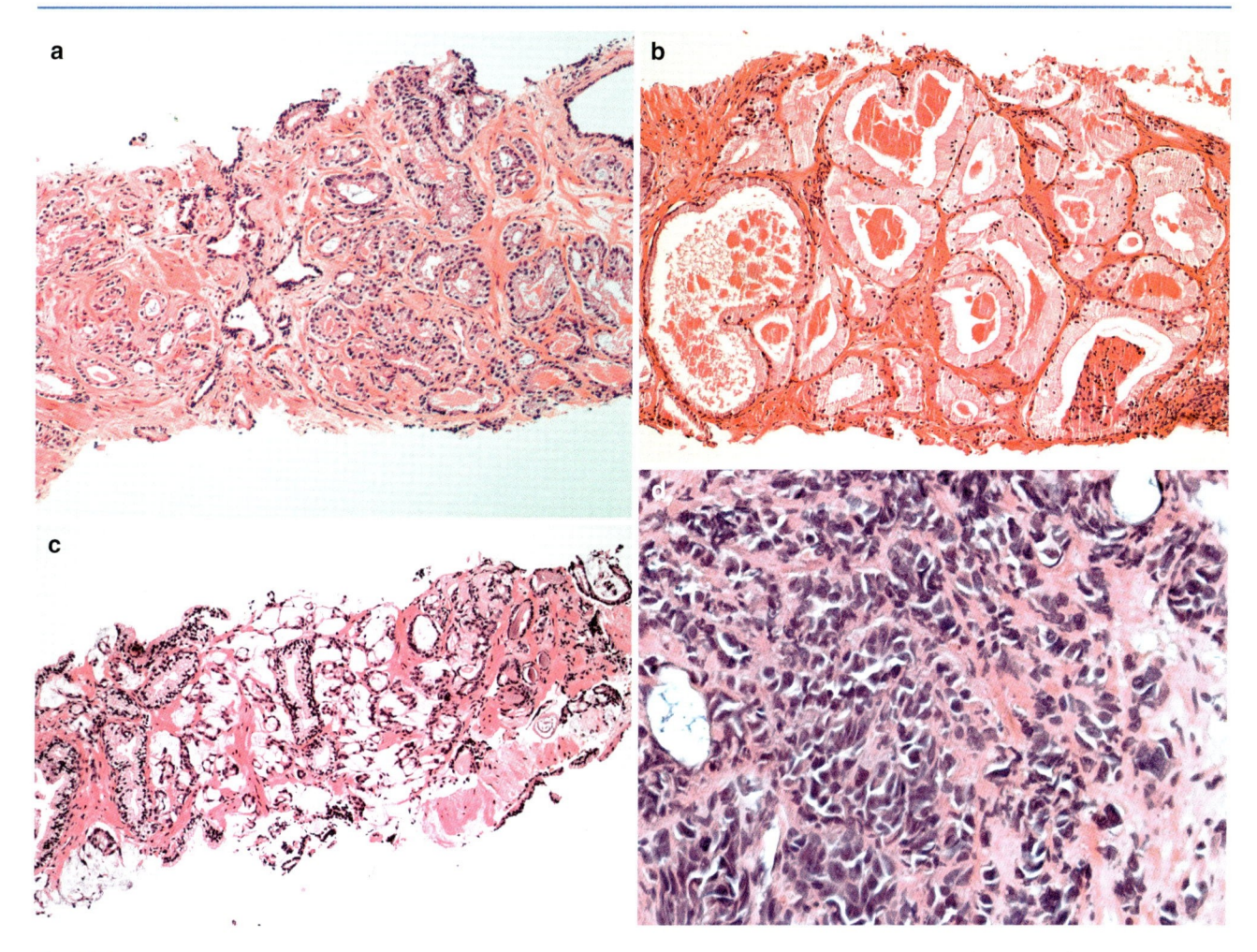

15.3 Adenocarcinoma of the Prostate

Fig. 15.4 Examples of conventional acinar carcinoma (**a**), foamy gland carcinoma (**b**), mucinous carcinoma (**c**), and small cell carcinoma (**d**). The overwhelming majority of prostate cancer is conventional acinar type and it is not necessary to specify such cancer as "acinar" or "conventional" type. Because morphological variations, including atrophic, pseudohyperplastic, and foamy gland cancer, bear no distinct clinical significance, they do not merit specific mentioning. Other morphological variants, including ductal, mucinous, signet ring cell, adenosquamous, sarcomatoid, and small cell carcinoma, may have diagnostic, prognostic, and therapeutic importance and should be diagnosed in prostate biopsies [13–18]. Diagnosis of "ductal," "mucinous," or "signet ring cell" carcinoma is reserved for radical prostatectomy or transurethral resection specimens in which a large amount of tissue can be evaluated. In needle biopsies, a diagnosis of prostate adenocarcinoma with "ductal," "mucinous," or "signet ring cell" features should suffice

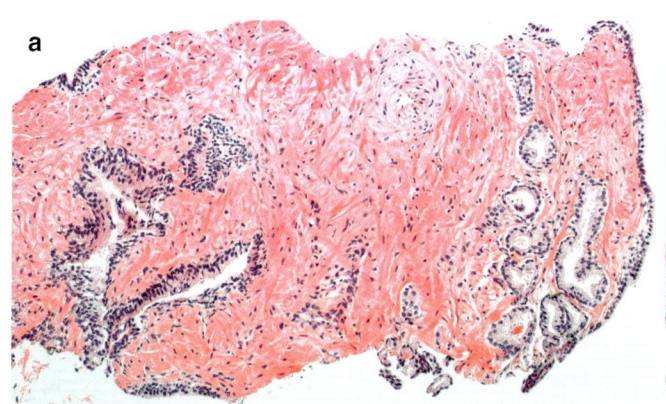

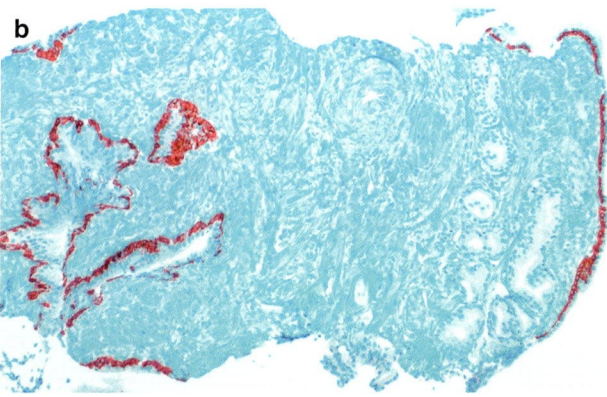

Fig. 15.5 Prostate biopsy containing a minute focus of cancer (**a**) that is negative for basal cell marker K903 (**b**). A common mistake is equating a minute focus of cancer to well-differentiated cancer and grading it as Gleason score 3 or 4. A small focus of cancer should be assigned a Gleason score of $3+3=6$ in most cases

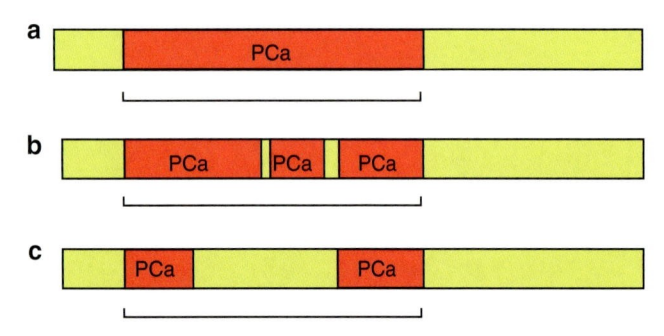

Fig. 15.6 Cancer volume measurement in prostate biopsy. Prostate cancer (PCa) involving biopsy core continuously (**a**), discontinuously with scant intervening benign glands (**b**), and discontinuously with abundant intervening benign glands (**c**). When estimating the tumor extent, one measures from one end of the tumor to the other end without excluding the intervening benign glands (*represented by brackets*). If two cancer foci are ≥ 3 mm apart on the same core (**c**), they may represent multifocal cancer. These cases can be signed out as "prostate cancer discontinuously involving X% of one core" to indicate such a possibility. The amount of cancer in needle cores is a very important prognostic factor [10, 19–21]. Many methods have been developed, including the number of biopsy cores involved by cancer, the linear length of cancer in millimeters in each core and total millimeters of cancer in all involved cores, percentage of each core involved by cancer, and total percentage of cancer in the entire biopsy. There is no consensus regarding the best method of reporting the tumor extent in needle biopsies. If applied consistently, these methods work equally well with a few caveats. Although a high cancer volume in needle biopsy in general correlates with a large-volume cancer in radical prostatectomy, a low volume in biopsy does not necessarily indicate a low volume cancer in radical prostatectomy. It is recommended that the report should include: (1) the number of the biopsy cores involved by cancer; (2) the measurement of each involved core by linear length of cancer in millimeters or percentage of each core involved by cancer. For a specimen with extremely fragmentary cores, an overall percentage of cancer over the entire specimen should be estimated

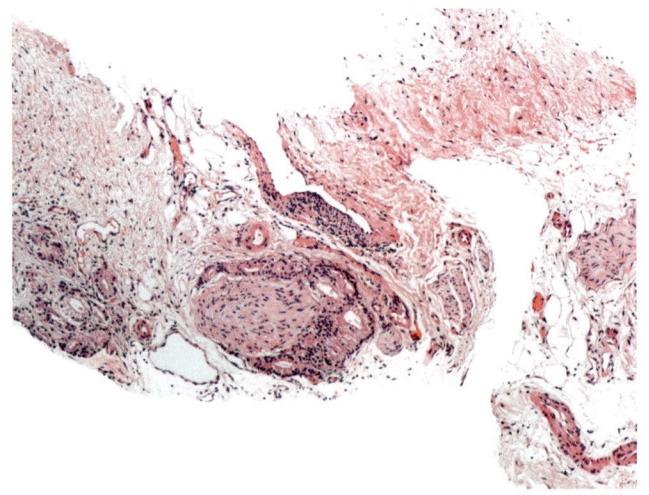

Fig. 15.7 Prostate cancer with extraprostatic extension in needle biopsy. Cancer glands encircle a nerve fiber (perineural invasion) and are present in the adipose tissue. Only in exceedingly rare cases is fat found in the prostate gland. Therefore, the presence of cancer glands in fat in a needle core can be interpreted safely as extraprostatic extension [22]. However, ganglion cells and skeletal muscle fibers can frequently be found within the prostate gland; therefore, involvement of these structures in needle cores should not be equated with extraprostatic extension [23]

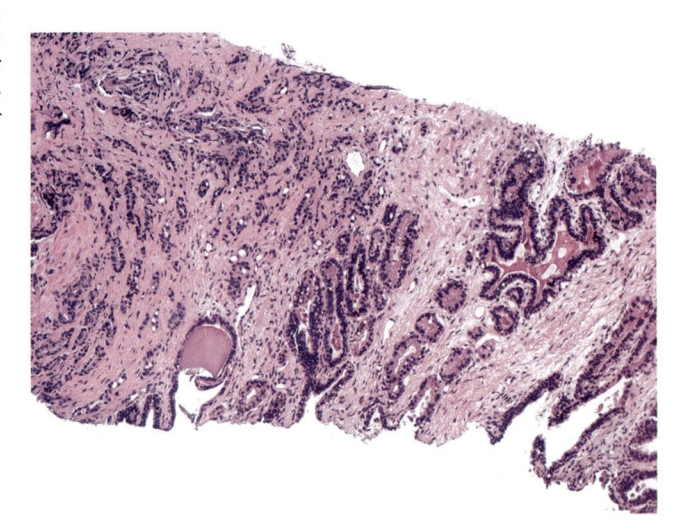

Fig. 15.8 Prostate cancer involving seminal vesicle/ejaculatory duct-like structure. Seminal vesicle can be distinguished in needle biopsy if its smooth muscle wall is present. In contrast, the ejaculatory duct has a rim of loose connective tissue rich in thin vessels. However, the distinction of the two is not always possible in biopsy with limited material. If so, the biopsy should be diagnosed as "cancer involving seminal vesicle/ejaculatory duct tissue" (*Image courtesy of* Dr. Cristina Magi-Galluzzi, Cleveland Clinic, Cleveland, OH)

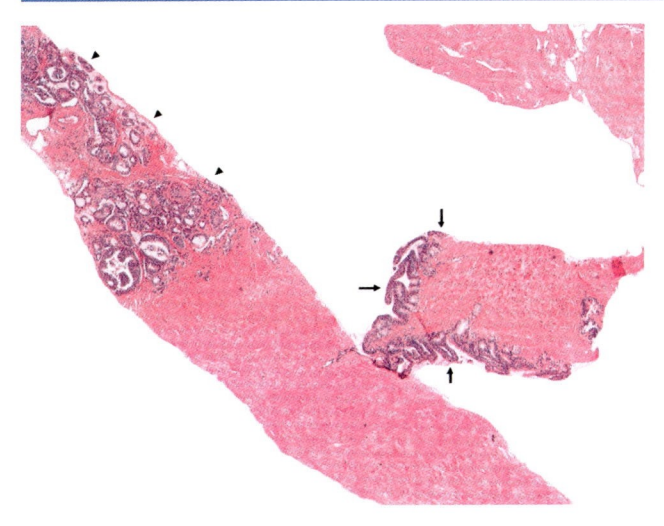

Fig. 15.9 A biopsy targeting the seminal vesicle. Urologists may perform a biopsy of the seminal vesicle to better stage prostate cancer before prostatectomy. A positive seminal vesicle biopsy confirms the presence of extraprostatic invasion and is the most significant predictor of pelvic lymph node metastases in men with clinically localized cancer [24, 25]. This biopsy specimen contains both seminal vesicle tissue (*arrows*) and cancer (*arrowheads*). Although present in this biopsy, the cancer glands do not involve the seminal vesicle. For such biopsies, the report should mention whether the seminal vesicle tissue is present and whether cancer involves the seminal vesicle tissue

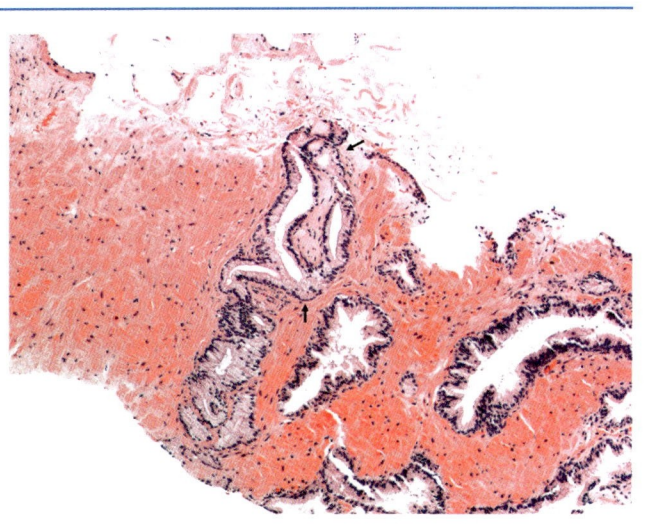

Fig. 15.11 Perineural invasion. Perineural invasion identified in needle biopsy (*arrows*) correlates with extraprostatic extension in radical prostatectomy [26]. This information may be used by surgeons to plan nerve-sparing surgery. Some radiation oncology studies suggest that it also independently predicts adverse outcomes after radiation therapy. However, it is considered a "category 3" prognostic factor (insufficient data to warrant prognostic utility). It can be reported if found in needle biopsies

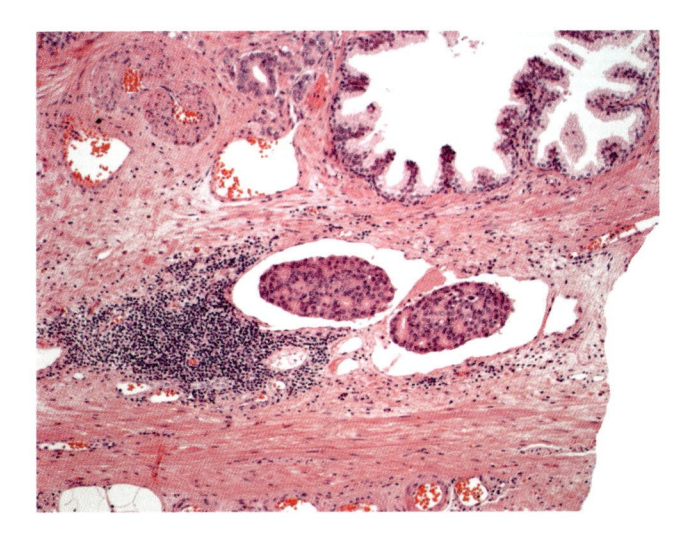

Fig. 15.10 Lymphovascular invasion. This finding is exceedingly rare in needle biopsy specimens and should be reported if definitively identified

FINAL DIAGNOSIS:

A. Prostate, Right Lateral Apex, Core Biopsy:
- Benign prostatic tissue.

B. Prostate, Right Lateral Mid, Core Biopsy:
- **ADENOCARCINOMA OF THE PROSTATE,** GLEASON SCORE 3+4=7, INVOLVING ONE CORE (10%, 2 MM).
- GLEASON PATTERN 4 ACCOUNTS FOR 30% OF THE TUMOR.
- No perineural invasion or tumor in extraprostatic adipose tissue are identified.

C. Prostate, Right Lateral Base, Core Biopsy:
- Benign prostatic tissue with chronic active inflammation.

D. Prostate, Right Apex, Core Biopsy:
- **ADENOCARCINOMA OF THE PROSTATE,** GLEASON SCORE 3+4=7, INVOLVING TWO CORES (20%, 2 MM, <5%, 0.1 MM).
- GLEASON PATTERN 4 ACCOUNTS FOR 10% OF THE TUMOR.
- No perineural invasion or tumor in extraprostatic adipose tissue are identified.

E. Prostate, Right Mid, Core, Biopsy:
- **ADENOCARCINOMA OF THE PROSTATE,** GLEASON SCORE 3+4=7, INVOLVING TWO CORES (40%, 6 MM, 5%, 1 MM).
- GLEASON PATTERN 4 ACCOUNTS FOR 30% OF THE TUMOR.
- No perineural invasion or tumor in extraprostatic adipose tissue are identified.

Fig. 15.12 A sample prostate biopsy report. (**a, b**) Three parts of this 12-part biopsy contain cancer. For each part that contains cancer, Gleason score, number of positive cores versus total number of cores, linear length of cancer in millimeters, and percentage of the core involved by cancer are included in the biopsy report. The inclusion of percentage of pattern 4/5 cancer glands, probability of pathological stage at radical prostatectomy (Partin Table in B), and preoperative prediction of remaining disease free after surgery (Han Table in B) may be included in the report to help patients and clinicians with therapeutic options. It is optional to include representative images of cancer or diagrams of cancer distribution, which seem to help patients and clinicians understand the biopsy reports

b

F. Prostate, Right Base, Core Biospy:
- Benign prostatic tissue.

G. Prostate, Left Lateral Apex, Core Biospy:
- Benign prostatic tissue.

H. Prostate, Left Lateral Apex, Core Biospy:
- HIGH GRADE PROSTATIC INTRAEPITHELIAL NEOPLASIA.

I. Prostate, Left Lateral Apex, Core Biospy:
- HIGH GRADE PROSTATIC INTRAEPITHELIAL NEOPLASIA.

J. Prostate, Left Apex, Core Biospy:
- HIGH GRADE PROSTATIC INTRAEPITHELIAL NEOPLASIA.

K. Prostate, Left Mid, Core Biospy:
- Benign prostatic tissue.

L. Prostate, Left Base, Core Biospy:
- Benign prostatic tissue.

Rajal Shah, Md
(Electronic Signature)
8:09AM 09 JUN 2010

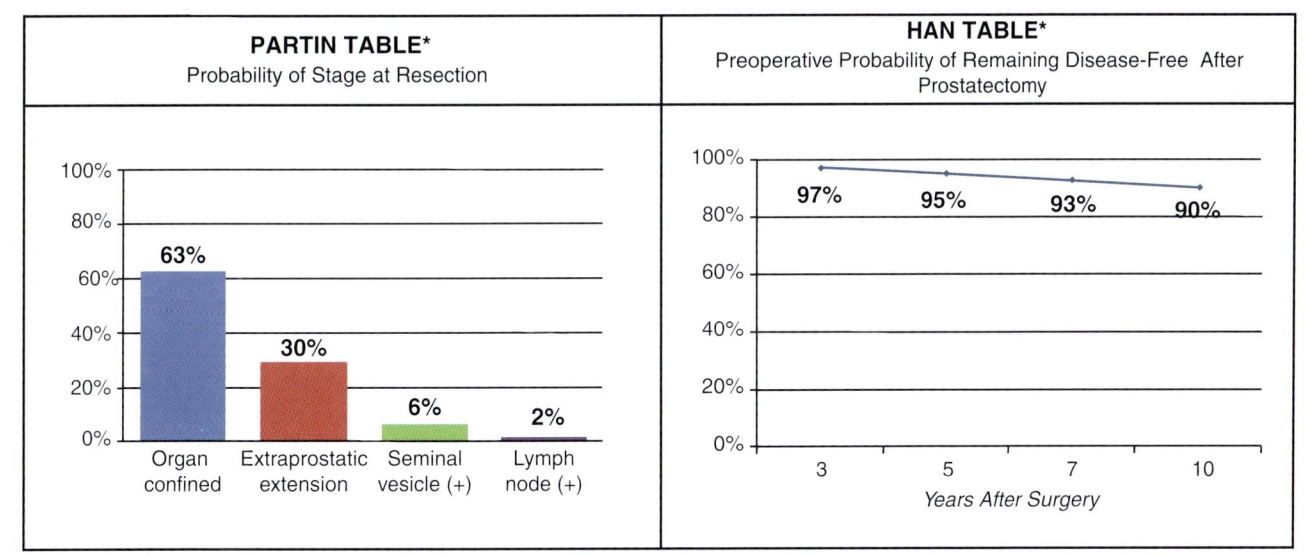

PARTIN TABLE*
Probability of Stage at Resection

- Organ confined: 63%
- Extraprostatic extension: 30%
- Seminal vesicle (+): 6%
- Lymph node (+): 2%

HAN TABLE*
Preoperative Probability of Remaining Disease-Free After Prostatectomy

Years After Surgery	3	5	7	10
Probability	97%	95%	93%	90%

* Partin and Han tables for the probability of post-prostatectomy pathologic stage and likehood of remaining disease free are based on clinical data present at the time of the biospy evaluation, PSA level, and pathogic grading (Gleason score). References: 1) Partin AW, et al. 277: 1445-51, 1997. 2) Partin AW, et al. Urology. 58: 843-8, 2001. 3) Han M, et al. Urol Clin North Am. 28: 555-65, 2001.

Fig. 15.12 (continued)

References

1. Epstein JI, Srigley J, Grignon D, Humphrey P (2007) Recommendations for the reporting of prostate carcinoma. Hum Pathol 38:1305–1309
2. Epstein JI, Srigley J, Grignon D, Humphrey P (2008) Recommendations for the reporting of prostate carcinoma: Association of Directors of Anatomic and Surgical Pathology. Am J Clin Pathol 129:24–30
3. Epstein JI, Srigley J, Grignon D et al (2007) Recommendations for the reporting of prostate carcinoma. Virchows Arch 451:751–756
4. Amin M, Boccon-Gibod L, Egevad L et al (2005) Prognostic and predictive factors and reporting of prostate carcinoma in prostate needle biopsy specimens. Scand J Urol Nephrol Suppl 216:20–33
5. Viglione MP, Potter S, Partin AW et al (2002) Should the diagnosis of benign prostatic hyperplasia be made on prostate needle biopsy? Hum Pathol 33:796–800
6. Rubin MA, Bismar TA, Curtis S, Montie JE (2004) Prostate needle biopsy reporting: how are the surgical members of the Society of Urologic Oncology using pathology reports to guide treatment of prostate cancer patients? Am J Surg Pathol 28:946–952
7. Merrimen JL, Jones G, Walker D et al (2009) Multifocal high grade prostatic intraepithelial neoplasia is a significant risk factor for prostatic adenocarcinoma. J Urol 182:485–490; discussion 490
8. Netto GJ, Epstein JI (2006) Widespread high-grade prostatic intraepithelial neoplasia on prostatic needle biopsy: a significant likelihood of subsequently diagnosed adenocarcinoma. Am J Surg Pathol 30:1184–1188
9. Badalament RA, Miller MC, Peller PA et al (1996) An algorithm for predicting nonorgan confined prostate cancer using the results obtained from sextant core biopsies with prostate specific antigen level. J Urol 156:1375–1380
10. Freedland SJ, Aronson WJ, Terris MK et al (2003) The percentage of prostate needle biopsy cores with carcinoma from the more involved side of the biopsy as a predictor of prostate specific antigen recurrence after radical prostatectomy: results from the Shared Equal Access Regional Cancer Hospital (SEARCH) database. Cancer 98:2344–2350
11. Koh H, Kattan MW, Scardino PT et al (2003) A nomogram to predict seminal vesicle invasion by the extent and location of cancer in systematic biopsy results. J Urol 170:1203–1208
12. Naya Y, Slaton JW, Troncoso P et al (2004) Tumor length and location of cancer on biopsy predict for side specific extraprostatic cancer extension. J Urol 171:1093–1097
13. Hansel DE, Epstein JI (2006) Sarcomatoid carcinoma of the prostate: a study of 42 cases. Am J Surg Pathol 30:1316–1321
14. Lane BR, Magi-Galluzzi C, Reuther AM et al (2006) Mucinous adenocarcinoma of the prostate does not confer poor prognosis. Urology 68:825–830
15. Mazzucchelli R, Morichetti D, Lopez-Beltran A et al (2009) Neuroendocrine tumours of the urinary system and male genital organs: clinical significance. BJU Int 103:1464–1470
16. Osunkoya AO, Nielsen ME, Epstein JI (2008) Prognosis of mucinous adenocarcinoma of the prostate treated by radical prostatectomy: a study of 47 cases. Am J Surg Pathol 32:468–472
17. Parwani AV, Kronz JD, Genega EM et al (2004) Prostate carcinoma with squamous differentiation: an analysis of 33 cases. Am J Surg Pathol 28:651–657
18. Samaratunga H, Delahunt B (2008) Ductal adenocarcinoma of the prostate: current opinion and controversies. Anal Quant Cytol Histol 30:237–246
19. D'Amico AV, Renshaw AA, Cote K et al (2004) Impact of the percentage of positive prostate cores on prostate cancer-specific mortality for patients with low or favorable intermediate-risk disease. J Clin Oncol 22:3726–3732
20. Maygarden SJ, Pruthi R (2005) Gleason grading and volume estimation in prostate needle biopsy specimens: evolving issues. Am J Clin Pathol 123:S58–S66
21. Rossi PJ, Clark PE, Papagikos MA et al (2006) Percentage of positive biopsies associated with freedom from biochemical recurrence after low-dose-rate prostate brachytherapy alone for clinically localized prostate cancer. Urology 67:349–353
22. Miller JS, Chen Y, Ye H et al (2010) Extraprostatic extension of prostatic adenocarcinoma on needle core biopsy: report of 72 cases with clinical follow-up. BJU Int 106:330–333
23. Ye H, Walsh PC, Epstein JI (2010) Skeletal muscle involvement by limited Gleason score 6 adenocarcinoma of the prostate on needle biopsy is not associated with adverse findings at radical prostatectomy. J Urol 184:2308–2312
24. Stone NN, Stock RG, Parikh D et al (1998) Perineural invasion and seminal vesicle involvement predict pelvic lymph node metastasis in men with localized carcinoma of the prostate. J Urol 160:1722–1726
25. Vallancien G, Bochereau G, Wetzel O et al (1994) Influence of preoperative positive seminal vesicle biopsy on the staging of prostatic cancer. J Urol 152:1152–1156
26. Harnden P, Shelley MD, Clements H et al (2007) The prognostic significance of perineural invasion in prostatic cancer biopsies: a systematic review. Cancer 109:13–24

Index

A

Absence of basal cells, 17, 19, 127
Adenoid cystic basal cell carcinoma, 57, 76, 94, 102
Adenoid cystic basal cell hyperplasia. *See* Basal cell hyperplasia
Adenosis, 43, 44, 82, 92–93, 108–109, 111
a-Methylacyl-CoA racemase (AMACR), 160
Amorphous intraluminal secretion, 21, 48
Androgen receptor (AR), 157
Apoptosis, 17, 22, 26, 68
Associated with HGPIN, 17, 22, 123, 127, 173
Atrophy
  classification, 86–87
  focal atrophy, 86–87, 91
  partial atrophy, 82, 86–91
  post atrophic hyperplasia, 82, 86–88, 90–91
Atypical adenomatous hyperplasia. *See* Adenosis
Atypical cribriform lesions of prostate
  approach to work up of atypical cribriform lesions in biopsy, 115, 119
  comparisons between cribriform HGPIN and intraductal carcinoma, 115, 118–120
  cribriform HGPIN, 115, 118–120
  intraductal carcinoma of prostate, 115–120
Atypical glands suspicious for cancer (ATYP)/atypical small acinar proliferation (ASAP)
  clinical significance
    cancer risk, 137
    incidence in prostate biopsy, 137
  histological features
    atrophic glands, 131
    crowded glands, 131, 133
    crush artifact obscuring morphology, 131, 132
    focal positive basal cell markers, 131
    HGPIN with adjacent small focus of atypical glands (PINATYP), 131, 135
    marked inflammation, 135
  reporting, 173
  work-up
    expert consultation, 137
    immunohistochemistry, 137

B

Bacillus Calmette-Guerin (BCG), 105, 106
Basal cell hyperplasia (BCH), 82, 94–97, 102
Basal cell lesions. *See also* Adenoid cystic basal cell carcinoma; Basal cell hyperplasia
  diagnostic approach, 97
Basal cell markers, 116, 117
BCG. *See* Bacillus Calmette-Guerin

BCH. *See* Basal cell hyperplasia
Benign mimics of prostate carcinoma
  atypical morphological features commonly encountered in benign mimics, 82
  classification, 79, 80
  histological features commonly associated with benign mimics, 81
  immunohistochemical features and ancillary studies, 82–88, 90, 92, 94, 98, 100, 102, 103, 105, 107–110
Benign prostate hyperplasia (BPH), 57, 59, 92, 94, 103, 104
Biomarkers
  diagnostic biomarkers, 157–165
  multiplex biomarkers, 161, 162
  prognostic biomarkers, 157–165
Biopsy, prostate. *See also* Needle core biopsy
  histological processing, 169
  number of needle cores, 170
  quality assurance measures, 172
  sectioning protocols, 170
  submission, handling and interpretation, 169–171
  tissue cuts per section, 170
Blue mucin, 17, 22, 26, 59, 61, 86, 94, 100, 101, 108, 108, 150
BPH. *See* Benign prostate hyperplasia

C

Cancer location reporting, 174
Cancer Volume measurement, 176
Carcinoid like prostate carcinoma, 69
Carcinosarcoma. *See* Sarcomatoid carcinoma
CD–68, 105, 107, 110, 111
Central zone glands, 102–103
Chromosomal translocations. *See* TMPRSS2:ETS gene fusions
Chronic lymphocytic leukemia (CLL), 107
Circulating microvesicles, 162
Clear cell adenocarcinoma, 100
Clear cell cribriform hyperplasia, 102–104
CLL. *See* Chronic lymphocytic leukemia
cMYC, 165
Colloid carcinoma. *See* Mucinous carcinoma
Cowper's glands, 57, 76, 84–86
Cribriform carcinoma, 44–48
Cribriform growth, 67, 79
Cribriform HGPIN, 115, 118–120
Cribriform proliferations of prostate, 102–104
  classification, 102
  differential diagnosis, 104
Crowded growth, 17, 24, 103, 134, 137
Crystalloids, 17, 22, 26, 92, 108
Cystic atrophy, 86, 87. *See also* Atrophy
Cytoplasmic amphophilia, 17, 59, 83, 102

D

Diffuse adenosis. *See* Adenosis
Ductal adenocarcinoma, 49, 57, 64–65

E

Early prostate cancer antigen (EPCA), 161
Ejaculatory duct epithelium, 82–83. *See also* Seminal vesicle
Enhancer of zeste homolog 2 (EZH2), 162
EPCA. *See* Early prostate cancer antigen
ERG *See* TMPRSS2:ERG and TMPRSS2:ETS gene fusions
ERG antibody, 160
ERG gene fusions. *See* TMPRSS2:ERG gene fusions
Extraprostatic extension, 9, 42, 43, 45, 76, 110, 127, 140, 174, 176, 177

EZH2. *See* Enhancer of zeste homolog 2

F

Fluorescence in situ hybridization (FISH), 160, 163, 164
Foamy gland carcinoma, 84, 86, 110
Foamy gland carcinoma of the prostate, 50, 57–58
Focal atrophy, 86–87, 91. *See also* Partial atrophy; Post atrophic hyperplasia

G

Gleason grading system
    biopsy and radical prostatectomy Gleason score correlation, 43, 52, 53
    clinical significance, 47, 48
    contemporary Gleason pattern 1, 44
    contemporary Gleason pattern 2, 44
    contemporary Gleason pattern 3, 45–46
    contemporary Gleason pattern 4, 46–47
    contemporary Gleason pattern 5, 48
    conventional system, 41, 43–46, 48
    current concepts, 44
    effect of tumor multifocality and sampling techniques, 53
    grading after therapy, 52
    grading of morphologic variants of prostate carcinoma, 50
    impact of modified International Society of Urologic Pathology (ISUP) system, 53
    modified ISUP system, 43, 53
    tertiary pattern 5 in biopsy, 41, 44, 52, 53
Glomerulation, or glomeruloid formation, 15, 16, 63
Glutathione s-transferase π 1(GSTP1), 159
Golgi phosphoprotein 2 (GOLPH2), 161, 162
Granulomatous inflammation. *See* Nonspecific granulomatous prostatitis
GSTP1. *See* Glutathione s-transferase π 1

H

Haphazard growth without accompanying benign glands, 18
Hereditary prostate cancer 1 (HPC1), 161
High-grade prostatic intraepithelial neoplasia (HGPIN), 82, 87, 94, 97, 102, 103, 111
    clinical significance
        cancer risk, 127
        incidence in prostate biopsy, 127
    diagnostic criteria, 122–126
    differential diagnosis
        basal cell hyperplasia, 127
        central zone glands, 127
        ductal adenocarcinoma, 127, 128
        intraductal carcinoma, 127, 129
        prostate carcinoma, 127
    histological features, 121, 127
    immunohistochemistry
        basal cell markers, 122
        ERG, 122
        α-methylacyl-CoA racemase (AMACR), 122
    reporting, 130
    vs. low grade PIN (LGPIN), 121, 127, 130
Histological features for and against cancer, 26
Histologic variants
    Gleason grading, 43
    types, 64, 66, 72, 76
    variant histology mimicking benign lesions, 57
Histological variants reporting, 29, 43, 57, 122
HPC1. *See* Hereditary prostate cancer 1

I

Immunohistochemistry
    basal cell markers
        basal cell marker cocktail, 30
        high-molecular-weight cytokeratin (HMWCK), 29–31, 38
        p63, 29–31, 33, 36–38
        prostate carcinoma lacks staining, 30
        types, 30, 38
    clinical utility, 29, 30, 34, 37, 38
    differential diagnosis, 38, 39
    ERG protein
        in high-grade prostatic intraepithelial neoplasia (HGPIN), 37
        in prostate cancer, 37
    α-methylacyl-CoA-racemase (AMACR)/P504S
        antibodies types, 34, 38
        antibody cocktails, 38
        apical cytoplasmic granular staining, 34
        expression in adenosis, 36
        expression in nephrogenic adenoma, 34
        heterogeneous, cancer glands, 34, 35
        positive staining, 34, 35, 38
        staining pattern in prostate cancer, 34, 35
    practical guidelines, 39
Infiltrative growth, 17, 17, 21, 25, 26, 61, 76, 76, 100, 105, 133, 149
Intracytoplasmic vacuoles, 49, 50
Intraductal carcinoma of prostate, 64, 72
    clinical significance, 115, 116
    molecular features, 116
    pathologic features, 120
    reporting recommendations, 120

L

Large duct carcinoma. *See* Ductal adenocarcinoma
Leiomyosarcoma, 139, 143, 145
Limited cancer diagnosis
    benign conditions that cause architectureal and cytological atypia
        adenosis, 23
        atrophy, 23
        inflammation, 23
        PINATYP, 24
    histological features considered specific for prostate cancer
        glomerulation, or glomeruloid formation, 15, 16
        incidence, 16
        mucinous fibroplasias/collegenous micronodule, 15, 16
        perineural invasion, 15, 16
            vs. perineural indentation by benign glands, 15, 16

histological features for and against cancer, 26
major cancer-associated histological features
   abnormal growth patterns
      cribriform architecture, 18
      infiltrative growth, 17
      soloid and single cells, 18
   absence of basal cells
      crushed cancer/stromal cells mimicking basal
         cells, 19
      immunohistochemistry, 17, 19
   nuclear atypia
      nuclear enlargement, 17, 20
      nuclear hyperchromasia, 17, 21
      prominent nucleoli, 17, 20
minor cancer-associated histological features
   other growth patterns
      amorphous intraluminal secretion, 21
      apoptosis, 17, 22
      associated with HGPIN, 17, 22
      blue mucin, 17, 22
      crowded growth, 17, 24
      crystalloids, 17, 22
      cytoplasmic amphophilia, 17, 21
      haphazard growth without accompanying benign
         glands, 18
      mitosis, 17, 22
   practical approaches, 36
   quantitative threshold, 24–25
Lipofuscin pigment, 82, 83
Lymphovasuclar invasion, 76, 174, 177

M
Malakoplakia, 107
Mesonephric remnant hyperplasia, 85–86
Michaelis-Gutman bodies, 107
Mitosis, 17, 22, 26, 68, 100, 122, 140
MUC–6, 82
Mucinous carcinoma, 49, 57, 66–67
Mucinous fibroplasias, or collegenous micronodule,
   15, 16, 16, 17, 49, 50, 66
Mucinous metaplasia, 57, 84, 86
Myoepithelial metaplasia, 108

N
Necrotizing squamous metaplasia, 74
Needle core biopsy, 170
   prostate
      biopsy location, 11–13
      biopsy method, 11–13
      cancer detection, 11–13
      number of needle cores, 13
Nephrogenic adenoma, 82, 100–102, 111
Nephrogenic metaplasia. See Nephrogenic adenoma
Neuroendocrine differentiation.
         See also Small cell carcinoma
   approach to differential diagnosis, 70
   carcinoid tumor, 69
Nonspecific granulomatous prostatitis, 105–107
Normal histological variations
   atrophy, 8
   basal cell hyperplasia, 8
   urothelial metaplasia, 8
   verumontanum mucosal gland hyperplasia, 7
Normal prostate gland

anatomic landmarks
   ejaculatory ducts, 1, 2
   urethra, 1, 2
anatomy of normal prostate gland
   relationship to bladder, 1
   relationship to rectum, 1
histology of non-prostate structures
   Cowper's glands, 6, 7
   irregular contour, 2, 3
   irregular prostateûperiprostatic interface, 8, 9
   paraganglia, 6, 7
   seminal vesicle/ejaculatory ducts, 6, 7
   skeletal muscle fibers, 8, 9
histology of normal prostate
   basal cells, 2, 3
   corpora amylacea, 2, 5
   lipofuscin pigment, 2, 5
   neuroendocrine cells, 5
   prostate epithelial cell types, 5
   secretory cells, 2, 3, 6
three zones of the prostate gland
   central zone, 1, 6
   disease preference, 1
   peripheral zone, 1, 6
   transition zone, 1, 6
Nuclear enlargement, 6, 17, 20, 23, 24, 25, 26, 36, 57, 58, 59, 61, 63,
   87, 88, 89, 91, 98, 102, 103, 116, 122, 126, 134, 135
Nuclear hyperchromasia, 53, 83

P
P27, 162
P53, 165
PAH. See Post atrophic hyperplasia
Papillary urothelial carcinoma, 100
Paraganglia, 109–110
Partial atrophy, 82, 86–91
PAX–2, 82, 100, 101
PAX–8, 82, 100, 101
PCA3. See Prostate cancer antigen 3
PCSA. See Prostate cell surface antigen
Perineural invasion
   In diagnosis, 17, 97, 127
   In reporting, 15
Phosphate and tensin homolog deleted on chromosome 10 (PTEN),
   157, 160, 161
Phyllodes tumor. See Specialized stromal tumors of prostate
Post atrophic hyperplasia (PAH), 82, 86–88, 90–91
Post radiation atypia, 98, 99
   morphology spectrum, 99
P63 positive prostate adenocarcinoma, 94
Practical approaches for diagnosis of cancer in biopsy, 26
Prominent nucleoli, 6, 17, 20, 26, 57, 58, 59, 59, 61, 63, 66, 83, 85,
   94, 95, 96, 98, 98, 100, 102, 103, 108, 108, 122, 122, 123,
   126, 127, 135, 137, 149, 150, 151
Prostate adenocarcinoma. See also Prostate carcinoma
   with atrophic features, 49, 57, 61–62
   with glomeruloid features, 49, 57, 63
   with mucinous features, 49, 66, 67
Prostate cancer, 57–76. See also Prostate carcinoma
   biomarkers, 157–165
   Gleason grading, 41–54
   model of prostate cancer progression, 158, 164, 165
   molecular biology, 157–165
   parameters that impact detection rate, 13
   prediction models, 42–43

Prostate cancer, 57–76. *See also* Prostate carcinoma (continued)
  recurrence categories, 42–43
  sampling techniques, 11–13
Prostate cancer antigen 3 (PCA3), 159, 162
Prostate carcinoma, 11–13, 41–54. *See also* Prostate cancer
  acinar carcinoma, 57, 61, 63, 64, 66–69, 71, 75
    benign mimics, 79–111
    histologic variants, 57–76
Prostate cell surface antigen (PCSA), 162
Prostate specific membrane antigen (PSMA), 162
Prostate stromal sarcoma (PSS), 139, 140, 142, 143
PSA
  derivatives, 157, 159
  types of measurement in clinical practice, 157, 158
Pseudohyperplastic carcinoma of prostate, 50, 57, 59–61
Pseudosignet ring cells, 75
PSMA. *See* Prostate specific membrane antigen
PSS. *See* Prostate stromal sarcoma
PTEN. *See* Phosphate and tensin homolog deleted on chromosome 10

Q

Quality assurance, 169–172
Quantitative threshold, 24–25

R

Radiation atypia. *See* Post radiation atypia
Reporting of prostate biopsy
  adenocarcinoma
    cancer volume measurement, 176
    extraprostatic extension, 174, 176, 177
    Gleason grading, 174
    histological variants, 174
    location, 174
    lymphovasuclar invasion, 174, 177
    perineural invasion, 174, 176, 177
    seminal vesicle/ejaculatory duct invasion, 174, 176, 177
    therapy-related changes, 174
  atypical glands suspicious for cancer (ATYP), 173
  benign diagnosis
    chronic and acute inflammation, 173
    stromal nodule, 173
  biopsy adequacy, 174
  high-grade prostatic intraepithelial neoplasia (HGPIN), 173, 179
Rhabdomyosarcoma, 139, 143, 145

S

Salvage radical prostatectomy. *See* Post radiation atypia
Sampling techniques
  extended biopsy, 11, 12
  future trends, 13
  impact on diagnosis, 11–13
  saturation biopsy, 11, 12
  sextant biospy, 11, 12
Sarcomatoid carcinoma, 49, 57, 71, 139, 140, 142
Sarcosine, 161
Sclerosing adenosis, 82, 108–109
Seminal vesicle, 82–83
Seminal vesicle/ejaculatory duct invasion, 174, 176, 177
Serine peptidase inhibitor, Kazal type (SPINK1), 162

SFT. *See* Solitary fibrous tumor
Signet ring cell carcinoma, 57, 75
Single cells, 18, 48, 48, 52, 53, 72, 75, 79, 99, 105, 108, 149, 149, 150
Small cell carcinoma, 57, 68–69
Small cell neuroendocrine carcinoma, 50, 57, 68–69
Small lymphocytic lymphoma, 107
Solitary fibrous tumor (SFT), 139, 142, 145
Soloid growth, 18
Specialized stromal tumors of prostate, 71
  stromal sarcoma, 140
  stromal tumors of uncertain malignant potential (STUMP), 140
Spindle cell lesions of the prostate
  classification, 139
  diagnostic approach, 144
  immunohistochemical characteristics, 145
SPINK1. *See* Serine peptidase inhibitor, Kazal type
Squamous and adenosquamous carcinoma, 57, 73–74
Stromal hyperplasia, 139–141
Stromal tumors of uncertain malignant potential (STUMP), 139–142, 145
STUMP. *See* Stromal tumors of uncertain malignant potential

T

Thrombomodulin, 116
TMPRSS2:ERG gene fusions, 116, 119, 160, 163, 164
TMPRSS2:ETS gene fusions, 157, 160, 164
  model of prostate cancer progression demonstrating role of ETS gene fusions, 164, 165
Transurethral prostate resection, recommendation for tissue submission, 172
Treatment effect in benign and malignant prostate tissue
  androgen pathway, 148
  anti-androgen therapy for prostate lesions, 148
  histological changes associated with cryotherapy
    basal cell hyperplasia, 154
    hemorrhage and hemosiderin, 154
    squamous cell metaplasia, 154
  histological changes associated with hyperthermia
    coagulative necrosis, 155
    granulation tissue, 155
  histological changes associated with radiation therapy
    benign prostate tissue
      basal cell hyperplasia, 152
      glandular atrophy, 151
      random atypical nuclei, 151
      vascular changes, 151, 152
    malignant porostate tissue
      atrophic changes, 151
      cytoplasmic vacuolation, 151
      nuclear pyknosis, 151, 153
    significance of postradiation biopsy, 151
  histologic changes following androgen-deprivation therapy
    benign prostate tissue
      basal cell hyperplasia, 149
      glandular atrophy, 149, 150
    malignant prostate tissue
      atrophic changes, 149
      bland cytology, 150
      glandular architecture, loss of, 149, 150
      Gleason grading, 147, 174
      histiocyte-like change, 150

Index

    individual cancer cells, 151
    mucinous degeneration, 149, 150
  reporting, 173
  treatment modalities for prostate lesions, 147
TTF1, 68

U
Urothelial carcinoma, 57, 64, 65, 72–74
  intraductal spread, 116, 118
  nested type, 100, 101
Urothelial carcinoma in situ, 98

V
Verumontanum mucosal gland hyperplasia, 83–84

X
Xanthogranulomatous prostatitis, 107
Xanthomatous inflammation, 57, 58, 110, 111

Printing: Ten Brink, Meppel, The Netherlands
Binding: Stürtz, Würzburg, Germany